Diabetes For Dummies®

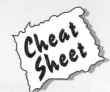
Cheat Sheet

Appropriate Standards for Continuing Diabetes Care

Following are guidelines for your diabetes care.

Frequency of visits:

- Daily if starting insulin
- Weekly for oral drugs
- Monthly if not stable
- Quarterly if stable

History at each visit:

- Frequency of hypoglycemia
- Results of blood glucose self-monitoring
- Changes in treatment
- Symptoms of complications
- Psychosocial issues
- New medications

Physical at each visit:

- Blood pressure
- Weight
- Foot exam if neuropathy is present

Physical at least annually:

- Dilated eye exam by eye doctor
- Filament test for foot sensation

Lab tests:

- Hemoglobin A1c every 3 months
- Fasting lipid profile yearly
- Microalbumin measurement yearly if urine protein negative

Frequency of blood glucose self-monitoring:

- Before meals and bedtime for person with type 1 diabetes
- Before breakfast and supper for person with type 2 diabetes
- Once daily for person with stable diabetes
- Before and 1 hour after meals for person with gestational diabetes or pregnant woman with type 1 diabetes

Ten Commandments for Great Diabetes Control

Follow these commandments, and your problems should be few and far between.

- Major monitoring (see Chapter 7)
- Devout dieting (see Chapter 8)
- Tenacious testing (see Chapter 7)
- Enthusiastic exercising (see Chapter 9)
- Lifelong learning (see Chapter 12)
- Meticulous medicating (see Chapter 10)
- Appropriate attitude (see Chapter 1)
- Preventive planning (see Chapter 8)
- Fastidious foot care (see Chapter 5)
- Essential eye care (see Chapter 5)

For Dummies: Bestselling Book Series for Beginners

Diabetes For Dummies®

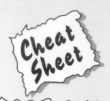

Cheat Sheet

Oral Drugs for Diabetes

The following table tells you what you need to know about some popular oral drugs.

Class	Brand Name	Generic Name	Average Dose	Range
Sulfonylureas	Orinase	tolbutamide	1,500 mg	500–3,000 mg
	Tolinase	tolazamide	250 mg	100–1,000 mg
	Diabinase	chlorpropamide	250 mg	100–500 mg
	Dymelor	acetohexamide	500 mg	250–1,500 mg
	Glucotrol	glipazide	10 mg	2.5–40 mg
	DiaBeta,	glyburide	7.5 mg	1.25–20 mg
	Glynase Amaryl	glimepiride	4 mg	1–8 mg
Meglitinides	Prandin	repaglinide	1 mg	0.5–4 mg
Biguanides	Glucophage	metformin	1,000 mg	500–2,000 mg
Thiazolidinediones	Actos	pioglitazone	30 mg	15–45 mg
	Avandia	rosiglitazone	4 mg	2–8 mg
Alpha-glucosidase inhibitors	Precose	acarbose	100 mg	50–250 mg
	Glyset	miglitol	50 mg	25–75 mg

Guidelines for Testing for Diabetes

These guidelines were developed by the American Diabetes Association to screen for diabetes at the earliest possible appropriate time:

People over age 45 should be tested every three years if normal.

People should be tested at a younger age and more often if they're:

- Obese
- Parent or siblings have diabetes
- From a high-risk group, such as African American, Hispanic, or Native American
- Delivered a baby over 9 pounds or had gestational diabetes
- Have high blood pressure
- Have low HDL cholesterol or high triglycerides

People with symptoms of thirst, frequent urination, and weight loss are tested immediately.

Copyright © 2002 Wiley Publishing, Inc.
All rights reserved.

Cheat Sheet $2.95 value. Item 5154-X.

For more information about Wiley Publishing, call 1-800-762-2974.

For Dummies: Bestselling Book Series for Beginners

Praise for Diabetes For Dummies

"As one of the country's leading endocrinologists, Alan Rubin could be expected to know a lot about diabetes. But the surprising thing about his new book is how well he says it, and his support of the glycemic index shows in particular that he is current with the latest thinking on how to deal with diabetes."

> — Rick Mendosa, Diabetes Journalist
> www.mendosa.com/diabetes.htm

"*Diabetes For Dummies* is a wonderfully written book and will become the companion book for all people with diabetes and their families. It is very clearly written so that it can be readily understood by younger diabetics as well as elderly diabetics, and it will be especially important for a newly diagnosed diabetic. It is also a must-read for diabetic educators."

> — Michael D. Goldfield, M.D.
> Assistant Clinical Professor of Psychiatry
> University of California Medical Center
> San Francisco, California

"At last, a diabetes book for everyone. Dr. Rubin is superb at translating the medical issues of diabetes into plain English. He does a terrific job of covering just about every conceivable aspect of diabetes in a clear, concise, and readable text with a touch of humor. A must-read."

> — G. Robert Hampton, M.D.
> Retinal Specialist on the American Academy of
> Ophthalmology's Public Information Committee
> Syracuse, New York

"Dr. Rubin provides a marvelous face-lift with the fun, very readable, and practical book. You'll learn ten myths about diabetes that you can forget along with hundreds of powerful tips that you'll long remember. Filled with wit and wisdom, this book will teach you the Ten Commandments of Diabetes Care which can add life to your years . . . and years to your life."

> — Dr. Joel Goodman
> Director, The HUMOR Project, Inc.
> Saratoga Springs, New York

"When it comes to diabetes, almost everyone is a dummy — including, alas, a number of health care professionals! This lively and lucid tell-it-all guide will provide you with the information you need to leap from the valley of diabetes ignorance to the peaks of understanding. (We particularly appreciate the extensive and inspiring list of famous people in all walks of life who have diabetes.)"

> — June Biermann and Barbara Toohey
> Founders and Editors-in-Chief of
> www.DiabetesWebsite.com

"I would recommend this book to parents, adolescents, and children with diabetes. It presents a clear, straightforward and honest discussion of diabetes and does this within the context of understanding developmental tasks and processes."

> — Sal Lomonaco, M.D.
> Associate Clinical Professor of Psychiatry
> Division of Child-Adolescent Psychiatry

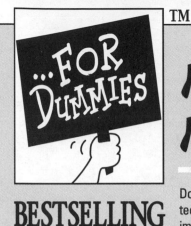

TM

...FOR DUMMIES

References for the Rest of Us! ®

BESTSELLING BOOK SERIES

Do you find that traditional reference books are overloaded with technical details and advice you'll never use? Do you postpone important life decisions because you just don't want to deal with them? Then our *For Dummies*® business and general reference book series is for you.

For Dummies business and general reference books are written for those frustrated and hard-working souls who know they aren't dumb, but find that the myriad of personal and business issues and the accompanying horror stories make them feel helpless. *For Dummies* books use a lighthearted approach, a down-to-earth style, and even cartoons and humorous icons to dispel fears and build confidence. Lighthearted but not lightweight, these books are perfect survival guides to solve your everyday personal and business problems.

Already, millions of satisfied readers agree. They have made For Dummies the #1 introductory level computer book series and a best-selling business book series. They have written asking for more. So, if you're looking for the best and easiest way to learn about business and other general reference topics, look to For Dummies to give you a helping hand.

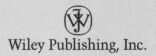

Wiley Publishing, Inc.

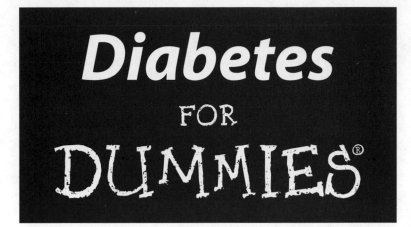

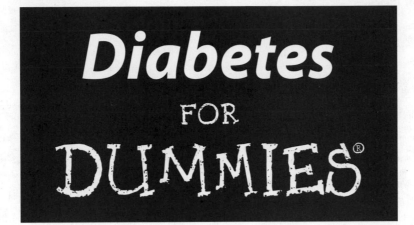

Diabetes
FOR
DUMMIES®

by Alan L. Rubin, M.D.

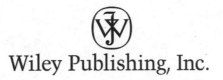

Wiley Publishing, Inc.

Diabetes For Dummies®

Published by
Wiley Publishing, Inc.
909 Third Avenue
New York, NY 10022
www.wiley.com

Copyright © 2001 by Wiley Publishing, Inc., Indianapolis, Indiana

Published simultaneously in Canada

For general information on our other products and services or to obtain technical support, please contact our Customer Care Department within the U.S. at 800-762-2974, outside the U.S. at 317-572-3993, or fax 317-572-4002.

Wiley also publishes its books in a variety of electronic formats. Some content that appears in print may not be available in electronic books.

Library of Congress Cataloging-in-Publication Data:

Library of Congress Control Number: 2001095568
ISBN: 0-7645-5154-X

Manufactured in the United States of America
18 17 16 15 14

About the Author

Alan L. Rubin, M. D., is one of the nation's foremost experts on diabetes. He is a professional member of the American Diabetes Association and the Endocrine Society and has been in private practice specializing in diabetes and thyroid disease for over 28 years. Dr. Rubin was Assistant Clinical Professor of Medicine at University of California Medical Center in San Francisco for 20 years. He has spoken about diabetes to professional medical audiences and non-medical audiences around the world. He has been a consultant to many pharmaceutical companies and companies that make diabetes products.

Dr. Rubin was one of the first specialists in his field to recognize the significance of patient self-testing of blood glucose, the major advance in diabetes care since the advent of insulin. As a result, he has been on numerous radio and television programs, talking about the cause, the prevention, and the treatment of diabetes and its complications.

Dedication

This book is dedicated to my wife Enid and my children, Renee and Larry. Their patience, enthusiasm, and encouragement helped to make the writing a real pleasure.

Author's Acknowledgments

The great acquisitions editor and midwife, Tami Booth, deserves great appreciation for helping to deliver this new baby. Her optimism and her ideas actually made this book possible. My project editor, Kelly Ewing, has made sure that this book follows the laws of grammar and is readable and understandable in the great *For Dummies* tradition. My thanks to Dr. Seymour Levin for the technical editing of this book.

Dietitian Nancy Bennett evaluated all the recipes, cooked them, tasted them, and put them into a form that could be followed by my readers. She also provided great food for thought about the role of the dietitian in diabetes care.

I want to thank ophthalmologist Dr. John Norris of Pacific Eye Associates in San Francisco for helping me to see the place of the eye physician in diabetes care. I also want to thank podiatrist Dr. Mark Pinter for helping me get a leg up on his specialty.

Librarians Mary Ann Zaremska and Nancy Phelps at St. Francis Memorial Hospital were tremendously helpful in providing the articles and books upon which the information in the book is based.

I want to thank Dr. Richard Bernstein of Marin County, California, for the many years of learning, collaboration, and enjoyment together.

Ronnie and Michael Goldfield should definitely be considered the godparents of this book.

My friends in the Dawn Patrol kept me laughing throughout the production of this book. Their willingness to follow me convinced me that others would be willing to read what I wrote.

My teachers are too numerous to mention, but one group deserves special attention. They are my patients over the last 28 years, the people whose trials and tribulations caused me to seek the knowledge that you will find in this book.

This book is written on the shoulders of thousands of men and women who made the discoveries and held the committee meetings. Their accomplishments cannot possibly be given adequate acclaim. We owe them big time.

Publisher's Acknowledgments

We're proud of this book; please send us your comments through our Online Registration Form located at www.dummies.com/register.

Some of the people who helped bring this book to market include the following:

Acquisitions, Editorial,
and Media Development

Project Editor: Kelly Ewing

Executive Editor: Tammerly Booth

Acquisitions Coordinator: Karen S. Young

Editorial Director: Kristin A. Cocks

Editorial Manager: Christine Meloy Beck

Editorial Administrator: Michelle Hacker

General Reviewer: Dr. Seymour Levin

Illustrator: Kathryn Born

Production

Project Coordinators: Dale White

Layout and Graphics: Stephanie Jumper, Jeremey Unger, Jacque Schneider, Erin Zeltner

Proofreaders: Andy Hollandbeck, Angel Perez, Marianne Santy, TECHBOOKS Production Services

Indexer: TECHBOOKS Production Services

Publishing and Editorial for Consumer Dummies

Diane Graves Steele, Vice President and Publisher, Consumer Dummies
Joyce Pepple, Acquisitions Director, Consumer Dummies
Kristin A. Cocks, Product Development Director, Consumer Dummies
Michael Spring, Vice President and Publisher, Travel
Brice Gosnell, Publishing Director, Travel
Suzanne Jannetta, Editorial Director, Travel

Publishing for Technology Dummies

Andy Cummings, Acquisitions Director

Composition Services

Gerry Fahey, Vice President, Production Services
Debbie Stailey, Director of Composition Services

Contents at a Glance

Cartoons at a Glance

By Rich Tennant

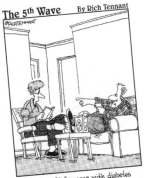

"C'mon, Darrel! Someone with diabetes shouldn't be lying around all day. Whereas someone with no life, like myself, has a very good reason."

page 265

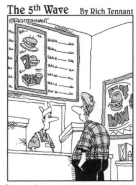

"Sorry sir—we don't currently offer a 'Happy Hemoglobin Meal'."

page 243

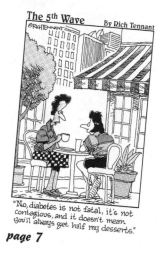

"No, diabetes is not fatal, it's not contagious, and it doesn't mean you'll always get half my desserts."

page 7

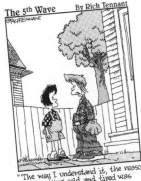

"The way I understand it, the reason I was getting cold and tired was because my body wasn't making enough insulation."

page 199

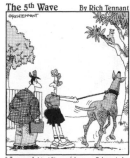

"I named him 'Glucose', because I have to keep him under control every day."

page 43

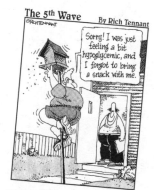

Sorry! I was just feeling a bit hypoglycemic, and I forgot to bring a snack with me.

page 101

Cartoon Information:
Fax: 978-546-7747
E-Mail: richtennant@the5thwave.com
World Wide Web: www.the5thwave.com

Table of Contents

Introduction

What's funny about diabetes? It's a disease, isn't it? Sure, it's a disease, but the people who have it at the beginning of the 21st century are the most fortunate group in history.

It reminds me of the story of the doctor who called his patient to give him the results of his blood tests. "I have bad news and worse news," said the doctor.

"My gosh," said the patient, "What's the bad news?"

"Your lab tests indicate that you have only 24 hours to live," said the doctor.

"What could be worse than that?" said the patient.

"I've been trying to reach you since yesterday," said the doctor.

Those of you with diabetes have a decade or more in which to avoid the long-term complications of this disease. In a sense, a diagnosis of diabetes is both good news and bad news. It is bad news because you have a disease you would happily do without. It is good news if you use it to make some changes in your lifestyle that can not only prevent complications but help you to live a longer and higher-quality life.

As for laughing about it, at times you will feel like doing anything but laughing. But scientific studies are clear about the benefits of a positive attitude. In a very few words: He who laughs, lasts. Another point is that people learn more and retain more when humor is part of the process.

If you have experienced something funny during the course of your diabetes care, I hope you share it with me. My goal is not to trivialize human suffering by being comic about it, but to lighten the burden of a chronic disease by showing that it is not all gloom and doom.

About This Book

The book is not meant to be read from cover to cover, although if you know nothing about diabetes, it might be a good approach. This book is to serve as a source for information about the problems that arise over the years. You can find the latest facts about diabetes and the best sources to discover any information that comes out after the publication of this edition.

Conventions Used in this Book

Diabetes, as you know, is all about sugar. But sugars come in many types. So doctors avoid using the words *sugar* and *glucose* interchangeably. In this book (unless I slip up), I use the word glucose rather than sugar. (You might as well get used to it, sweetie.)

What You Don't Have to Read

Throughout the book, you find shaded areas, which I call sidebars. These sidebars contain material that is interesting but not essential. I hereby give you permission to skip them if the material inside them is of no particular interest to you. You will still understand everything else.

Foolish Assumptions

The book assumes that you know nothing about diabetes. You will not suddenly have to face a term that is not explained and that you never heard of before. For those who already know a lot about diabetes, you can find more in-depth explanations. You can pick and choose how much you want to know about a subject, but the key points are clearly marked.

How This Book Is Organized

This book is divided into six parts to help you find out all you can about the topic of diabetes.

Part 1: Dealing with the Onset of Diabetes

To slay the dragon, you have to be able to identify it. This part clears up the different types of diabetes, how you get them, and if you can give them to others.

In this part, you find out how to deal with the emotional and psychological consequences of the diagnosis and what all those big words mean. You also find out how to prevent the complications of diabetes.

Part II: How Diabetes Affects Your Body

In medical history, there have been a few diseases that seem to affect every part of the body. If you understand diabetes, you will have a pretty good grasp of how other illnesses can change the state of your health.

In this part, you find out what you need to know about both the short- and long-term complications of diabetes. You also find out about some sexual problems related to diabetes and the problems of a diabetic pregnancy.

Part III: Managing Diabetes: The "Thriving with Diabetes" Lifestyle Plan

In this part, you discover all the tools available to treat diabetes. You find out about the kinds of tests that you should be doing as well as the tests your doctor should be ordering in order to get a clear picture of the severity of your diabetes, what to do about it, and how to follow the success of therapy.

You also discover the dietary changes that you need to make to control your blood glucose and how to get the most out of your exercise routine and medications.

Finally, you find out about the huge amount of help out there for you and your family. It is yours for the taking, and you definitely should take advantage of it.

Part IV: Special Considerations for Living with Diabetes

The way that diabetes develops is different for each age group. In this part, you hear about those differences and how to manage them. You also find out about some of the special economic problems of people with diabetes, which relate to jobs and insurance.

Lastly, this part covers all the new developments in diagnosing, monitoring, and treating diabetes and helps correct a lot of misinformation about diabetes treatment.

Part V: The Part of Tens

This part presents some key suggestions, the stuff you most need to know as well as the stuff you least want to know.

You discover the ten commandments of diabetes care and the myths that confuse many diabetic patients. You also find out how to get others to help you in your efforts to control your diabetes.

Part VI: Appendixes

This part of the book contains even more information about diabetes. Two special appendixes help you improve your diet by giving you recipes and diabetic exchanges. Another appendix points out hot spots to visit on the Internet. And in case you forget what a term means, you can quickly flip to the handy glossary in the back of this book.

Icons Used in This Book

The icons tell you what you must know, what you should know, and what you might find interesting but can live without.

This icon marks whenever I tell a story about patients.

This icon marks paragraphs where I define terms.

When you see this icon, it means the information is essential and you should be aware of it.

This icon points out when you should see your doctor (for example, if your blood glucose level is too high or you need a particular test done).

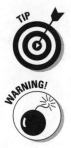

This icon marks important information that can save you time and energy.

This icon warns against potential problems (for example, if you don't treat something).

Part I
Dealing with the Onset of Diabetes

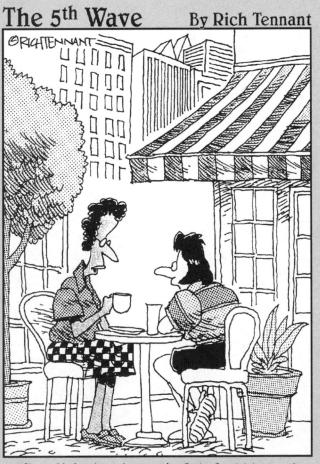

The 5th Wave   By Rich Tennant

"No, diabetes is not fatal, it's not contagious, and it doesn't mean you'll always get half my desserts."

In this part . . .

Y ou have found out that you or a loved one has
diabetes. What do you do now? This part helps you
deal with all the emotions that arise when you discover
that you will not live forever — from wondering whether
the diagnosis is correct to avoiding the complications
associated with diabetes.

Chapter 1

Dealing with Diabetes

· ·

· ·

As a person with diabetes, you are more than the sum of your blood glucose levels. You have feelings, and you have a history. The way that you respond to the challenges of diabetes determines whether the disease will be a moderate annoyance or the source of major sickness.

One of my patients told me that she was working at her first job out of college, where the employee tradition was to have a birthday cake and celebration for all birthdays. She came to the first celebration and was urged to eat cake. She refused and refused, until finally she had to say, "I can't eat the cake because I am diabetic." The woman urging her said, "Thank God. I thought you just had incredible willpower." Twenty years later, my patient clearly remembers being told that having diabetes is better than having willpower. Another patient told me this: "The hardest thing about having diabetes is having to deal with doctors who do not respect me." Several times over the years, she had followed her doctor's recommendations exactly, but her glucose control had not been satisfactory. The doctor blamed her for this "failure."

And unless you live alone on a desert island, your diabetes doesn't affect just you. Your family, friends, and coworkers are affected by how you deal with your diabetes and by their desire to help you. This chapter shows you some coping skills to help you deal with diabetes and deal with your important relationships.

You Are Not Alone

Are you as pretty as Nicole Johnson, the 1999 Miss America? Are you as funny as Jackie Gleason or Jack Benny? Are you an actor with the talent of James Cagney, Spencer Tracy, or Elizabeth Taylor? Can you hit a tennis ball like Arthur Ashe? Can you paint like Paul Cézanne? Do you have the charisma of Gamel Abdel-Nasser? Can you write like Ernest Hemingway or H. G. Wells? Can you sing like Ella Fitzgerald or Elvis Presley? Do you have the inventive powers of Thomas Alva Edison? You have at least one thing in common with all of these famous people. You all have diabetes.

Diabetes is a common disease, so it's bound to occur in some very uncommon people. The list of people with diabetes is long, and you may be amazed at some of the people who you find have diabetes. The point is that every one of them lives or lived with this chronic illness, and every one of them was able to do something special with his or her life.

Politicians seem to be a group with a lot of diabetes. Maybe politicians eat too many of those fund-raising dinners full of alcohol, starchy foods, and calorie-rich desserts. (See Chapter 4 for the place of diet in the onset of diabetes.) In any case, among the Russian premiers who have had diabetes are Yuri Andropov, Nikita Krushchev, and Mikhail Gorbechev. Israeli Prime Minister Menachem Begin had diabetes. Balancing him on the Arab side is King Fahd of Saudi Arabia. Winnie Mandela of South Africa has it. President Clinton's mother, Virginia Kelley, a politician by association, had diabetes. Rounding off the list are Clinton Anderson, a U.S. Senator from New Mexico, Fiorello LaGuardia, a New York mayor, and Josip Tito, former ruler of Yugoslavia.

Jackie Gleason probably leads the list of actors and comedians with diabetes for his motto, "How Sweet It Is!" Could he have been referring to his diabetes or his blood glucose? Among the other great talents with diabetes are these: Halle Berry, with type 1 diabetes; Mary Tyler Moore, also with type 1; Kate Smith, who sang "God Bless America;" and Mae West, who told men to "Come up and see me sometime."

Walt Kelly, who drew the *Pogo* comic strip, joins Paul Cézanne as artists with diabetes. Mario Puzo, author of The *Godfather*, joins Ernest Hemingway and H.G. Wells among the great writers. In business, Ray Kroc founded the McDonald's chain while dealing with his diabetes.

The singers and musicians group contains some of the greatest voices you will ever hear. Besides Ella and Elvis, musicians with diabetes include Jerry Garcia of the Grateful Dead, Johnny Cash, Carol Channing of *Hello Dolly* fame, jazz musician Dizzy Gillespie, and gospel singer Mahalia Jackson. The great composer of operas, Giacomo Puccini, also had diabetes.

Diabetes doesn't prevent the achievement of great records in sports. It didn't stop Arthur Ashe from winning the U.S. Open Tennis Tournament more than once. Jackie Robinson lived with type 1 diabetes all of his life — and, unfortunately, at a time when doctors didn't possess the tools to control diabetes that we have today. Catfish Hunter could strike out many a batter, even when his glucose was a little off. The great Ty Cobb got plenty of hits despite his diabetic condition. Billie Jean King put women's tennis on the map when she beat Bobby Riggs. Her diabetes certainly didn't slow her serve. (If you want to know the role of sports and other activities in your life, see Chapter 9.)

The names in the preceding paragraphs are just a partial list of those with diabetes who have achieved greatness. The point of these many examples is this: *Diabetes shouldn't stop you from doing what you want to do with your life.* You must follow the rules of good diabetic care, as I describe in Chapters 7 through 12. But if you follow those rules, you will actually be healthier than people without diabetes who smoke, overeat, under exercise, or combine these and other unhealthy habits. If you follow the rules of good diabetes care, you will be just as healthy as the person without diabetes.

Perhaps the many people with diabetes who achieved greatness used the same personal strengths to overcome the difficulties associated with diabetes and to excel at their particular callings. Or maybe their diabetes forced them to be stronger, more perseverant, and therefore more successful. Chapter 15 shows you a few areas (such as piloting a commercial flight) in which certain people with diabetes can't participate — due to the ignorance of some legislators. These last few blocks to complete freedom of choice for those with diabetes will come down as you show that you can safely and competently do anything that a person without diabetes can do.

Dealing with the Diagnosis of Diabetes

Do you remember what you were doing when you found out that you or a loved one had diabetes? Unless you were too young to understand, the news was quite a shock. Suddenly you had a condition from which people die. Many of the feelings that you went through were exactly those of a person learning that he or she is dying. The following sections describe the normal stages of reacting to a diagnosis of a major medical condition such as diabetes.

The stage of denial

You probably began by denying that you had diabetes, despite all the evidence. Your doctor may have helped you to deny by saying that you had just "a touch of diabetes," which is an impossibility equivalent to "a touch of pregnancy." You probably looked for any evidence that the whole thing was a mistake. Ultimately, you had to accept the diagnosis and begin to gather the information needed to start to help yourself. But perhaps you neglected to take your medication, follow your diet, or perform the exercise that is so important to maintaining your body.

Hopefully, you not only accepted the diabetes diagnosis yourself, but you also shared the news with your family, friends, and people close to you. Having diabetes isn't something to be ashamed of, and it isn't something that you should hide from anyone. You need the help of everyone in your environment, from your coworkers who need to know not to tempt you with treats that you can't eat, to your friends who need to know how to give you glucagon, a treatment for low blood glucose, if you become unconscious from a severe insulin reaction.

Your diabetes isn't your fault — nor is it a form of leprosy or other diseases that historically or currently carry a social stigma. Diabetes isn't contagious, and no one can catch it from you.

When you're accepting and open about having diabetes, you'll find that you're far from alone in your situation. (If you don't believe me, read the section "You Are Not Alone," earlier in this chapter.) For example, one of my patients told me about an uplifting experience that she had. She arrived at work one morning and was very worried when she realized that she had forgotten her insulin. But she quickly found a source of comfort when she remembered that she could go to a diabetic coworker and ask to borrow some insulin. Another time, she left the crowd at a party and stepped into a friend's bedroom to take a shot of insulin, and she found a man there doing the same thing.

The stage of anger

When you've passed the stage of denying that you or a loved one has diabetes, you may become angry that you're saddled with this "terrible" diagnosis. But you'll quickly find that diabetes isn't so terrible and that you can't do anything to rid yourself of the disease. Your anger only worsens your situation, and it's detrimental in the following ways:

- ✔ If your anger becomes targeted at a person, he or she is hurt.
- ✔ You often feel guilty that your anger is harming you and those close to you.
- ✔ Anger often keeps you from successfully managing your diabetes.

As long as you're angry, you are not in a problem-solving mode. Diabetes requires your focus and attention. Turn your anger into creative ways to manage your diabetes. (For ways to manage your diabetes, see Part III.)

The stage of bargaining

The reactions of anger that you may experience often lead to a stage when you or your loved one becomes increasingly aware of the loss of immortality and bargain for more time. At this point, most people with diabetes realize that they have plenty of life ahead of them, but they start to be overwhelmed by the talk of complications, blood tests, and pills or insulin. You may experience depression, which makes good diabetic care all the more difficult.

Studies have shown that people with diabetes suffer from depression at a rate that is two to four times higher than the rate for the general population. Those with diabetes also experience anxiety at a three to five times higher rate than people without diabetes.

If you suffer from depression, you may feel that your diabetic situation creates problems for you that justify being depressed. You may rationalize your depression in the following ways:

- Diabetes hinders you as you try to make friends.
- As a person with diabetes, you don't have the freedom to choose your leisure activities.
- You may feel that you're too tired to overcome difficulties.
- You may dread the future and possible diabetic complications.
- You don't have the freedom to eat what you want.
- All the minor inconveniences of dealing with diabetes may produce a constant level of annoyance.

All of the preceding concerns are legitimate, but they also are all surmountable. How do you handle your many concerns and fend off depression? The following are a few important methods:

- Try to achieve excellent blood glucose control.
- Begin a regular exercise program.
- Recognize that every abnormal blip in your blood glucose is not your fault.

The final stage: Moving on

If you can't overcome the depression brought on by your diabetic concerns, you may need to consider therapy or antidepressant drugs. But you probably won't reach that point. You may experience the various stages of reacting to your diabetes in a different order than I describe in the previous sections. Some stages may be more prominent, and others may be hardly noticeable.

Don't feel that any anger, denial, or depression is wrong. These are natural coping mechanisms that serve a psychological purpose for a brief time. But allow yourself to have these feelings — and then drop them. Move on and learn to live normally with your diabetes.

Maintaining a High Quality of Life

You may assume that a chronic disease like diabetes will lead to a diminished quality of life for you. But must this be the case? Several studies have been done to evaluate this question.

A very recent study, in the *Journal of the American Medical Association* on November 4, 1998, lasting only 12 weeks, looked at the difference in the perceived quality of life between a group that had good diabetic control and a group that had poor diabetic control. The well-controlled group had lower distress from symptoms, a perception that they were in better health, and a feeling that they could think and learn more easily. This translated into greater productivity, less absenteeism, and fewer days of restricted activity.

Most of the other studies of quality of life for people with diabetes have been long-term studies. In one study of more than 2,000 people with diabetes, receiving many different levels of intensity of treatment, the overall response was that quality of life was lower for the person with diabetes than for the general population. But several factors separated those with the lower quality of life from those who expressed more contentment with life.

One factor that contributed to a lower quality of life rating is a lack of physical activity. This is one negative factor that you can alter immediately. Physical activity is a habit that you must maintain on a lifelong basis. (See Chapter 9 for advice on exercise.) The problem is that making a long-term change to a more physically active lifestyle is difficult; most people maintain their activity for awhile but eventually fall back into inactive routines.

Another study demonstrated the tendency for people with diabetes (and for people in general) to abandon exercise programs after a certain length of time. This was reported in the *New England Journal of Medicine* on July 18, 1991. In this study, a group of people with diabetes received professional support for two years to encourage them to increase physical activity. For the first six months, the study participants responded well and exercised regularly, with the result that their blood glucose, their weight, and their overall health improved. After that, participants began to drop out and not come to training sessions. At the end of the two-year study, most participants had regained their weight and slipped back into poor glucose control. It is noteworthy that the few who didn't stop their exercise maintained the benefits and continued to report an improved quality of life.

Perhaps you're afraid that intensified insulin treatment, which involves three or four daily shots of insulin and frequent testing of blood glucose, will keep you from doing the things that you want to do and will diminish your daily quality of life. (See Chapter 10 for more information about intensified insulin treatment.) Another study in *Diabetes Care* in November 1998 explored whether the extra effort and time consumed by such diabetes treatments had an adverse effect on people's quality of life. The study compared people with diabetes to people with other chronic diseases, such as gastrointestinal disease and hepatitis (liver infection), and then compared all of those groups to a group of people who had no disease. The diabetic group reported a higher quality of life than the other chronic illness groups. The people in the diabetic group were not so much concerned with the physical problems of diabetes, such as intense and time-consuming tests and treatments, as they were concerned with the social and psychological difficulties.

Many other studies have examined the different aspects of diabetes that affect a person with diabetes' quality of life. The following studies had some useful findings:

- **Family support:** People with diabetes greatly benefit from their family's help in dealing with their disease. But do people with diabetes in a close family have better diabetic control? One study in *Diabetes Care* in February 1998 attempted to answer this question and found some unexpected results. Having a supportive family didn't necessarily mean that the person with diabetes in the study would maintain better glucose control. But a supportive family did make the person with diabetes feel more physically capable in general and much more comfortable with his or her place in society.

- **Insulin injections for adults:** Do adults with diabetes who require insulin shots experience a diminished quality of life? A report in *Diabetes Care* in June 1998 found that insulin injections don't reduce the quality of life; the person's sense of physical and emotional well-being remains the same after beginning insulin injections as it was before injections were necessary.

- **Insulin injections for teenagers:** Teenagers who require insulin injections don't always accept the treatment as well as adults do, so teenagers more often experience a diminished quality of life. Even teenagers who successfully control their diabetes with injections feel that diabetes is negatively affecting their lives. They are often depressed and struggle with their diabetic control, although they usually maintain good control.

- **Quality of life over the long term:** How does a person's perception of quality of life change over time? As they age, do most people with diabetes feel that their quality of life increases, decreases, or persists at a steady level? The consensus of studies is that most people with diabetes experience an increasing quality of life as they get older. People feel better about themselves and their diabetes after dealing with the disease for a decade or more. This is the healing property of time.

Putting all this information together, what can you do to maintain a high quality of life with diabetes? Here are the steps that accomplish the most for you:

- Keep your blood glucose as normal as possible (see Part III)
- Make exercise a regular part of your lifestyle
- Get plenty of support from family, friends, and medical resources
- Stay aware of the latest developments in diabetes care
- Maintain a healthy attitude. Remember that some day you will laugh about things that bug you now, so why wait?

SEE YOUR DOCTOR

When you're having trouble coping

You wouldn't hesitate to seek help for your physical ailments associated with diabetes, but you may be very reluctant to seek help when you can't adjust psychologically to diabetes. The problem is that sooner or later, your psychological maladjustment will ruin any control that you have over your diabetes. And, of course, you won't lead a very pleasant life if you're in a depressed or anxious state all the time. The following symptoms are indicators that you're past the point of handling your diabetes on your own and may be suffering from depression:

- You can't sleep.
- You have no energy when you are awake.
- You can't think clearly.
- You can't find activities that interest or amuse you.
- You feel worthless.
- You have frequent thoughts of suicide.
- You have no appetite.
- You find no humor in anything.

If you recognize several of these symptoms as features of your daily life, you need to get some help. Your sense of hopelessness may include

the feeling that no one else can help you — and that simply isn't true. Your primary physician or endocrinologist is the first place to go for advice. He or she may help you to see the need for some short-term or long-term therapy. Well-trained therapists — especially therapists who are trained to take care of people with diabetes — can see solutions that you can't see in your current state. You need to find a therapist whom you can trust, so that when you're feeling low you can talk to this therapist and feel assured that he or she is very interested in your welfare.

Your therapist may decide that your situation is appropriate for medication to treat the anxiety or depression. Currently, many drugs are available that are proven safe and free of side effects. Sometimes a brief period of medication is enough to help you adjust to your diabetes.

You can also find help in a support group. The huge and continually growing number of support groups shows that positive things are happening in these groups. In most support groups, participants share their stories and problems, which helps everyone involved to cope with their own feelings of isolation, futility, or depression.

Chapter 2

It's the Glucose

The Greeks and Romans knew about diabetes. Fortunately, the way they tested for the condition — by tasting the urine — has gone by the wayside. In this way, the Romans discovered that the urine of certain people was *mellitus*, the Latin word for *sweet*. The Greeks noticed that when people with sweet urine drank, the fluids came out in the urine almost as fast as they went in the mouth, like a siphon. They called this by the Greek word for *siphon — diabetes*. This is the origin of the modern name for the disease, diabetes mellitus.

In this chapter, I cover the not-so-fun stuff about diabetes — the big words, the definitions, and so on. But if you really want to understand what's happening to your body when you have diabetes — and I know I would — then you won't want to skip this chapter despite the technical words.

Recognizing Diabetes

The sweetness of the urine comes from *glucose*, also known as blood sugar. Many different kinds of sugars are in nature, but glucose is the sugar that has the starring role in the body, providing a source of instant energy so that muscles can move and important chemical reactions can take place. Sugar is a carbohydrate, one group of the three sources of energy in the body. The others are protein and fat, which I discuss in greater detail in Chapter 8.

Table sugar, or *sucrose*, is actually two different kinds of sugar — glucose and fructose — linked together. Fructose is the type of sugar found in fruits and vegetables. It is sweeter than glucose, which makes sucrose sweeter than glucose as well. Your taste buds require less sucrose or fructose to get the same sweetening power of glucose.

Diabetes mellitus is not the only condition associated with thirst and frequent urination. Another condition in which fluids go in and out of the body like a siphon is called *diabetes insipidus*. Here, the urine is not sweet. Diabetes insipidus is an entirely different disease that you should not mistake for diabetes mellitus.

The standard definition of diabetes mellitus is excessive glucose in a blood sample. For years, doctors set this level fairly high. The standard level for a normal glucose was lowered in 1997 because too many people were experiencing complications of diabetes even though they did not have the disease by the then-current standard. After much discussion, many meetings, and the usual deliberations that surround a momentous decision, the American Diabetes Association published the new standard for diagnosis, which includes any one of the following three criteria:

- ✔ **Casual plasma glucose** concentration greater than or equal to 200 mg/dl along with symptoms of diabetes (see the section "Losing control of glucose," later in this chapter). Mg/dl stands for *milligrams per deciliter*. The rest of the world uses the International System (SI), where the units are mmol/L, which is *millimoles per liter*. To get mmol/L, you divide mg/dl by 18. Therefore, 200 mg/dl is 11.1 mmol/L.

- ✔ **Fasting plasma glucose (FPG)** of greater than or equal to 126 mg/dl or 7 mmol/L. *Fasting* means that the patient has consumed no food for eight hours prior to the test.

- ✔ **Blood glucose** of greater than or equal to 200 mg/dl (11.1 mmol/L), when tested two hours (2-h PG) after ingesting 75 grams of glucose by mouth. This test has long been known as the Oral Glucose Tolerance Test. Although this test is rarely done because it takes time and is cumbersome, it remains the gold standard for the diagnosis of diabetes.

If one of the preceding criteria is positive one time, that is not enough. Any one of the tests must be positive on another occasion to make a diagnosis of diabetes. More than one patient has come to me with a diagnosis of diabetes who had been tested only once. When I did one of the tests for confirmation, I didn't find diabetes.

Putting it another way:

- ✔ FPG less than 110 mg/dl (6.1 mmol/L) is a normal fasting glucose.

- ✔ FPG greater than or equal to 110 mg/dl but less than 126 mg/dl (7.0 mmol/L) is impaired fasting glucose.

✔ FPG equal to or greater than 126 mg/dl (7.0 mmol/L) gives a provisional diagnosis of diabetes.

✔ 2-h PG less than 140 mg/dl (7.8 mmol/L) is normal glucose tolerance.

✔ 2-h PG greater than or equal to 140 mg/dl but less than 200 mg/dl (11.1 mmol/L) is impaired glucose tolerance.

✔ 2-h PG equal to or greater than 200 mg/ dl gives a provisional diagnosis of diabetes.

In order to understand the symptoms of diabetes, you need to know a little about the way the body normally handles glucose and what happens when things go wrong. The following sections explain the fine line that your body toes between control and lack of control of its glucose levels.

Controlling glucose

A hormone called *insulin* finely controls the level of glucose in your blood. A *hormone* is a chemical substance made in one part of the body that travels (usually through the bloodstream) to a distant part of the body where it performs its work. In the case of insulin, that work is to act like a key to open the inside of a cell, such as muscle, fat, or other cells, so that glucose can enter. If glucose can't enter the cell, it can provide no energy to the body.

Insulin is essential for growth. In addition to providing the key to entry of glucose into the cell, scientists consider insulin the builder hormone. It enables fat and muscle to form; it promotes storage of glucose in a form called *glycogen* for use when fuel is not coming in. It blocks breakdown of protein. Without insulin, you do not survive for long. With this fine-tuning, the body manages to keep the level of glucose pretty steady at about 60 to 115 milligrams per deciliter (mg/dl) (3.3 to 6.4 mmol/L) all the time.

Losing control of glucose

Your glucose starts to rise in your blood when insulin is either not present in sufficient quantity or is not working effectively. Once your glucose rises above 180 mg/dl (10.0 mmol/L), glucose begins to spill into the urine and make it sweet. Up to that point, the kidney, the filter for the blood, is able to extract the glucose before it enters your urine. It is the loss of glucose into the urine that leads to many of the short-term complications of diabetes. (See Chapter 4 for more on short-term complications.)

The following list contains the most common early symptoms of diabetes and how they occur. One or more of the following symptoms may be present when diabetes is diagnosed:

- ✔ **Frequent urination and thirst:** The glucose in the urine draws more water out of the blood, so more urine forms. More urine in your bladder makes you feel the need to urinate more frequently during the day and to get up at night to empty the bladder, which keeps filling up. As the amount of water in your blood declines, you feel thirsty and drink much more frequently.

- ✔ **Fatigue:** Because glucose can't enter cells that depend on insulin as a key for glucose (the most important exception is the brain, which does not need insulin), glucose can't be used as a fuel to move muscles or to facilitate the many other chemical reactions that have to take place to produce energy. The person with diabetes often complains of fatigue and feels much stronger once treatment allows glucose to enter cells again.

- ✔ **Weight loss:** Weight loss is common among some people with diabetes because they lack insulin, which is the builder hormone. When insulin is lacking for any reason, the body begins to break down. You lose muscle tissue. Some of the muscle converts into glucose even though it cannot get into cells. It passes out of your body in the urine. Fat tissue breaks down into small fat particles that can provide an alternate source of energy. As your body breaks down and you lose glucose in the urine, you often experience weight loss. However, most people with diabetes are heavy rather than skinny. (I explain why in Chapter 3.)

- ✔ **Persistent vaginal infection among women:** As blood glucose rises, all the fluids in your body contain higher levels of glucose, including the sweat and body secretions such as semen in men and vaginal secretions in women. Many bugs, such as bacteria and fungi, thrive in the high glucose environment. Women begin to complain of itching or burning, an abnormal discharge from the vagina, and sometimes an odor.

Discovering Ways to Treat Diabetes

A condition that must have been diabetes mellitus appears in the writings of China and India more than 2,000 years ago. The description is the same one that the Greeks and Romans reported — urine that tasted sweet. Scholars from India and China were the first to describe frequent urination. But it wasn't until 1776 that researchers discovered the cause of the sweetness — glucose. And it wasn't until the 19th century that doctors developed a new chemical test. Later discoveries showed that the pancreas produced a crucial substance, called insulin, that controlled the glucose in the blood. (For more on insulin, see the "Controlling glucose" section, earlier in the chapter.) Since that time, insulin has been extracted and purified enough to save many lives. Oral drugs to reduce blood glucose have become available only in the last 40 years.

Once insulin was discovered, diabetes specialists, led by Elliot Joslin and others, recommended three basic treatments for diabetes that are as valuable today as they were in 1921:

- Diet (see Chapter 8)
- Exercise (see Chapter 9)
- Medication (see Chapter 10)

The discovery of insulin did not solve the problem of diabetes, although it immediately saved the lives of thousands of very sick individuals for whom the only treatment had been starvation. As these people aged, they were found to have unexpected complications in the eyes, the kidneys, and the nervous system (see Chapter 5). And insulin did not address the problem of the much larger group of people with diabetes now known as type 2 (see Chapter 3). Their problem was not lack of insulin but resistance to its actions. Fortunately, doctors do have the tools now to bring the disease under control.

The next major discovery was the group of drugs called *sulfonylureas* (see Chapter 10), the first drugs that could be taken by mouth to lower the blood glucose. But the only way to know the level of the blood glucose was still by testing the urine, which was entirely inadequate for good diabetic control (see Chapter 7).

Around 1980, the first portable meters for blood glucose testing became available. Now it became possible, for the first time, to relate treatment to a measurable outcome. This has led, in turn, to discovery of other great drugs for diabetes like metformin, rosiglitazone, and others yet to come.

If you are not using these wonderful tools for your diabetes, you are missing the boat. You can find out exactly how to use them in Part III.

Typical Patient Stories

The numbers that are used to diagnose diabetes don't begin to reflect the human dimensions of the disease. People end up with these tests after days to months (or even years) of minor discomforts that reach the point where they can no longer be tolerated. The next few stories of real (though renamed) patients can help you understand that diabetes is a disease that happens to people — people who are working, relaxing, travelling, sleeping, and doing many other things that make life so complex.

Tracking diabetes around the world

Diabetes is a global health problem. A 1994 study estimated that approximately 100 million people around the world have diabetes and that by the year 2010, the number would rise to more than 215 million. These estimates were made before the current, more inclusive definition of diabetes was accepted in 1997. Under the new definition, prevalence of diabetes in the world was more like 140 million in 1994 and will be 300 million in 2010. Diabetes is concentrated where food supplies allow people to eat more calories than they need so that they develop obesity, a condition of excessive fat. There are actually several different types of diabetes, but the type usually associated with obesity, called type 2 diabetes (see Chapter 3), far outweighs the other types.

Diabetes is also increasing throughout the world because the age of the population is increasing. Age is a major risk factor for diabetes along with obesity. (See Chapter 3 for more risk factors.) As other diseases are controlled and the population gets older, more diabetes is being diagnosed.

One very interesting study traces people of Japanese ancestry as they went from living in Japan to living in Hawaii and finally the United States mainland. Those in Japan, where people customarily maintain a normal weight, tended to have a very low incidence of diabetes. As they moved to Hawaii, the incidence of diabetes began to rise along with their average weight. On the mainland, where food is most available, these Japanese had the highest rate of diabetes of all.

Not only the number of calories but the composition of the diet changes as people migrate. Before they migrate, they tend to consume a low-fat, high-fiber diet. Once they reach their new destination, they adopt the local diet that tends to be higher in fat and lower in fiber. The carbohydrates in the new diet are from high-energy foods, which do not tend to be filling, promoting more caloric intake.

The Japanese provide another interesting lesson about the place of obesity as a factor in the onset of diabetes. Japanese Sumo wrestlers have to gain enormous quantities of weight in order to fight in a certain weight class. Even while they are still fighting, they demonstrate a high frequency of diabetes. Once they become more sedentary, the frequency goes up to 40 percent, a huge prevalence.

Another group that shows the consequences of switching from a moderate calorie, relatively nutritious diet to a higher calorie diet is the North American Indian. Some tribes, such as the Pima Indians, have a prevalence of diabetes as high as one out of two people. In contrast, the finding of diabetes in South American Indian tribes, such as in Chile where they have maintained a more traditional diet, is extremely rare.

In China, as the country becomes more affluent, doctors are seeing a significant increase in the incidence of diabetes. Migrant Chinese populations show even higher rates, especially where the environment allows them to gain more weight and be more sedentary.

In the United States there were about 20 million people with diabetes in the year 2000. This represents about 7 to 8 percent of the population. Currently only half the people with diabetes are aware that they have the condition. The big project for the next two years is to get people to know their blood glucose level just like they know their cholesterol, and to seek treatment.

ANECDOTE

Jane Fein was a 46-year-old woman who worked in a computer company and had to do a lot of standing. She noticed that she had been having some tingling in her feet but thought it was due to all the standing. However, she had gained 22 pounds in the last six years and couldn't seem to shed them. She was beginning to wake up a few times at night to go to the bathroom. She thought this might be associated with her menopause, which was just beginning. She decided to see her gynecologist, who told her everything was fine but suggested a urinalysis because she was waking up so much. To everyone's surprise, glucose was present in her urine, and the gynecologist sent her to an internist. The internist did a random glucose in the lab. It was 225 mg/dl (12.5 mmol/L). He did a fasting blood glucose the next morning, and it was 163 mg/dl (9.0). He made a diagnosis of type 2 (see Chapter 3) diabetes and started Jane on a program of diet and exercise.

The Steadmonsons — John, Mary, daughter Rachel, 9, and son Lyle, 5 — were on a trip to the California desert in June. The heat made everyone extremely thirsty and forced them to drink lots of fluids. Lyle was also urinating a lot, but no one thought much about it. However, when they returned home, Lyle continued to complain of thirst and urinate excessively. He seemed to eat a lot of sweets but did not gain weight. Then Lyle wet his bed, which had not happened for years. Mary felt she should take him to the pediatrician because he did not seem like his usual active self. The doctor did a random blood glucose, which was 468 mg/dl (26 mmol/L). A repeat random blood glucose was 392 mg/dl (21.2 mmol/L). The doctor told Mary and John that Lyle had type 1 diabetes. This was the beginning of a lot of changes in the Steadmonson household.

Leslie Law was a 28-year-old woman who had just started a new job. She was eating well but losing weight. She noticed increased thirst and urination, which caused her boss to comment upon the frequent absences in the middle of work. She decided to stop drinking so many beverages, but the urination continued and she began to feel very weak. One afternoon, she fainted at the office, and an ambulance was called. At the hospital, she was found to have a blood glucose of 683 mg/dl (37.9 mmol/L). A repeat blood glucose after receiving fluids because of her very dehydrated state was 592 (32.9 mmol/L). She was started on insulin treatment and rapidly regained her weight and her strength and returned to work after a few days.

Sal Renolo was a 46-year-old black belt judo instructor. Despite his very active lifestyle, he was not careful about his diet and had gained 16 pounds in the last few years. He was more fatigued than he had been in the past but blamed this on his increasing age. His mother had diabetes, but he assumed that his physical fitness would protect him from this condition. He was finding that he could barely get through a one-hour class without excusing himself for a bathroom break. One of his new students had diabetes, and he seemed to have more energy than Sal and never left the class during the lesson. He suggested to Sal that he ought to have the problem checked, but Sal insisted that he could not possibly have diabetes with all his activity. The symptoms of fatigue and frequent urination got worse, and he finally made an appointment with the doctor. Blood tests revealed a random blood glucose of 264 mg/dl (14.7 mmol/L). The following week, another random blood glucose was 289 (16.0 mmol/L). The doctor told Sal he had diabetes, but Sal refused to believe it. He left the doctor's office in an angry mood but vowed to lose weight and did so successfully. On a repeat visit to the doctor, a random glucose was 167 mg/dl (9.3 mmol/L). He told the doctor that he knew he did not have diabetes, but the resolve to eat carefully did not last and he was back six weeks later with a glucose of 302 mg/dl (16.8 mmol/L). Finally, he accepted the diagnosis and started treatment. He rapidly returned to his usual state of health, and the fatigue disappeared.

Debby O'Leary's active sex life with her husband was continually being interrupted by vaginal yeast infections, which resulted in an unpleasant odor and redness and itching. She would go to the drugstore and purchase an over-the-counter preparation, which promptly cured the condition but it rapidly returned. Finally, after three of these infections in two months, she decided to see her gynecologist. The gynecologist told her she needed a prescription drug and gave it to her. The cure lasted a little longer, but the infection promptly returned. On a return visit, the gynecologist did a urinalysis and found glucose in her urine. A random blood test showed a glucose of 243 mg/dl (13.5 mmol/L). He sent her to an internist, who ordered a variety of tests including a fasting blood glucose which was 149 mg/dl (8.3 mmol/L). The doctor told her she had diabetes and recommended exercise and diet to start with. This not only lowered her blood glucose to the point that she no longer developed yeast infections, but the resulting weight loss and return of energy that she did not know was missing, made her sex life with her husband even more satisfying.

Chapter 3

What Type of Diabetes Do You Have?

*Y*ou may not think that having a personal relationship with one of your body organs is possible or even desirable. But don't disregard your pancreas, a shy little organ that can rear its lovely head at entirely unexpected moments. (You probably didn't even know that your pancreas has a head and a tail, but it does. Now you've broken the ice!) Most of the time, your pancreas hides behind your stomach quietly doing its work, helping with digestion first and then helping to make use of the digested food. The information in this chapter should put you on closer terms with your pancreas, which is good, because you need it as much as it needs you. In one way or another, the pancreas plays a role in all of the various types of diabetes.

You can prevent diabetes, but not quite as easily as you may like. (Hopefully, you weren't looking for quack doctor platitudes, such as "You need surgery, but if you can't afford it, I can touch up your x-rays for half the price!") Your best method for preventing diabetes would be to pick your parents carefully, but that's a little bit impractical, even with modern technology.

In general, you can prevent a disease if it meets two requirements. First, you have to be able to identify individuals who are at high risk for getting the disease. Second, the disease must have at least some treatments or actions that you can take to definitely reduce the occurrence of the disease. You can meet both of these requirements in an effort to prevent diabetes. This chapter shows you how to identify whether you're at risk for type 1 or type 2 diabetes, and it covers definite actions that you can take to prevent both of these types of diabetes.

This chapter also helps you get a clear understanding of your type of diabetes, how it relates to the other types of diabetes, and how the failure of your friendly pancreas to do its assigned job can lead to a host of unfortunate consequences. (I cover these consequences in greater detail in Part II.)

Getting to Know Your Pancreas

You don't see your pancreas very often, but you hear from it all the time. It has two major functions. One is to produce digestive enzymes, which are the chemicals in your small intestine that help to break down food. The *digestive enzymes* don't have much relation to diabetes, so I won't spend much time talking about them in this book. Your pancreas's other function is to produce and secrete directly into the blood a hormone of major importance, *insulin*. Figure 3-1 shows the microscopic appearance of the pancreas. The insulin-producing pancreas cells are found in groups called *Islets of Langerhans*.

If you understand only one hormone in your body, insulin should be that hormone (especially if you want to understand diabetes). Over the course of your life, the insulin that your body produces or the insulin that you inject into your body (as I describe in Chapter 10) affects whether or not you control your diabetes and avoid the complications of the disease.

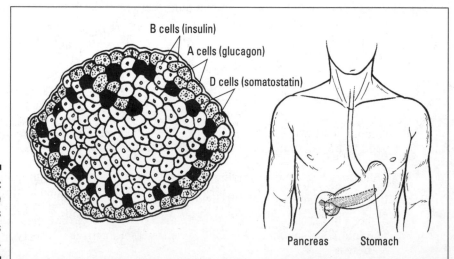

Figure 3-1:
The pancreas and its parts.

B cells (insulin)
A cells (glucagon)
D cells (somatostatin)

Pancreas   Stomach

Think of your insulin as an insurance agent, who lives in San Francisco (which is your pancreas) but travels from there to do business in Seattle (your muscles), Denver (your fat tissue), Los Angeles (your liver), and other places. This insulin insurance agent is insuring your good health.

Wherever insulin travels in your body, it opens up the cells so that glucose can enter them. After glucose enters, the cells can immediately use it for energy, store it in a storage form of glucose (called *glycogen*) for rapid use later on, or convert it to fat for use even later as energy.

After glucose leaves your blood and enters your cells, your blood glucose level falls. Your pancreas can tell when your glucose is falling, and it turns off the release of insulin to prevent unhealthy low levels of blood glucose called *hypoglycemia* (see Chapter 4). At the same time, your liver begins to release glucose from storage and makes new glucose from amino acids in your blood.

If your insurance agent (insulin, remember? — stick with me here!) doesn't show up when you need him (meaning that you have an absence of insulin, as in type 1 diabetes) or he does a poor job when he shows up (such as when you have a resistance to insulin, as in type 2 diabetes), your insurance coverage may be very poor (in which case, your blood glucose starts to climb). High blood glucose is the beginning of all your problems.

Doctors have proven that high blood glucose is bad for you and that keeping the blood glucose as normal as possible prevents the complications of diabetes (which I explain in Part II). Most treatments for diabetes are directed at restoring the blood glucose to normal.

You Have Type 1 Diabetes

John Phillips, a 6-year-old boy, was always very active, and his parents became concerned when the counselors at summer camp told them that he seemed not to have much energy. When he got home from camp, John's parents noticed that he was thirsty all the time and running to the bathroom. He was very hungry but seemed to be losing weight, despite eating more than enough. John's parents took him to the pediatrician, who did several blood glucose tests and told them that their son has *type 1 diabetes mellitus*, which used to be called *juvenile diabetes* or *insulin-dependent diabetes*.

This story has a happy ending because John's parents, though quite upset, were willing to do the necessary things to bring John's glucose under control. John is just as energetic as ever, but he has had to get used to a few inconveniences in his daily routine. (I cover such daily lifestyle changes in Part III.) The following sections detail the symptoms and causes of this type of diabetes.

Identifying the symptoms of type 1 diabetes

Before your doctor actually diagnoses you with diabetes, you may notice that you have some of the major signs and symptoms of type 1 diabetes. If you experience the following symptoms, take time to ask your doctor about the possibility that you have diabetes:

- **Frequent urination:** You experience frequent urination because your kidneys can't return all the glucose to your bloodstream when your blood glucose level is greater than 180 mg/dl (10 mmol/L). (See Chapter 7 for all the details on blood glucose level testing.) The large amount of glucose in your urine makes the urine so concentrated that water is drawn out of the blood and into the urine to reduce the concentration of glucose in the urine. This water and glucose fill up the bladder repeatedly.

- **Increase in thirst:** Your thirst increases as you experience frequent urination, because you lose so much water in the urine that your body begins to dehydrate.

- **Weight loss:** You lose weight as your body loses glucose in the urine and your body breaks down muscle and fat looking for energy.

- **Increase in hunger:** You notice that you're increasingly hungry. Your body has plenty of extra glucose in the blood, but your hunger is a result of your cells becoming malnourished because you lack insulin to allow the glucose to enter into your cells. Your body is going through "hunger in the midst of plenty."

- **Weakness:** You feel weak because your muscle cells and other tissues do not get the energy that they require from glucose.

Type 1 diabetes used to be called *juvenile* diabetes because it occurs most frequently in children. However, so many cases are found in adults that doctors don't use the term *juvenile* any more. Some children are diagnosed early in life, and other children have a more severe onset of the disease as they get a little older. With older children, the early signs and symptoms of diabetes may have been missed by parents, camp counselors, or teachers. These kids have a great deal of fat breakdown in their bodies to provide energy, and this fat breakdown creates other problems. *Ketone bodies*, products of the breakdown of fats, begin to accumulate in the blood and spill into the urine. Ketone bodies are acidic and lead to nausea, abdominal pain, and sometimes vomiting.

At the same time, the child's blood glucose rises higher. Levels as high as 400 to 600 mg/dl (22.2 to 33.3 mmol/L) are not uncommon, but levels as low as 300 (16.6 mmol/L) are possible. The child's blood is like thick maple syrup and doesn't circulate as freely as normal. The large amount of water leaving the body with the glucose depletes important substances such as sodium and potassium. The vomiting causes the child to lose more fluids and body substances. All these abnormalities cause the child to become very drowsy and possibly lose consciousness. This situation is called *diabetic ketoacidosis*, and if it isn't identified and corrected soon, the child can die. (See Chapter 4 for more details on the symptoms, causes, and treatments of ketoacidosis.)

A few special circumstances affect the symptoms that you may see in persons with type 1 diabetes. Remember the following factors:

- **The "honeymoon" period** is a time after the diagnosis of diabetes, when the person's insulin needs decline for one to six months and the disease seems to get milder. The honeymoon period is longer when a child is older at the time of diagnosis, but the apparent diminishing of the disease is always temporary.
- **Males and females** get type 1 diabetes to an equal degree.
- **Warm summer months** are associated with a decrease in the occurrence of diabetes compared to the winter months, particularly in older children. The probable reason for this is that a virus is involved in bringing on diabetes, and viruses spread much more when children are learning and playing together inside in the winter.

Investigating the causes of type 1 diabetes

When your doctor diagnoses you with type 1 diabetes, you almost immediately begin to wonder what could have caused you to acquire the disease. Did someone with diabetes sneeze on you? Did you eat so much sugary food that your body reacted by giving you diabetes? Well, rest assured that the causes of diabetes aren't so simple or easily avoidable.

Type 1 diabetes is an *autoimmune disease*, meaning that your body is unkind enough to react against — and, in this case, destroy — a vital part of itself, namely the insulin-producing beta cells of the pancreas. One way that doctors discovered that type 1 diabetes is an autoimmune disease is by measuring proteins in the blood, called *antibodies*, which are literally substances directed against your body — and, in particular, against your islet cells. (These specific antibodies are called *islet cell antibodies*.) Doctors find the islet cell antibodies in relatives of those who have type 1 diabetes and in the people with diabetes themselves for a few years before the disease begins.

Another clue that type 1 diabetes is an autoimmune disease is that treatments to reduce autoimmunity also delay the onset of type 1 diabetes. Also, type 1 diabetes tends to occur in people who have other known autoimmune diseases.

You may wonder how doctors can know in advance that certain people will develop diabetes. The method of predicting isn't 100 percent accurate, but people who get type 1 diabetes more often have certain abnormal characteristics on their genetic material, their *chromosomes*, that are not present in people who don't get diabetes. Doctors can look for these abnormal characteristics on your DNA and wait to see whether you develop diabetes.

But having these abnormal characteristics on your chromosomes isn't enough to guarantee that you'll get diabetes. Many people who have these specific abnormalities never get diabetes, so doctors need to consider other factors in addition to your DNA. Another essential factor in predicting whether you will develop diabetes is your exposure to something in the environment, most likely a virus. If this virus infiltrates your body, it can cause diabetes by attacking your pancreas directly and diminishing your ability to produce insulin, which quickly creates the diabetic condition in your body. The virus can also cause diabetes if it is made up of a substance that is also naturally present in your pancreas. If the virus and your pancreas possess the same substance, the antibodies that your body produces to fight off the virus will also attack the shared substance in your pancreas, leaving you in the same condition as if the virus itself attacked your pancreas.

Researchers haven't identified one particular virus that they can blame for type 1 diabetes. Research on patients who are at the beginning stages of type 1 diabetes has uncovered many different viruses that could be the culprit. The type 1 diabetes virus may be the same as a virus that causes the common cold.

Getting type 1 diabetes

You may get type 1 diabetes if you have certain factors on your *chromosomes*, the DNA in each cell in your body that determines your physical characteristics. If you have several of these factors, your chance of getting type 1 diabetes is much greater than that of a person who has none of these factors. But just having these factors is not enough. You have to come in contact with something in your environment that triggers the destruction of your *beta cells*, the cells that make insulin. Doctors think that this environmental trigger is probably a virus, and they've identified several viruses that may be to blame. Doctors think they are the same viruses that cause the common cold. Persons with type 1 diabetes probably get the virus just like any cold virus — from someone else who has the virus who sneezes on them. But because they also have the genetic tendency, they get type 1 diabetes.

A small number (about 10 percent) of patients with type 1 diabetes don't seem to need an environmental factor to trigger the diabetes. In them, the disease is entirely an autoimmune destruction of the beta cells. If you fall into this category of people with diabetes, you may have other autoimmune diseases such as autoimmune thyroid disease.

How likely are you to get type 1 diabetes if your brother or sister gets it? Studies of many families have provided fairly good answers to this question. If one of your parents has type 1 diabetes, the odds are only 3 to 4 percent that you will get it. You get half of your total genetic material from each parent. If you and your sibling (brother or sister) have exactly the same genetic material, you are identical twins. The identical twin of a person with type 1 diabetes has about a 20 percent chance of also getting type 1 diabetes. If you have only half of your genetic material in common with your sibling who has type 1 diabetes, your chance of getting type 1 diabetes drops to 5 percent. If none of the genetic material associated with diabetes is the same as your sibling with type 1 diabetes, your chance of developing type 1 diabetes is less than 1 percent. These relatively low chances of both siblings — even for identical twins — getting diabetes clearly show that more factors than your genetic inheritance from your parents are involved in acquiring type 1 diabetes. Otherwise, identical twins would both have type 1 diabetes almost 100 percent of the time.

Preventing type 1 diabetes

In order to prevent diabetes, you have to undergo preventive treatments before the disease starts, which is a method called *primary prevention*. Preventive treatment given to a person with diabetes after the disease is triggered but before the disease makes the person sick is called *secondary prevention*. In order to try secondary prevention, the doctor must be able to recognize that diabetes has begun, even though the patient is not sick. And months to years must pass between diagnosis and onset of symptoms in order to have enough time for the treatment to prevent sickness. Type 1 diabetes is an excellent candidate for both primary and secondary prevention.

Doctors can analyze the genetic material (DNA) of a person who has a family history of diabetes to see whether that person has the genetic material most often found in people who have diabetes. Then the person could receive primary prevention to block the disease.

An example of primary prevention for type 1 diabetes would be vaccination against the viruses that may be associated with diabetes. Unfortunately, doctors haven't yet pinpointed the exact virus or viruses, so vaccinations aren't practical at the present time. Doctors have tried vaccinations in countries (such as Finland) where type 1 diabetes occurs most often, but the vaccinations didn't stop the number of new cases of type 1 diabetes from rising.

Doctors also have considered giving antiviral agents to people who are at high risk of acquiring diabetes, but this approach has been successful only in animal testing so far.

You may think that all the recent scientific advances in gene research would enable doctors to change people's genetic material to prevent the onset of type 1 diabetes. Although scientists have made great strides in identifying the genes associated with diabetes, they haven't quite reached the point where they can change those genes. Such methods for primary prevention of type 1 diabetes are something for the future.

Some doctors believe that certain chemicals in cow's milk bring on type 1 diabetes. Researchers are comparing breast-fed babies who are susceptible to type 1 diabetes to susceptible babies who are given cow's milk. They haven't yet determined whether cow's milk is a factor that causes type 1 diabetes.

On the other hand, lots of trials of secondary prevention are under way, though most show only partial success. Most of these trials make use of doctors' knowledge that patients whose bodies produce autoantibodies have type 1 diabetes and that the antibodies are gradually destroying their insulin-producing beta cells. In these patients, full-blown type 1 diabetes may take a couple of years to appear and create major problems, so the doctor has time to intervene. The most prevalent methods of secondary prevention for type 1 diabetes attempt to block the autoimmune disease from destroying all of your pancreas's beta cells. The following list shows some of the more promising secondary prevention trials and techniques:

- **Steroid drugs:** You can take steroid drugs such as prednisone to block autoimmune conditions. When doctors find islet cell antibodies in a person with type 1 diabetes, they give the person these steroids, which reduce the amount of islet cell antibodies and seem to prolong the period between the development of the antibodies and the onset of symptoms such as excessive thirst and urination. But this approach isn't 100-percent successful, and steroids have many side effects — especially in small children, who are the usual victims of type 1 diabetes. Small children who use steroids suffer from growth problems, infections, and other unwanted side effects. If diabetes becomes active, the reason may be the failure of the steroid to prevent the autoimmune destruction of the pancreas as well as the glucose abnormalities caused by the steroid itself.

- **Cytotoxic drugs:** Another group of drugs that doctors use to increase the time between antibodies and disease are the so-called *cytotoxic drugs,* which act against the cells that may participate in the destruction of the pancreatic beta cells. Again, studies have shown only a slowing down of the time between antibodies and symptoms. Cytotoxic drugs destroy various types of cells — and not just the bad cells. Studies of cytotoxic drugs have all been complicated by side effects that were severe and damaging to some of the patients.

- ✓ **Nicotinamide:** In animal studies, nicotinamide (a B vitamin) protects the beta cells of mice that are diabetes-prone. A similar trial in humans was somewhat successful, showing that 20 percent of patients using nicotinamide didn't develop symptoms of diabetes and didn't lose as many beta cells. Doctors are surprised that a drug known to raise plasma glucose (see Chapter 2) could prevent diabetes.

- ✓ **Insulin:** In another study, small amounts of insulin were given to people who have islet cell antibodies, in an attempt to prolong the time between antibodies and symptoms. This approach initially showed some promise, but further into the study, there has been no difference in the development of diabetes between those given insulin and those who did not receive it.

The most important study of prevention ever done for type 1 diabetes is called the Diabetes Control and Complications Trial (DCCT), published in 1993. The DCCT showed that keeping very tight control over your blood glucose is possible but difficult. The difficult part of keeping your blood glucose close to normal is that you increase your risk of having low blood glucose, or hypoglycemia (see Chapter 4). The DCCT study showed that you can prevent the complications of diabetes — including eye disease, kidney disease, and nerve disease — by keeping your blood glucose as normal as possible. If you already suffered from such complications, improving your blood glucose control very significantly slowed the progression of the complications. Since the DCCT, doctors generally treat type 1 diabetes by keeping the patient's blood glucose as close to normal as possible and practical.

You Have Type 2 Diabetes

ANECDOTE

Edythe Fokel, a 46-year-old woman, has gained about ten pounds in the last year, so that her 5-foot 5-inch body now weighs about 155 pounds. Edythe doesn't do much exercise. She has noticed that she feels more fatigued recently, but she blames her age and approaching menopause for this. One reason that Edythe is more tired is that she gets up several times a night to urinate, which is unusual for her. She is especially disturbed because her vision is blurry, and she does a lot of work on a computer. Finally, Edythe went to her gynecologist because she developed a rash and discharge in her vagina. When Edythe described her symptoms, her gynecologist decided to do a blood glucose test and referred her back to her primary physician when Edythe's blood glucose level registered at 220 mg/dl (12.2 mmol/L).

Edythe's primary doctor asked her whether other members of her family have had diabetes, and she replied that her mother and a sister are both being treated for it. The doctor also asked Edythe about any tingling in her feet, and she admitted that she noticed some tingling for the past few months but didn't think it was important. The primary doctor repeated the random blood glucose test, which came back at 260 mg/dl (14.4 mmol/L), and told Edythe that she had type 2 diabetes.

The signs and symptoms that Edythe manifests in this scenario, along with the results of the two blood glucose tests, provide a textbook picture of type 2 diabetes. (Type 2 diabetes used to be known as *adult onset diabetes* or *non-insulin dependent diabetes*.) But be aware that people with type 2 diabetes may have few or none of these symptoms. That is why it is so important for your doctor to check your blood glucose level on a regular basis. (I discuss how often you should do this test in Chapter 7.)

Type 2 diabetes begins around age 40 and increases in frequency as you get older. Because the symptoms are so mild at first, you may not notice them. You may ignore these symptoms for years before they become bothersome enough to consult your doctor. So type 2 diabetes is a disease of gradual onset rather than the severe emergency that can herald type 1 diabetes. No autoimmunity is involved in type 2 diabetes, so no antibodies are found. Doctors believe that no virus is involved in the onset of type 2 diabetes.

Recent statistics show ten times more people with type 2 diabetes than type 1 throughout the world. Although type 2 is the much more prevalent type of diabetes, those with type 2 diabetes seem to have milder severity of complications (such as eye disease and kidney disease) from diabetes. (See Part II for details about the possible complications of diabetes. See Part III for treatments that can help you prevent these complications.)

Identifying the symptoms of type 2 diabetes

A fairly large percentage of the population of the United States (approximately 16 to 18 million people) has type 2 diabetes. The following signs and symptoms are good indicators that you have type 2 diabetes. If you experience many of these symptoms, check with your doctor:

- **Fatigue:** Type 2 diabetes makes you tired because your body's cells aren't getting the glucose fuel that they need. Even though there is plenty of insulin, your body is resistant to its actions. (See the "Getting to Know Your Pancreas" section for more explanation.)

- **Frequent urination and thirst:** You find yourself urinating more frequently than usual, which dehydrates your body and leaves you thirsty.

✔ **Blurred vision:** The lenses of your eyes swell and shrink as your blood glucose levels rise and fall. Your vision blurs because your eye can't adjust quickly enough to these changes in the lens.

✔ **Slow healing of skin, gum, and urinary infections:** Your white blood cells, which help with healing and defend your body against infections, don't function correctly in the high-glucose environment present in your body when it has diabetes. Unfortunately, the bugs that cause infections thrive in the same high-glucose environment. So diabetes leaves your body especially susceptible to infections.

✔ **Genital itching:** Yeast infections also love a high-glucose environment. So diabetes is often accompanied by the itching and discomfort of yeast infections.

✔ **Numbness in the feet or legs:** You experience numbness because of a common long-term complication of diabetes, called neuropathy. (I explain the details of neuropathy in Chapter 5.) If you notice numbness and neuropathy along with the other symptoms of diabetes, you probably have had the disease for quite a while, because neuropathy takes more than five years to develop in a diabetic environment.

✔ **Heart disease:** Heart disease occurs much more often in type 2s than in the nondiabetic population. But the heart disease may appear when you are merely glucose-intolerant (which I explain in the next section), before you actually have diagnosable diabetes.

✔ **Obesity:** If you're obese, you are considerably more likely to acquire diabetes than you would be if you maintained your ideal weight. (See Chapter 8 for the details on how to figure out your weight classification.) But not all obese people become diabetic, so obesity isn't a definite sign that you have diabetes.

The signs and symptoms of type 2 diabetes are similar in some cases (such as high blood glucose) to the symptoms of type 1 diabetes (which I cover in the "Identifying the symptoms of type 1 diabetes" section, earlier in this chapter), but in many ways they are different. The following list shows some of the differences between symptoms in type 1 and type 2 diabetes:

✔ **Age of onset:** Those with type 1 diabetes are usually younger than those with type 2 diabetes.

✔ **Body weight:** Those with type 1 diabetes are thin or normal in weight, but obesity is a common characteristic of those with type 2 diabetes.

✔ **Level of glucose:** Those with type 1 diabetes have higher glucose levels at onset of the disease. Those with type 1 diabetes usually have blood glucose levels of 300 to 400 mg/dl (16.6 to 22.2 mmol/L), and those with type 2 diabetes usually have blood glucose levels of 200 to 250 mg/dl (11.1 to 13.9 mmol/L).

✔ **Severity of onset:** Type 1 diabetes usually has a much more severe onset, but type 2 diabetes gradually shows its symptoms.

Investigating the causes of type 2 diabetes

Although type 2 diabetes doesn't appear in your body until late in your life (as opposed to the early onset of type 1 diabetes), you're probably nonetheless shocked and curious about why you developed the disease. Doctors have learned quite a bit about the causes of type 2 diabetes. For example, they know that type 2 diabetes runs in families. Usually, people with type 2 diabetes can find a relative who has had the disease. Therefore, doctors consider type 2 diabetes to be much more of a genetic disease than type 1 diabetes. In studies of identical twins, when one twin has type 2 diabetes, the likelihood that type 2 diabetes will develop in the other twin is nearly 100 percent.

Those with type 2 diabetes have plenty of insulin in their bodies (unlike people with type 1 diabetes, who have none of their own insulin in their bodies), but their bodies respond to the insulin in abnormal ways. Those with type 2 diabetes are *insulin-resistant*, meaning that their bodies resist the normal, healthy functioning of insulin. This insulin resistance, combined with not enough insulin to overcome the insulin resistance, causes type 2 diabetes, just like the absent insulin causes type 1 diabetes.

Before obesity or lack of exercise (or diabetes for that matter) is present, future type 2 patients already show signs of insulin resistance. First of all, the amount of insulin in the blood of these people is elevated compared to normal people. Secondly, a shot of insulin doesn't reduce the blood glucose in these insulin-resistant people nearly as much as it does in people without insulin resistance. (See Chapter 10 to find out more about insulin shots in diabetes.)

When your body needs to make extra insulin just to keep your blood glucose normal, your insulin is, obviously, less effective than it should be — which means that you have *impaired glucose tolerance*. Your body goes through impaired glucose tolerance before you actually have diabetes, because your blood glucose is still lower than the levels needed (see Chapter 2) for a diagnosis of diabetes. When you have impaired glucose tolerance and you add other factors such as weight gain, a sedentary lifestyle, and aging, your pancreas can't keep up with your insulin demands and you become diabetic.

Another factor that comes into play when doctors make a diagnosis of type 2 diabetes is the release of sugar from your liver, known as your *hepatic glucose output*. Why is your glucose high in the morning after you've fasted all night? You would think that your glucose would be low because you didn't eat any sugar to increase your body's glucose. In fact, your liver is a storage bank for a lot of glucose, and it can make even more from other substances in the body. As your insulin resistance increases, your liver begins to release glucose inappropriately and your fasting blood glucose rises.

People often think that the following factors cause type 2 diabetes, but they actually have nothing to do with the onset of the disease:

- ✔ **Sugar:** Eating excessive amounts of sugar does not cause diabetes, but it may bring out the disease to the extent that it makes you fat. Eating too much protein or fat will do the same thing.

- ✔ **Emotions:** Changes in your emotions do not play a large role in the development of type 2 diabetes, but may be very important in dealing with diabetes mellitus and subsequent control.

- ✔ **Stress:** Too much stress isn't a major factor that causes diabetes.

- ✔ **Antibodies:** Antibodies against islet cells are not a major factor in type 2 diabetes. Type 2 diabetes isn't an autoimmune disease like type 1.

- ✔ **Gender:** Males and females are equally as likely to develop type 2 diabetes. Gender doesn't play a role in the onset of this disease.

- ✔ **Diabetic ketoacidosis:** Type 2 diabetes isn't generally associated with diabetic ketoacidosis (see Chapter 4). People with type 2 diabetes are ketosis resistant, except under extremely severe stress caused by infections or trauma. (See Chapter 4 for a discussion of *hyperosmolar syndrome,* a related condition in which people with type 2 diabetes have extremely high glucose but don't have the fat breakdown that leads to acidosis.)

Getting type 2 diabetes

Genetic inheritance causes type 2 diabetes, but environmental factors such as obesity and lack of exercise trigger the disease. People with type 2 diabetes are insulin-resistant before they become obese or sedentary. Later, aging, poor eating habits, obesity, and failure to exercise combine to bring out the disease. Inheritance seems to be a much stronger factor in type 2 diabetes than in type 1 diabetes. The chance that a parent with type 2 diabetes will have a child with type 2 diabetes (assuming that the other parent doesn't have the disease) is about 10 percent. An identical twin of a person with type 2 diabetes will eventually get the disease much more often than 50 percent of the time. If you are a nonidentical brother or sister of someone with type 2 disease, you will get it about 40 percent of the time. These are much higher figures than for type 1 diabetes.

A number of early warning signs appear in the population that is most expected to develop type 2 diabetes. People with type 2 diabetes often have a history of malnutrition at a young age. Perhaps these people didn't make enough insulin-producing cells when they were young, because they didn't need them for their reduced food intake. When these people are presented with ample supplies of food at an older age, their pancreases may not have enough insulin-producing cells to handle the load.

In developing countries, where people often don't get enough food, people whose genetic makeup enables their bodies to use carbohydrates in a very efficient manner have an advantage over the rest of the population because they can survive on the low food and calorie supplies. When these people finally receive ample supplies of food, their bodies are overwhelmed and they're likely to become fat and sedentary and develop diabetes. This may explain why people in developing countries are the most at risk to develop type 2 diabetes. Population studies show that the incidence of diabetes is greatest in developing countries such as China and India.

Preventing type 2 diabetes

Doctors can predict type 2 diabetes years in advance of its actual diagnosis by studying the close relatives of people who already have the condition. This early warning period offers plenty of time to try techniques of primary prevention (which I explain in the "Preventing type 1 diabetes" section, earlier in this chapter). After doctors find high blood glucose in a person and diagnose type 2 diabetes, complications such as eye disease and kidney disease (see Chapter 5) take ten or more years to develop in that person. During this time, doctors can apply secondary prevention techniques (the various treatments I discuss in Part III).

Because so many people suffer from type 2 diabetes, doctors have had a wealth of people to study in order to determine the most important environmental factors that turn a genetic predisposition to type 2 diabetes into a clinical disease. The following are the major environmental factors:

✔ **High body mass index:** The *body mass index (BMI)* is the way that doctors look at weight in relation to height. BMI is a better indicator of a healthy weight than just weight alone, because a person who weighs 150 pounds and is 62 inches tall is overweight, but a person who weighs 150 pounds and is 70 inches tall is thin. You can easily determine your BMI by using the following formula: Your weight (in pounds) x 705, divided by your height (in inches). Divide that result by your height again (in inches). If you use the metric system, you simply divide your weight in kilograms by your height in meters and divide that result by your height in meters again. Using this formula, the person with a height of 62 inches has a BMI of 27.5 while the person with the height of 70 inches has a BMI of 21.6. The result is expressed in kilograms per meter squared (kg/m2).

The new definition of BMI states that a person with a BMI from 25 to 29.9 is overweight, and a person with a BMI of 30 or greater is obese. A BMI between 20 and 25 is considered normal weight.

Many studies have verified the great importance of the level of the BMI in determining who will get diabetes. A large study of thousands of nurses in the United States showed that the nurses with a BMI of greater than 35 had diabetes almost 100 times more often than nurses with a BMI of less than 22. Even among the women in this study considered to be lean, those with the higher BMI, though still in the category of lean, had three times the prevalence of diabetes compared to more lean nurses. Also, a large study of physicians in the U.S. found the same relationship of high BMI to high levels of type 2 diabetes. The same study also showed that the length of time that you're obese is important, because men who were obese ten years earlier more often had diabetes than men who weren't obese at that time.

✔ **Physical inactivity:** Physical inactivity has a high association with diabetes, as evidenced in many studies. Former athletes have diabetes less often than nonathletes. The same study of nurses' health that I cite in the preceding bullet item showed that women who were physically active on a regular basis had diabetes only two-thirds as often as the couch potatoes. The preceding study of physicians' health showed the same thing. In a study in Hawaii, the occurrence of diabetes was greatest for the nonexercisers, and none of the people in the study were obese, so that was not a factor.

✔ **Central distribution of fat:** When people with diabetes become fat, they tend to distribute the extra weight as centrally distributed fat, also known as *visceral fat.* You check your visceral fat when you measure your waistline, because this type of fat stays around your midsection. So a person with visceral fat is more apple-shaped than pear-shaped. Visceral fat also happens to be the type of fat that probably comes and goes most easily on your body, and it is relatively easy to lose when you diet. Visceral fat seems to cause more insulin resistance than fat in other areas, and it is also correlated with the occurrence of coronary artery disease. If you have a lot of visceral fat, losing just 5 to 10 percent of your weight may very dramatically reduce your chance of diabetes or a heart attack.

If you are 40 or younger and your waistline measures 39.5 inches (100 centimeters) or greater, or you are between the ages of 40 and 60 and your waistline measures 35.5 inches (90 centimeters) or more, you have a significantly increased risk of a heart attack.

✔ **Low intake of dietary fiber:** Populations with a high prevalence of diabetes tend to eat a diet that is low in fiber. Dietary fiber seems to be protective against diabetes, because it slows down the rate at which glucose enters the bloodstream.

If you recognize any of the preceding factors in your body or lifestyle, you can correct them. Type 2 diabetes allows the high-risk individual or the diagnosed person the time to work toward prevention or control of the disease. In Part III, I show you specific ways to reduce your weight, increase your exercise, improve your diet, and prevent or reverse diabetes and diabetic complications.

Prevention research: Possibilities for future prevention of diabetes

Researchers have performed many valuable studies on the prevention of type 2 diabetes. The results of these studies suggest that you can prevent diabetes, but probably only by making major lifestyle changes and sticking to them over a long period of time. Here are some important conclusions based on prevention research:

- Taking drugs that don't treat your insulin resistance doesn't help to prevent your diabetes or its complications.

- If you exercise regularly, you can delay the onset of diabetes.

- If you maintain a proper diet and exercise regularly, you can delay the onset of diabetes and slow the complications that may occur.

- Controlling your blood pressure and your blood glucose both have substantial benefits for preventing the complications of diabetes.

A study reported in the New England Journal of Medicine in July 1991 confirmed the preceding conclusions by looking at obese people who had close relatives with type 2 diabetes — which meant that these people were highly likely to develop diabetes. For six months, the researchers gave the participants extensive training in exercise routines and maintaining proper diet. Many of the participants lost significant amounts of weight, improved their overall health, and staved off the development of diabetes. But after six months, many of the people being studied were no longer participating as fully and sticking as closely to the diet and exercise regimens. By the time that 12 months of the study had passed, more of the participants were straying farther from the diet and exercise that they needed, and they were regaining some of the weight that they had lost. The researchers found that the people who were able to maintain the proper diet and exercise — which helped them not to gain weight — were least likely to develop diabetes. The main point that this study proves is the importance (and, for many people, the difficulty) of maintaining a program of diet and exercise for a long period of time.

You Have Gestational Diabetes

If you're pregnant (yes, that excludes you men) and you've never had diabetes before, during the course of your pregnancy you could acquire a form of diabetes called *gestational diabetes*. If you already have diabetes when you become pregnant, that is called *pregestational diabetes*. As Chapter 6 shows you, the difference between pregestational diabetes and gestational diabetes is very important in terms of the consequences for both mother and baby. Gestational diabetes occurs in about 2 percent of all pregnancies.

During your pregnancy, you can acquire gestational diabetes because the growing fetus and the placenta create various hormones to help the fetus grow and develop properly. Some of these hormones have other characteristics, such as anti-insulin properties, that decrease your body's sensitivity to insulin, increase glucose production, and therefore cause diabetes.

At approximately your 20th week of pregnancy, your body produces enough of these hormones to block your insulin's normal actions and cause diabetes. After you give birth, the fetus and placenta are no longer in your body, so their anti-insulin hormones are gone and your diabetes disappears.

 Be aware that, even though your diabetes subsides after you give birth, type 2 diabetes develops within 15 years after the pregnancy in more than half of the women who had gestational diabetes. This high likelihood of type 2 diabetes probably results from a genetic susceptibility to diabetes in these women that is magnified by the large amount of anti-insulin hormones in their bodies during pregnancy.

Your obstetrician should do a test for gestational diabetes around the 24th to the 28th week of your pregnancy.

Could You Have Another Type of Diabetes?

Cases of diabetes other than type 1, type 2, or gestational are rare and usually don't cause severe diabetes in the people who have them. But occasionally one of these other types of diabetes is responsible for a more severe case of diabetes, so you should know that they exist. The following list gives you a brief rundown of the symptoms and causes for other types of diabetes:

✓ **Diabetes due to loss or disease of pancreatic tissue:** If you have a disease such as cancer that necessitates the removal of some of your pancreas, you lose your pancreas's valuable insulin-producing beta cells and your body becomes diabetic. This form of diabetes isn't always severe because you lose *glucagon,* another hormone found in your pancreas, after your pancreatic surgery. Glucagon blocks insulin action in your body, so when your body has less glucagon, it can function with less insulin, leaving you with a milder case of diabetes.

✓ **Diabetes due to other diseases:** Your body has a number of hormones that block insulin action or have actions that are opposed to insulin's actions. You produce these hormones in glands other than your pancreas. If you get a tumor on one of these hormone-producing glands, the gland sometimes produces excessive levels of the hormones that act in opposition to insulin. Usually, this gives you simple glucose intolerance rather than diabetes, because your pancreas makes extra insulin to combat the hormones. But if you have a genetic tendency to develop diabetes, you may develop diabetes in this case.

✔ **Diabetes due to hormone treatments for other diseases:** If you're receiving hormones to treat a disease other than diabetes, those hormones could cause diabetes in your body. The hormone that is most likely to cause diabetes in this situation is hydrocortisone (similar drugs are prednisone and dexamethasone), an anti-inflammatory agent used in diseases of inflamation (such as arthritis). If you're taking hydrocortisone and you have the symptoms of diabetes listed in earlier sections of this chapter, talk to your doctor.

✔ **Diabetes due to other drugs**: If you're taking other commonly used drugs, be aware that some of them raise your blood glucose as a side effect. Some antihypertensive drugs, especially hydrochlorothiazide, raise your blood-glucose level. Niacin, a drug commonly used for lowering cholesterol, also raises your blood glucose. If you have a genetic tendency toward diabetes, taking these drugs may be enough to give you the disease.

Conditions and hormones that can lead to diabetes

The following is a partial list of hormones caused by tumors and their associated conditions:

✔ Excessive adrenal gland hormone (hydrocortisone) is present in *Cushing's Syndrome.* Hydrocortisone stimulates the liver to put out more glucose while it blocks the uptake of glucose by muscle tissue.

✔ Excessive prolactin is present in a *Prolactin Secreting Tumor of the Pituitary Gland.* It blocks insulin action and glucose intolerance results.

✔ Excessive growth hormone is made by a tumor of the pituitary gland resulting in *acromegaly.* Growth hormone reduces insulin sensitivity and forces the pancreas to make much more insulin.

✔ Excessive epinephrine is made by a *pheochromocytoma* (a tumor of another part of the adrenal gland). It causes increased liver production of glucose, while it blocks insulin secretion.

✔ Excessive aldosterone is made by still another part of the adrenal gland in a condition called *primary hyperaldosteronism.* This condition causes glucose intolerance

in a different way — by facilitating the loss of body potassium, which has a negative effect on insulin production.

✔ Excessive thyroid hormone found in *hyperthyroidism* causes the liver and other organs to produce excessive quantities of glucose. Hyperthyroidism is also a disease of autoimmunity, which may play a role in the loss of glucose tolerance.

✔ A *Glucagon Secreting Tumor of the Pancreas* can create excessive glucagon. Glucagon has many properties that are opposite to insulin. This condition is rare, and only around 100 cases of it have been described in medical literature, so don't think you have it.

✔ A *Somatostatin Secreting Tumor of the Pancreas* can create excessive somatostatin. Somatostatin is another hormone made in a cell present in the Islets of Langerhans. Somatostatin actually blocks insulin from leaving the beta cell, but it also blocks glucagon and other hormones, so the diabetes is very mild. This condition occurs even less often than the Glucagon Secreting Tumor.

Part II
How Diabetes Affects Your Body

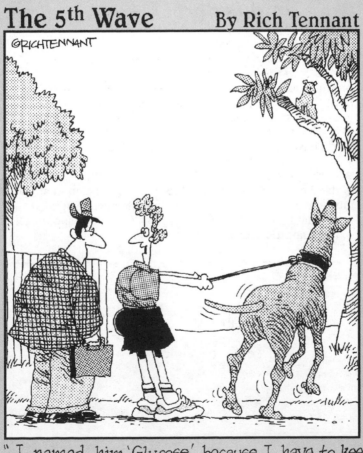

"I named him 'Glucose', because I have to keep him under control every day."

In this part . . .

Diabetes, if not treated properly, can have profound effects on your body. This part explains these effects, how they occur, the kinds of symptoms they produce, and what you and your doctor need to do to treat them. You may be surprised at how many parts of your body can be affected by diabetes. Remember that everything I describe in this part is preventable, and even if you have not been able to prevent it, it is very treatable.

With the pace of discovery in diabetes, most of the effects of the disease will be fit for exhibition in an ancient history museum in the not-too-distant future. Meanwhile, it is important that you know about the effects and respond to them appropriately.

Chapter 4

Battling Short-Term Complications

· ·

· ·

Chapters 2 and 3 tell you all about how doctors make a diagnosis of diabetes and how they determine which type of diabetes you have. Those
chapters cover some of the signs and symptoms of diabetes, which you could
consider to be the shortest of the short-term complications of the disease
because they're generally mild and begin to subside when you start treatment. This chapter covers the more serious forms of short-term complications of diabetes, which occur when your blood glucose is out of control —
reaching dangerously high or low levels.

Solving Short-Term Complications

Although the complications that I cover in this chapter are called short term,
you may experience them at any time during the course of your diabetes.
Short term simply means that these complications arise rapidly in your body,
as opposed to the long-term complications that take ten or more years to
develop. (See Chapter 5 for all the details about long-term complications.)
Short-term complications develop in days or even hours, and fortunately
they respond to treatment just as rapidly.

Generally, you experience the severe short-term complications associated
with high blood glucose when you aren't monitoring your blood glucose
levels. Small children and older folks who live alone or have illnesses are
susceptible to lapses in glucose monitoring and, therefore, to short-term
complications. If you suffer an acute illness or trauma, you should monitor
your glucose even more frequently than usual because you're more vulnera-
ble to short-term complications.

Most importantly, with the exception of *hypoglycemia* (low blood glucose), you should treat all the complications in this chapter as medical emergencies. Don't try to treat these complications at home. Keep in touch with your doctor and go to the hospital promptly if your blood glucose is uncontrollably high or you're unable to hold down food. You may need a few hours in the emergency room or a day or two in the hospital to reverse your problems.

The short-term complications of diabetes affect your ability to function normally. So you may have trouble driving your car properly. If you're a student, you may have difficulty studying or taking tests. You may find that the Bureau of Motor Vehicles and the Federal Aviation Association are extra careful about giving you, and all people with diabetes, a driver's license or a pilot's license. Potential employers may question your ability to perform certain jobs. But most companies and government agencies are very enlightened about diabetes and do everything possible to accommodate you in these situations. (Chapter 15 shows you how to overcome some challenges that you may face with employment and insurance.)

You don't have to feel limited in what you can do. You can have control over your diabetes, and all of the short-term complications are avoidable. If you take your medication at the appropriate time, eat the proper foods at the proper times, and monitor your blood glucose regularly, you're unlikely to suffer from any severe forms of the short-term complications. As you closely monitor and control your blood glucose, it may drop to lower than normal levels, but monitoring quickly alerts you to the drop and you can treat it before it affects your mental and physical functioning. (See Chapter 7 for all the details on glucose monitoring and other testing.)

Understanding Hypoglycemia

The condition of low blood glucose is known as *hypoglycemia*. If you have diabetes, you can get hypoglycemia only as a consequence of your diabetes treatment. As a person with diabetes, you're in constant combat with high blood glucose, which is responsible for most of the long-term and short-term complications of the disease. Your doctor prescribes drugs and other treatments in an effort to fine-tune your blood glucose as it would be in someone else's body. (Part III explains many techniques that help you control your blood glucose levels.) But, unfortunately, these drugs and treatments aren't always perfect. If you take too much of a drug, exercise too much, or eat too little, your blood glucose can drop to the low levels at which symptoms develop. The following sections explain more about hypoglycemia's symptoms, causes, and treatment.

Symptoms of hypoglycemia

Your body doesn't function well when you have too little glucose in your blood. Your brain needs glucose to run the rest of your body, as well as for intellectual purposes. Your muscles need the energy that glucose provides in much the same way that your car needs gasoline. So, when your body detects that it has low blood glucose, it sends out a group of hormones that rapidly raise your glucose. But those hormones have to fight the strength of the diabetes medication that has been pushing down your glucose levels.

At what level of blood glucose do you develop hypoglycemia? Unfortunately, the level varies for different individuals, particularly depending on the length of time that the person has had diabetes. But most experts agree that a blood glucose of 60 mg/dl (3.3 mmol/L)or less is associated with signs and symptoms of hypoglycemia in most people.

Doctors traditionally put the symptoms of hypoglycemia into two major categories:

- **Symptoms that are due to your brain not receiving enough fuel so that your intellectual function suffers.** This first category of symptoms is called *neuroglycopenic* symptoms, which is medicalese for "not enough (*penic*) glucose (*glyco*) in the brain (*neuro*)." (If your brain could speak, it would just say, "Whew, I'm ready for a meal!")

- **Symptoms due to the side effects of the hormones (especially epinephrine) that your body sends out to counter the glucose-lowering effect of insulin.** The second category of symptoms is called *adrenergic* symptoms, because epinephrine comes from your adrenal gland.

Adrenergic symptoms occur most often when your blood glucose falls rapidly. The following adrenergic symptoms may tip you off that you're hypoglycemic:

- Whiteness, or pallor, of your skin
- Sweating
- Rapid heartbeat
- Palpitations, or the feeling that your heart is beating too fast
- Anxiety
- Sensation of hunger

Neuroglycopenic symptoms occur most often when your hypoglycemia takes longer to develop. The symptoms become more severe as your blood glucose drops lower. The following neuroglycopenic symptoms are often signs that you're becoming (or already are) hypoglycemic:

- ✔ Headache
- ✔ Loss of concentration
- ✔ Visual disorders, such as double vision
- ✔ Fatigue
- ✔ Confusion
- ✔ Convulsions
- ✔ Coma, or an inability to be awakened

Intelligent people lose their ability to think clearly when they become hypoglycemic. They make simple mistakes, and other people often assume that they are drunk.

One of my patients was driving on a highway when another driver noticed that she was weaving back and forth in her lane and reported her to the highway patrol. A patrolman stopped her, concluded that she was drunk, and took her to jail. Fortunately, someone noticed that she was wearing a diabetic medical bracelet. After promptly receiving the nutrition that she needed, she rapidly recovered. No charges were filed, but clearly this is a situation that you want to avoid. Always test your blood glucose level to make sure that it's satisfactory before driving your car.

If you take insulin or a *sulfonylurea drug*, which squeezes more insulin out of your reluctant pancreas, for your own safety you need to wear or carry with you some form of identification, in case you unexpectedly develop hypoglycemia. (See Chapter 10 for a full explanation of the insulin and sulfonylurea medications.)

Causes of hypoglycemia

Hypoglycemia results from elevated amounts of insulin driving down your blood glucose to low levels, but an extra high dose of insulin or sulfonylurea isn't always the culprit that elevates your insulin level. The amount of food you take in, the amount of fuel (glucose) that you burn for energy, the amount of insulin circulating in your body, and your body's ability to raise glucose by releasing it from the liver or making it from other body substances all affect your blood glucose level.

When you take insulin shots, you have to time your food intake to raise your blood glucose as the insulin is taking effect. Chapter 10 explains the different kinds of insulin and the proper methods for administering them. But remember that the different types of insulin are most potent at differing amounts of time (minutes or hours) after you inject them. If you skip a meal or take your insulin too early or too late, your glucose and insulin levels won't be in sync and you'll develop hypoglycemia. If you go on a diet and don't adjust your medication, the same thing happens.

If you take sulfonylurea drugs, you need to follow similar restrictions. You and your doctor must adjust your dosage when your calorie intake falls. Other drugs don't cause hypoglycemia by themselves, but when combined with sulfonylureas they may lower your glucose enough to reach hypoglycemic levels. (Chapter 10 talks more about these other drugs.)

Your diet plays a major role in helping you avoid hypoglycemia if you take medication. You're better off to have a snack in the middle of the morning and in the afternoon — in addition to your usual breakfast, lunch, and dinner — especially if you take insulin. A properly timed snack provides you with a steady source of glucose to balance the insulin that you're taking. Chapter 8 gives much greater detail about proper diet.

Exercise generally lowers your blood glucose as well. Obviously, exercise burns more of your body's fuel, which is glucose. Some people with diabetes use exercise in place of extra insulin to get their high blood glucose down to a normal level. But if you don't adjust your insulin dose or food intake to match your exercise, exercise can result in hypoglycemia.

One of my patients is dedicated to exercise. He has taken insulin shots for years but requires very little insulin to control his glucose because he burns so much glucose through exercise. He avoids hypoglycemia by measuring his blood glucose level many times a day — especially before vigorous exercise. If his level is low at the beginning of exercise, he eats extra carbohydrates before he starts. Chapter 8 tells you which foods to eat (and when) in order to have the intended effect on your glucose levels.

People who exercise regularly require much less medication and generally can manage their diabetes more easily than nonexercisers can. Chapter 9 covers much more about the benefits of exercise.

Several drugs that you may take unrelated to your diabetes can lower your blood glucose. One important and widely used drug, which you may not even think of as a drug, is alcohol in the form of wine, beer, and other spirits. Alcohol can block your liver's ability to release glucose. It also blocks hormones that raise blood glucose and increases the glucose-lowering effect of insulin. If you're malnourished for some reason or you simply haven't eaten in a while and you drink alcohol before going to bed, you may experience severe fasting hypoglycemia the next morning.

If you take insulin or sulfonylurea drugs, don't drink alcohol without eating some food at the same time. Food counteracts some of the glucose-lowering effects of alcohol.

Also, be aware that aspirin (and all of the drugs related to aspirin, called *salicylates*) can lead you to hypoglycemia. In adults who have diabetes, aspirin can increase the effects of other drugs that you're taking to lower your blood glucose. In diabetic children, aspirin has an especially profound effect on lowering blood glucose to hypoglycemia levels.

Treatment of hypoglycemia

The vast majority of hypoglycemia cases are mild. You (or a friend or relative) notice that you have the symptoms of hypoglycemia. You can treat the problem with a small quantity of glucose in the form of sugar cubes, two or three glucose tablets, a small amount of a sugary soft drink, or anything that has about 15 grams of glucose in it. (Glucose tablets are available in any drugstore, and any person with diabetes who may develop hypoglycemia should carry them.) Eight ounces of milk or six ounces of orange juice work very well. Sometimes you need a second treatment. Approximately 20 minutes after you try one of these solutions, measure your blood glucose to find out whether your level has risen sufficiently.

Because your mental state may be mildly confused when you have hypoglycemia, you need to make sure that your friends or relatives know in advance what hypoglycemia is and what to do about it. Inform people about your diabetes and about how to recognize hypoglycemia. Don't keep your diabetes a secret. The people close to you will be glad to know how to help you.

If you can't sit up and swallow properly when you have hypoglycemia, people shouldn't try to feed you. Anyone who is trying to treat your condition can try several other options. One option is to use an emergency kit, such as the kit called "Glucagon for Emergencies." This kit includes a syringe with 1 mg of glucagon, one of the major hormones that raises glucose, which your helper should inject into your muscle. The injection of glucagon raises your blood glucose so that you regain consciousness within 20 minutes. You need to get a prescription from your doctor for this type of glucagon kit. Also make sure that the kit doesn't become outdated if you haven't used it for a long time. Glucagon corrects your hypoglycemic condition for about an hour after you receive an injection. If your hypoglycemia recurs shortly after you receive glucagon or doesn't respond to the glucagon, someone needs to make an emergency call to 911 for you. (Sulfonylurea drugs most often cause such a severe case of hypoglycemia.) The emergency crew checks your blood glucose and gives you an intravenous (IV) dose of high-concentration glucose. Most likely, you will continue the IV in the emergency room until you show stable and normal blood glucose levels.

Combating Ketoacidosis

Chapter 3 talks about the tendency of people with type 1 diabetes to suffer from a severe diabetic complication called *ketoacidosis*, or very high blood glucose with large amounts of acid in the blood. The prefix *keto* refers to *ketones* — substances that your body makes as fat breaks down during ketoacidosis. *Acid* is part of the name because your blood becomes acidic from the presence of ketones.

Occasionally, ketoacidosis is the symptom that alerts doctors that you have type 1 diabetes, but more frequently it occurs after you already know that you have the disease. Although ketoacidosis occurs mostly in people with type 1 diabetes (who develop diabetes at an early age), the person is usually 40 or more years old when ketoacidosis actually begins.

Ketoacidosis occurs mostly in people with type 1 diabetes because they have no insulin in their bodies except what they inject as medication. Those with type 2 diabetes (or with other forms of the disease) rarely get ketoacidosis because they have some insulin in their bodies, even though the insulin usually isn't fully active due to insulin resistance. People with type 2 diabetes get ketoacidosis mainly when they have severe infections or traumas that put their bodies under great physical stress.

The following sections explain ketoacidosis's symptoms, causes, and treatments.

Symptoms of ketoacidosis

The symptoms of ketoacidosis regularly alert doctors to type 1 diabetes in children. But ketoacidosis more often occurs in adults with type 1 diabetes, so they should also keep an eye out for the following symptoms:

- **Nausea and vomiting:** You experience these symptoms because of the buildup of acids and the loss of important body substances.

- **Rapid breathing:** (This is also known as *Kussmaul breathing,* after the man who first described it.) You experience rapid breathing when your blood is so acidic that your body attempts to blow off some of the acid through the lungs. Your breath has a fruity smell due to acetone.

- **Extreme tiredness and drowsiness:** You're tired because your brain is bathed in very thick blood, like syrup, and is missing the essential substances you've lost in the urine.

- **Weakness:** You become weak because your muscle tissue is unable to get its fuel, namely glucose.

In this age of self-monitoring for blood glucose levels, ketoacidosis is becoming more rare, but it still occurs. (See Chapter 7 for more on self-monitoring.) If you use a source of insulin that can be interrupted, you could unexpectedly develop ketoacidosis. For example, if you rely on an insulin pump, which pushes insulin under your skin automatically (as I describe in Chapter 10), the pump could stop for some reason; then your insulin delivery would cease, your glucose level would rise, and ketoacidosis would develop if you don't notice the interruption soon enough.

You may notice that you have some symptoms of ketoacidosis and begin to suspect that you have this complication. But that diagnosis is best made by a doctor — preferably in the hospital, where you can begin treatment at once. Doctors make a diagnosis of ketoacidosis when they see the following abnormalities:

- High blood glucose, usually more than 300 mg/dl (16.6 mmol/L)
- Acid condition of your blood
- Excessive levels of ketones in your blood and urine
- Dry skin and tongue, indicating dehydration
- Deficiency of potassium in your body
- An acetone smell on your breath

When your doctor finds these abnormalities, he or she will want to begin treatment immediately.

Causes of ketoacidosis

The most common causes of ketoacidosis are interruption of your insulin treatment or an infection. Your body can't go for many hours without insulin activity before it begins to burn fat for energy and begins to make extra glucose that it can't use. The process of burning fat creates ketones in your blood, which are responsible for your ketoacidosis. (Refer to the earlier section "Combating Ketoacidosis.")

If you go on a strict diet to lose weight, your body burns some of its fat stores and produces ketones, similar to how it burns fat when you lack insulin. But in this case, your glucose remains low and (unless you have type 1 diabetes) you have sufficient insulin to prevent excessive production of new glucose or release of large amounts of glucose from your liver. So a strict diet doesn't generally lead to ketoacidosis.

Treatment of ketoacidosis

Ketoacidosis is a serious condition that requires professional treatment. But even though you leave the treatment to a professional rather than trying to manage it yourself, you should know the treatment processes so that you understand what's happening to you or to your loved one.

The basis of ketoacidosis treatment is to restore the proper amount of water to your body, reduce the acid condition of your blood by getting rid of the ketones, restore substances such as potassium that you've lost, and return your blood glucose to its normal level of around 80 to 120. All of these improvements should happen simultaneously after you begin treatment.

Your doctor sets up a flowchart to keep track of your levels of glucose, acid, potassium, and ketones, along with other parameters. Although you've lost a lot of potassium, for example, the initial blood reading of potassium on your flowchart may look normal. As your treatment progresses, more potassium goes into your cells to replenish losses there, so your blood potassium may fall. If that happens, the doctor administers more potassium to fix the problem.

Obviously, because your lack of insulin got you into this ketoacidosis situation, your doctor gives you insulin intravenously to restore your insulin levels and reverse the abnormalities in your body. At some point, your blood glucose may fall toward hypoglycemia. If it does, your doctor gives you another IV made up of glucose and a solution of salt, potassium, and water.

After you receive insulin, your body stops breaking down fat for energy because your cells can use glucose for energy as they're supposed to. Soon, your body rids itself of the ketones in your bloodstream that caused your complication and your body takes on a more normal condition.

Your doctor gives you large volumes of a saltwater solution intravenously to replace the six or more liters of fluids that you lose during ketoacidosis. Replenishing your body's fluids relieves the nausea and vomiting that you've endured, and you're now able to keep down liquid and solid foods again. Hopefully, you notice your normal mental functioning returning, which means that you'll soon be ready to resume self-administering your insulin and controlling your own diet. By this time, the doctor has probably found and corrected a malfunctioning insulin pump or an infection that was a factor in causing your ketoacidosis.s

Ketoacidosis may not sound like a walk in the park, but you may think that your doctor can control it with little or no risk to you. For the most part, that's true, but be aware that ketoacidosis is fatal for 10 percent of people with diabetes who get it — mostly elderly people with diabetes and those with other illnesses that complicate treatment. Recognizing the symptoms early and seeking treatment quickly greatly enhance your chances of an uneventful recovery from ketoacidosis.

Managing the Hyperosmolar Syndrome

The highest blood glucose condition that you may find yourself in is called the *hyperosmolar syndrome*. Like ketoacidosis, the hyperosmolar syndrome is a medical emergency that needs to be treated in a hospital.

The hyperosmolar syndrome is also like ketoacidosis in its effects on your body. The hyperosmolar syndrome creates ketones in your blood, but it doesn't make your blood as acidic as ketoacidosis does. It also raises your blood glucose levels considerably higher than ketoacidosis does. (See the "Combating Ketoacidosis" section for more information.)

The name *hyperosmolar syndrome* refers to the excessive levels of glucose in the blood. *Hyper* means "larger than normal," and *osmolar* has to do with concentrations of substances in the blood. So hyperosmolar, in this situation, means that the blood is simply too concentrated with glucose. Other hyperosmolar syndromes occur when other substances are at fault.

The following sections explain hyperosmolar syndrome's symptoms, causes, and treatments.

Symptoms of the hyperosmolar syndrome

Because the hyperosmolar syndrome complication is so similar to ketoacidosis, it has many of the same symptoms as ketoacidosis. The main difference is that with hyperosmolar syndrome, you don't experience the rapid Kussmaul breathing, because your blood isn't overly acidic as a part of this complication. Also, the symptoms of the hyperosmolar syndrome develop over many days or weeks, unlike ketoacidosis's quick and acute development in your body.

If you measure your blood glucose on a daily basis, you should never develop the hyperosmolar syndrome because you'll notice that your blood glucose is getting high before it reaches the critical complication level.

The most important signs and symptoms of the hyperosmolar syndrome are as follows:

- Frequent urination
- Thirst
- Weakness
- Leg cramps

✔ Sunken eyeballs and rapid pulse, due to dehydration

✔ Decreased mental awareness or coma

✔ Blood glucose of 600, or higher if you wait longer to see your doctor

You may also develop more threatening symptoms with this complication. Your blood pressure may be low. Your nervous system may be affected with paralysis of the arms and legs, but these respond to treatment. You may have high counts of potassium, sodium, and other blood constituents (such as white blood cells and red blood cells), but these counts usually fall rapidly and your doctor will replace these elements in your blood as water is restored to your body.

Causes of the hyperosmolar syndrome

The hyperosmolar syndrome afflicts mostly the elderly with diabetes who live alone or in nursing homes where they're not carefully monitored. Age and usually some neglect combine to increase the likelihood that a person with diabetes will lose large quantities of fluids through vomiting or diarrhea and then not replace those fluids. These people tend to have mild type 2 diabetes, and sometimes their diabetes is undiagnosed and untreated.

Age is also a contributing cause of the hyperosmolar syndrome because your kidneys gradually become less efficient as you age. When your kidneys are in their prime, your blood glucose level needs to reach only 180 mg/dl before your kidneys begin to remove some excess glucose through your urine. But as your kidneys grow older and slower, they require a gradually higher blood glucose level before they start to send excess glucose to your urine. If you're at an age (usually 70 or older for people in average health) when your kidneys are really laboring to remove the excess glucose from your body and you happen to lose a large amount of fluids from sickness or neglect, your blood volume decreases, which makes it even harder for your kidneys to remove glucose. At this point, your blood glucose level begins to skyrocket. If you don't replace some of the lost fluids soon, your glucose rises even higher.

If you allow your blood glucose to rise and don't get the fluids that you need, your blood pressure starts to fall and you get weaker and weaker. As the concentration of glucose in your blood continues to rise, you become increasingly confused, and your mental state diminishes as the glucose concentration rises until you eventually fall into a coma.

Other factors — such as infection, failure to take your insulin, and taking certain medications — can raise your blood glucose to the hyperosmolar syndrome levels, but not replacing lost body fluids is the most frequent cause.

Treatment of the hyperosmolar syndrome

Even more so than ketoacidosis (see the section "Treatment of ketoacidosis," earlier in this chapter), the hyperosmolar syndrome requires immediate and skilled treatment from a doctor. By no means should you try to treat the hyperosmolar syndrome yourself. In fact, you should avoid doctors who are not experienced in treatment of this condition. You need the proper treatment from an experienced doctor — and you need it fast. The death rate for the hyperosmolar syndrome is high because most people who suffer from it are elderly and often have other serious illnesses that complicate treatment. When you arrive at your doctor's office or emergency room with the hyperosmolar syndrome, your doctor must accomplish the following tasks fairly rapidly:

✔ Restore large volumes of water to your body

✔ Lower your blood glucose level

✔ Restore other substances that your body has lost, such as potassium, sodium, chloride, and so on

Your doctor creates a chart to monitor your levels of glucose, blood concentration (osmolarity), potassium, sodium, and other tests, which are measured hourly in some cases. You may think that you need to receive large amounts of insulin to lower your high glucose level, but the large doses of fluids that your doctor gives you to replenish your body fluids do so much to lower your glucose that you need only smaller doses of insulin. As your body fluids return to normal, your kidneys begin to receive much more of the blood that they need in order to rid your body of the excess glucose.

Chapter 5

Preventing Long-Term Complications

· ·

In This Chapter

▶ Getting long-term complications

▶ Dealing with kidney disease

▶ Handling eye disease

▶ Battling nerve disease

▶ Understanding diabetes's effect on the heart

▶ Encountering diabetic peripheral vascular disease and cerebrovascular disease

▶ Coping with the diabetic foot

▶ Identifying skin problems

· ·

*Y*ou may think that diabetes has made your life more complicated. But you'll long for the good old, complicated days if you ever develop one of the severe complications that I describe in this chapter. The complications in this chapter are the problems that occur if you permit your blood glucose to rise and remain high over many years. The point that I stress throughout this book is that you have a choice. Working with your doctor and other helpers, you can keep your blood glucose near normal, and you'll never have to deal with the long-term complications covered in this chapter.

Your struggle to live an uncomplicated life with diabetes is similar to the struggle of a commercial airplane pilot who took the airplane down for a very rough landing. The pilot stood at the exit, as was his custom, waiting for passengers to make nasty comments about the landing, but none of the passengers mentioned it. Finally, a little old lady walked to the exit with her cane and said to the pilot, "Tell me, did we land, or were we shot down?"

The choice is yours: You can have a smooth landing, free of complications, that goes relatively unnoticed by you and those around you. Or you can have the feeling that you have been shot down.

How Long-Term Complications Develop

Doctors aren't sure of the precise reason that long-term complications of diabetes develop. They have lots of theories, many of them strongly based on findings in animals and human beings. For most long-term complications except heart disease — such as kidney disease, eye disease, and nerve disease — doctors believe that years of high blood glucose levels initiate the complications. (In the case of heart disease, high blood glucose levels may make the disease worse or more complicated but not actually cause it.) Most long-term complications require ten or more years to develop, which seems like a long time, until you consider that many people with type 2 diabetes have it for five or more years before a doctor diagnoses it.

Often the long-term complication itself (rather than a high blood glucose level) is the clue that leads a doctor to diagnose diabetes in a patient. Therefore, doctors need to look for long-term complications immediately after diagnosing diabetes, because the diabetes and any long-term complications may have been with the patient for quite some time already. Because of the possibility of long-term complications being present at the diagnosis of diabetes, your doctor also must immediately take steps to control your glucose levels.

Kidney Disease

Your kidneys rid your body of many harmful chemicals and other compounds produced during the process of normal metabolism. Your kidneys act like a filter through which your blood pours, trapping the waste and sending it out in your urine, while the normal contents of the blood go back into your bloodstream. They also regulate the salt and water content of your body. When kidney disease (also known as *nephropathy*) causes your kidneys to fail, you must either use artificial means, called *dialysis*, to cleanse your blood and control the salt and water or receive a new working donor kidney, called a *transplant*.

In the United States today, half the patients who require long-term dialysis require it because of diabetes. Fortunately, this number is on the decline because of the increasing awareness among people that they need to control their blood glucose. Although the incidence of kidney disease is only about 5 percent among people with type 2 diabetes, compared to 30 percent among people with type 1 diabetes, the absolute number of patients with kidney disease is about the same for the two groups because type 2 diabetes is ten times as common as type 1.

JARGON ALERT

How high glucose leads to complications

Although doctors aren't certain about the causes of most long-term complications, I mention the current theories about the causes of the complications as I explain each complication in the following sections of this chapter. But all long-term complications share several common characteristics, described in the following list:

✔ Advanced glycated end products (AGEs) are one of the substances that damage tissues. AGEs can damage the eyes, the kidneys, the nervous system, and other organs in your body. You always have glucose in your blood, and some of that glucose attaches to other substances in your bloodstream to form glycated (glucose-attached) products. In this way, hemoglobin, which carries oxygen through your blood to cells and tissues throughout your body, attaches to glucose to form hemoglobin A1c. Albumin, a protein in blood, forms glycated albumin. Glucose can attach to red blood cells and white blood cells as well as to other cells and molecules in the bloodstream. When these normal body substances attach to glucose, they no longer work normally.

✔ When glucose attaches to other substances and cells, it alters their functions, usually in a negative fashion. For example, hemoglobin A1c holds on to oxygen more strongly than hemoglobin, so the cells that need oxygen don't get it as easily. Red blood cells that are glycated do not last as long in your blood circulation. Glycated white blood cells can't fight infection as well as unglycated white cells can.

✔ Your body handles a certain level of glycated substances. But when your blood glucose is elevated for prolonged periods of time, the level of glycated cells and substances becomes excessive, and the complications I describe in this chapter result.

✔ The Polyol Pathway is another major source of damage to the body in diabetes. Polyol Pathway refers to one direction, or pathway, that glucose can take as it is metabolized (broken down). For example, the common pathway is to form carbon dioxide and water as energy is produced. When you have a lot of glucose in your blood, an abnormal amount is metabolized to become a product called sorbitol. Sorbitol is a member of a class of substances called polyols. Sorbitol accumulates in many tissues where it can damage them in various ways:

✔ Damage from swelling: Body water enters the cells to make the concentration of substances equal outside and inside, because sorbitol does not pass out of the cell. This causes damage and destruction of cells.

✔ Damage from chemical reactions: During the production of sorbitol, other compounds are produced that chemically damage the cells and tissues.

Diabetes and your kidneys

Your kidneys contain a structure called the *glomerulous*, which is responsible for cleansing your blood (see Figure 5-1). Each kidney has hundreds of thousands of glomeruli. Your blood passes through the tiny glomerular capillaries, which are in intimate contact with tubules through which your filtered blood travels. As the filtered blood passes through the tubules, most of the water and the normal contents of the blood are reabsorbed and sent back into your body, while a small amount of water and waste passes from the kidney into the ureter and then into the bladder and out through the urethra.

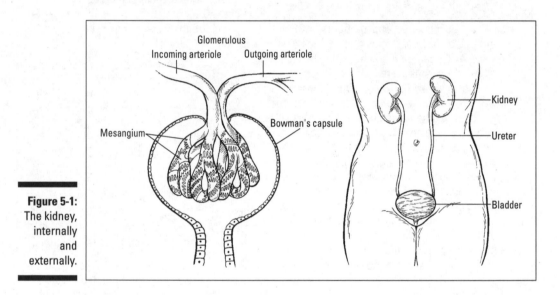

Figure 5-1:
The kidney,
internally
and
externally.

When you first get diabetes, your kidneys are enlarged and seem to function abnormally well, judging by how fast they clear wastes from your body. Your kidneys seem to function so well because you have a large amount of glucose entering your kidneys, which draws a lot of water with it and causes an increase in the pressure inside each glomerulous. This more rapid transit of blood through the kidneys is known as an increased *glomerular filtration rate* (GFR). Early in the development of your diabetes, the membrane surrounding your glomeruli, called the *glomerular basement membrane*, thickens, as do other adjacent structures. These expanding membranes and structures begin to take up the space occupied by the capillaries inside the glomeruli so that the capillaries are unable to filter as much blood.

Fortunately, you have many more glomeruli than you really need. In fact, you can lose a whole kidney and still have plenty of reserve to clean your blood. If your kidney disease goes undetected for about 15 years, damage may become so severe that your blood shows measurable signs of the beginning of kidney failure, called *azotemia*. If the neglect of the disease reaches 20 years, your kidneys may fail entirely. (For more on the timing of kidney failure, see the sidebar "Time course of kidney failure.")

Not every person with diabetes is at equal risk for kidney disease and kidney failure. It seems to be more common in certain families and among certain racial groups, especially African-Americans, Mexican Americans, and Native Americans. It is certainly more common when high blood pressure is present. Although we believe that high blood glucose is the major factor leading to nephropathy, only half of the people who have been poorly controlled go on to develop nephropathy.

Earliest changes

If the kidneys are going to be damaged by diabetic nephropathy, very early on there is a characteristic finding in the urine called *microalbuminuria*. A healthy kidney permits only a tiny amount of *albumin*, a protein in the blood, to enter the urine. A kidney that is being damaged by nephropathy is unable to hold back as much albumin, and the level in the urine increases. In the early stages, however, the amount is less than that required to trigger a positive test when the traditional urine dipstick is used. It is necessary to do a more sophisticated test for microalbuminuria. This can be done by collecting a 24-hour urine specimen, by a random urine, or by the collection of a specimen over a certain time period, usually four hours. If the level of albumin is abnormally high, it needs to be checked once again to be certain, because some things like exercise can trigger a false positive test. A second positive test should lead to some action to protect the kidneys. Microalbuminuria is found about five years before the urine becomes dipstick positive. Treatment during the stage of microalbuminuria can reverse the kidney disease. Once macroalbuminuria (a positive urine dipstick) is found, the disease can be slowed but not stopped.

If you have had type 1 diabetes for five years or more or at the initial diagnosis of type 2 diabetes, **your doctor must check for microalbuminuria** unless you already have dipstick-positive proteinuria. If negative, it should be checked annually.

Progressive changes

After five years of poorly controlled diabetes, there is significant expansion of the *mesangial tissue*, the cells between the capillaries. The amount of microalbuminuria is very consistent with the amount of mesangial expansion. Thickening of the glomerular basement membrane is taking place at the same time but does not correlate as well with the amount of microalbuminuria.

Over the next 15 to 20 years, the open capillaries and tubules are squeezed shut by the encroaching tissues and appear like round nodules, known by the names of their discoverers as Kimmelstiel-Wilson nodules and diagnostic of diabetic nephropathy. As the glomeruli are replaced by nodules, less and less filtration of the blood can take place. The blood urea nitrogen begins to rise, ultimately ending in uremia when the kidneys are not doing any cleansing.

Other factors besides high blood glucose contribute to the continuing destruction of the kidneys. They include

- **High blood pressure,** which may be almost as important as the glucose level. If the blood pressure is controlled by drugs, the damage to the kidneys slows very significantly. This is shown by the occasional person with diabetes who has hypertension but has disease of one of the arteries to a kidney so that this kidney does not feel the force of the blood pressure. While the other kidney goes on to develop nephropathy, this kidney is protected and does not develop it.

- **Factors of inheritance,** because certain families and ethnic groups have a higher incidence of diabetic nephropathy.

- **Abnormal blood fats,** because it has been shown that elevated levels of certain cholesterol-containing fats promotes enlargement of the mesangium.

- **Cigarette smoking,** because heart disease is greatly increased in diabetic nephropathy. Cigarettes are clearly linked to increased occurrence of heart disease.

Time course of kidney failure

If the patient is going to have kidney failure, the time course is as follows:

- At the time of onset of diabetes, the kidneys are large and the glomerular filtration rate is increased.

- By about two years, the glomerular basement membrane and mesangium are beginning to thicken.

- For 10 to 15 years, there is a silent period when there are no clinical signs that the kidneys are failing.

- After 15 years, it becomes obvious that the kidneys are failing because there are elevations of measurable waste products in the blood — the blood urea nitrogen, or BUN, and the creatinine. In addition, a test of the urine reveals large amounts of protein, which should not be found normally.

- By 20 years, the patient will either begin dialysis or have a kidney transplant.

Diabetic nephropathy does not occur alone. Other complications develop at a faster or slower rate. They include

✔ **Diabetic eye disease:** At the time of complete failure of the kidneys, called *end stage renal disease,* diabetic retinopathy (eye disease) is always present (see the section "Eye Disease," later in this chapter). As kidney disease gets worse, retinopathy accelerates. But only half the people with retinopathy also have nephropathy. Once microalbuminuria is present, all the patients will also have some retinopathy. Therefore, if you have diabetes and have microalbuminuria and retinopathy is not present, your doctor should look for another cause of kidney disease besides diabetes.

✔ **Diabetic nerve disease, or neuropathy:** There is not as great an association between nephropathy and neuropathy. Fewer than 50 percent of patients with nephropathy will have neuropathy. Neuropathy gets worse as kidney disease gets worse, but once dialysis is started, some of the neuropathy disappears so that part of the neuropathy may be due to wastes that are retained because of the failing kidney rather than true damage to the nervous system. (For more on this condition, see the section "Nerve Disease, or Neuropathy" later in this chapter.)

✔ **Hypertension:** Hypertension plays an important role in accelerating the kidney damage. Once there is overt proteinuria, which means it is dipstick positive, one-third of the patients will have high blood pressure. As the blood tests for kidney failure begin to rise, two-thirds of patients are hypertensive. With end stage renal disease, almost all have high blood pressure.

✔ **Edema:** *Edema,* or water accumulation, in the feet and legs occurs as the amount of protein in the urine exceeds one or two grams a day.

Treatment

Happily, all the inconvenience and discomfort associated with diabetic nephropathy can be avoided. Following are a few key treatments that you can do to prevent the disease or significantly slow it down once it begins:

✔ **Control your blood glucose:** This has been shown to avoid the onset of nephropathy and slow it down once it starts. Both the Diabetes Control and Complications Trial in the United States, which studied glucose control in type 1 diabetes, and the United Kingdom Prospective Diabetes Study Groups in type 2 diabetes have shown this clearly. If you keep your blood glucose close to normal, you will not develop diabetic nephropathy. (For information on controlling your blood glucose, see Part III.)

- ✔ **Control your blood pressure:** This protects the kidneys from rapid deterioration. Treatment begins with a low-salt diet, but drugs are usually needed. High blood pressure can be controlled by a variety of drugs, but one class of drugs seems particularly valuable in nephropathy. It's a class called the *angiotensin converting enzyme inhibitors,* or ACE inhibitors. (For more on ACE inhibitors, see the sidebar.)

- ✔ **Control the blood fats:** Because abnormalities of blood fats seem to make the kidney disease worse, it is important to lower the bad, or LDL, cholesterol and raise the good, or HDL, cholesterol while lowering the other fat that is damaging, namely, the triglycerides. A number of excellent drugs, in a class called *statins,* can do this. The ACE inhibitors also seem to help the levels of fats. (See the sidebar on ACE inhibitors for more information.)

- ✔ **Avoid other damage to the kidneys:** People with diabetes tend to have more urinary tract infections, which damage the kidneys. Urinary tract infections must be looked for and treated. People with diabetes also have nerve damage to the nerves that control the bladder, producing a neurogenic bladder. (See the section "Disorders of automatic (autonomic) nerves" in this chapter.) When the nerves that detect a full bladder fail, proper emptying of the bladder is inhibited and can lead to infections. When there is disease in the urinary system, the doctor often does an *intravenous pyelogram* (IVP), a study to observe the appearance and function of the kidney and the rest of the urinary tract. People with diabetes with some kidney failure are at high risk for complete failure of the kidneys as a result of an IVP. Other types of studies that do not put the kidneys at risk should be used.

- ✔ **Conduct dialysis if preventive treatment fails:** If dialysis is done, two techniques are currently in use: *hemodialysis* and *peritoneal dialysis.*

  - • With **hemodialysis,** the patient's artery is hooked into a tube that runs through a filtering machine that cleanses the blood and then sends it back into the patient's bloodstream. When the patient is moderately well, hemodialysis is done three times a week in a hospital-like setting. However, there is the potential for many complications, including infection, low blood pressure, and so on. In addition, with failure of the kidneys, a main source for the breakdown of insulin is gone, and the patient requires much less or no insulin, so control of the blood glucose may actually get easier.

  - • **Peritoneal dialysis** consists of the insertion of a tube into the body cavity that contains the stomach, liver, and intestines, called the *peritoneal cavity.* A large quantity of fluid is dripped into the cavity, and it draws out the wastes, which are then removed as the fluid drains out of the cavity. Peritoneal dialysis is done at home, often on a daily basis. Peritoneal dialysis requires the use of sugar in the fluid so that people with diabetes may have very high blood glucose levels unless insulin is added to the bags of dialysis fluid. Peritoneal dialysis is also associated with a high rate of infection where the tube enters the peritoneal cavity.

Little difference exists in the long-term survival of patients treated with hemodialysis compared with peritoneal dialysis, so the choice becomes one of convenience and whether one is covered by insurance more than the other. People with diabetes do not tolerate kidney failure well, so dialysis tends to be done earlier in them than in people without diabetes.

✔ **Receive a kidney transplant if preventive treatment fails:** Patients who receive a kidney transplant do seem to do better than dialysis patients, but in the United States, because of a lack of kidneys, 80 percent of patients have dialysis and 20 percent have a transplant. The transplant is foreign to the person with diabetes who receives it, and the person's body tries to reject it, requiring the use of antirejection drugs, some of which make diabetic control more complicated. The kidney that is least rejected is the one from a donor who is most closely related to the patient. Once a healthy kidney enters the body of a person with diabetes, it is subject to the damage done by elevated glucose levels so that control of the glucose becomes even more important.

ACE inhibitors to the rescue

ACE inhibitors have long been known to lower blood pressure, but recent studies show that they lower the pressure inside the glomerulous. The result is a 50 percent reduction in death due to diabetic nephropathy and an equal reduction in the need for dialysis or transplantation.

Treatment should begin when the blood pressure is 140/90 or higher. The target blood pressure is 120/80 and even lower in younger people. ACE inhibitors can even be used when there is microalbuminuria without hypertension, because the microalbuminuria suggests that there is increased pressure within the kidney. Once ACE inhibitors are used, the excretion of albumin begins to fall, and this can be used to monitor their effectiveness if the blood pressure is normal.

ACE inhibitors are not perfect treatment because an incidence of cough exists, which some people find hard to tolerate, but the choice of a particular ACE inhibitor may solve this problem. In addition, ACE inhibitors tend to raise the potassium in the blood. This is already a problem with failing kidneys, so a higher potassium level may add to the problem. A very high potassium level can cause abnormalities in the heart.

Other drugs used for high blood pressure include the calcium channel blockers, which may be as useful as ACE inhibitors. Other antihypertensives that have been standards in the past for hypertension may cause unacceptable side effects. Water pills (diuretics such as hydrochlorothiazide) will raise the blood glucose. Beta blockers like propranolol will make the abnormal fats worse. They also cause a difficulty in recognizing when the blood glucose has gone down to very low levels.

Eye Disease

The eyes are the second major organ of the body affected by diabetes over the long term. Some eye diseases, such as glaucoma and cataracts, also occur in the nondiabetic population, though they appear at a higher rate and earlier in people with diabetes. Glaucoma and cataracts respond to treatment very well. Diabetic retinopathy, however, is limited to the diabetic population and may lead to blindness. In the past, blindness was inevitable, but this result is far from the case today.

In order to understand how diabetes affects the eyes, Figure 5-2 shows you the different parts of the eye.

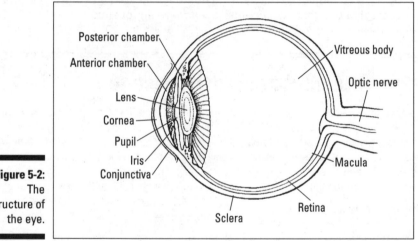

Figure 5-2:
The
structure of
the eye.

Light enters the eye through the lens, where it is bent and focused upon the retina. The place in the retina where the lens focuses is called the macula. The retina collects an image and transfers it to the optic nerve, which carries it to the brain where the image is interpreted. Between the lens and the retina is a transparent material called the *vitreous body*. Many more structures are within the eye, but they're not important for my purposes in this chapter. The eye muscles surround the eye on all sides and are attached to it. These muscles permit you to look up, down and sideways without moving your head. These eye muscles are important in the discussion of diabetic nerve damage, called neuropathy. (For more on this condition, see the section "Nerve Disease, or Neuropathy," later in this chapter.)

Following is a list of common eye diseases found in people with diabetes.

- ✔ **Cataracts:** These opaque areas of the lens can block vision if they're large enough. Cataracts tend to be more common in people with diabetes, even at a young age, both as a result of advanced glycation end products, which form within the lens, and as a result of the increased concentration of sorbitol in the lens. Cataracts can be surgically removed by a fairly routine operation. The entire lens is removed, and an artificial lens is put in its place. With removal, you have an excellent chance for the restoration of your vision.

- ✔ **Glaucoma:** This high pressure inside the eye is enough to do damage to the optic nerve. Glaucoma is found more often in people with diabetes than in the nondiabetic population. If unchecked, the high pressure can destroy the optic nerve and vision along with it. Fortunately, medical treatment can lower the eye pressure and save the eye. Eye doctors check for glaucoma on a routine basis.

- ✔ **Retinopathy:** *Diabetic retinopathy* refers to a number of changes that are seen on the retina of the eye. These changes indicate that the patient has been exposed to high levels of blood glucose over time. If untreated at the appropriate time, retinopathy can lead to blindness. The first changes are seen after ten years of diabetes in both type 1 and 2. Because retinopathy is much more complicated and less treatable than the other two conditions, I discuss it in much more detail in the next section.

You must get an annual eye examination by an ophthalmologist or optometrist to preserve vision in diabetes. This is a situation where an expert is definitely needed. Doctors who are not ophthalmologists or optometrists diagnose retinopathy correctly only 50 percent of the time, while ophthalmologists and optometrists are correct more than 90 percent of the time. If you haven't been doing so already, you need to get an eye examination at the time of the diagnosis of type 2 diabetes or five years after the diagnosis of type 1 diabetes and every year after that.

Retinopathy

Ophthalmologists break down retinopathy into two major types, according to their potential to cause visual loss:

- ✔ *Background retinopathy* is usually benign but can be a predictor of worse problems. The first changes noted by the ophthalmologist are *retinal aneurysms,* which are the result of weakening of the capillaries of the eye with production of outpocketing of the capillaries. These aneurysms appear as small red dots on the back of the eye. They are benign and disappear over time. The weakened capillaries also rupture sometimes and release blood to form *retinal hemorrhages* and *hard exudates.* The hard exudates, which are yellowish and appear round and sharp, are scars from the hemorrhage. If they extend into the macular area, they reduce vision. If the capillaries in the retina allow fluid and other things to flow into the macula, you get macular edema and again loss of vision. These exudates and hemorrhages can last for years. As the capillaries close, you have a decreased blood supply to the retina, and *cotton wool spots* or *soft exudates* appear. These represent destruction of the nerve fiber layer because of the lack of blood.

These changes usually do not cause loss of vision, but in about 50 percent of cases, they go on to the more serious proliferative retinopathy.

✔ *Proliferative retinopathy* ends up with vision loss if untreated. Just as in many other parts of the body when the blood supply is reduced, new blood vessels form to carry more blood to the retina. When this happens, the patient is entering the stage of proliferative retinopathy. This is where some visual loss becomes more certain. The growth of blood vessels takes place into the vitreous. Hemorrhage into the vitreous blocks vision. As the hemorrhage forms a clot and contracts, it may pull up the retina to produce *retinal detachment*. Because the lens can no longer focus the light on to the macula, you have a complete loss of vision.

Retinopathy, like nephropathy, has a number of important associations:

✔ Certain ethnic groups are at very high risk for retinopathy. These include certain American Indian groups like the Pima Indians as well as Mexican Americans. It is uncertain if African Americans are at higher risk.

✔ Specific genetic material, if found in a person with diabetes, increases the incidence of retinopathy. This can be found by doing a chemical analysis of a person's chromosomes, the material in each cell that holds the genes. If the genetic material is found, that person has a higher likelihood of developing retinopathy.

✔ Males and females get retinopathy equally.

✔ Greater duration of diabetes results in more eye disease.

✔ High blood pressure worsens the eye disease.

✔ Nephropathy occurs along with the eye disease.

✔ Smoking and alcohol use probably worsen retinopathy (but the final word on this is not in).

✔ Patients with severe diabetic retinopathy are at increased risk for heart attacks.

No drugs are currently available to treat retinopathy, but laser surgery is an excellent treatment option. And the use of laser surgery to create many burns in the retina has been shown to save many eyes. The original studies used one eye as the untreated or control eye and the other as the treated eye. The risk of severe visual loss is reduced to less than half as often when laser treatment is used to preserve the eye. Because the retina is being burned, you have some minor loss of vision. You also have a mild decrease in night vision and a minor decrease in the size of the field that your eye can take in at one time. The procedure is done outside the hospital. It is used for treating macular edema with success as well.

Laser surgery cannot treat a detachment that has already occurred. To do so, a surgical procedure called *vitrectomy* is used. This operation, done under general anesthesia, involves the removal of the vitreous body and its replacement with a sterile solution. Attachments to the retina are cut, and the retina returns to its place. Any hemorrhages in the vitreous are removed at the same time. Vitrectomy is successful in restoring some vision about 80 to 90 percent of the time. If a retinal detachment is also present, the amount of improvement depends upon the extent and duration of the retinal attachment with restoration of vision occurring about 50 to 60 percent of the time.

Resources for the blind and visually impaired

A search for resources for the blind and visually impaired must begin in the World Wide Web. Using a search engine, you can come up with more than 8,000 sites that have something to do with loss of vision and blindness. One of the first sites is the Blindness Resource Center, which contains a huge list of other sources of information sponsored by the New York Institute for Special Education. It is at `www.nyise.org/text/blindness.htm`. Of note is that it is a large-print version, easily read by the sight impaired.

The Blindness Resource Center is filled with useful information. Just to give you the flavor of what is available, here are some of the other sites described and to which you can link from this site:

- Blind Net, which contains useful and factual information about blindness at `www.blind.net/blindind.htm`
- Blind Related Mailing Lists at `www.redwhiteandblue.org/blists.html`
- Blind Links, extensive links to services for the blind at `seidata.com/~marriage/rblind.html`
- Cornucopia of Disability Information, a large collection of documents related to disability at `codi.buffalo.edu/`
- Dialogue Magazine, written specifically for the blind at `www.teleport.com/~blindskl/`
- Narrative Television Network, an effort to open the world of entertainment to the blind at `www.narrativetv.com/`
- The Internet Phone Book of Blind Users and Services at `www.redwhiteandblue.org/pmenu.html`

Undoubtedly, one of its best links is to the American Foundation for the Blind at www.afb.org/. It would take a good part of a lifetime to read all of the resource materials that the AFB provides on thousands of pages. The AFB is the organization that Helen Keller devoted her life to, and it has every imaginable resource — and some that are unimaginable. Just a few of the AFB's reports and fact sheets include

- ✔ A profile of the blind and visually impaired audience for television and video
- ✔ Adding audio description to television science programs: impact on legally blind viewers
- ✔ National aging and vision network
- ✔ Fact sheet on Braille
- ✔ Synthetic speech systems
- ✔ Catalog houses that sell specialty products
- ✔ Information on accommodating the applicant or employee who is blind or visually impaired
- ✔ Art for and by the blind bibliography

The World Wide Web is an enormous resource for the visually handicapped and should be utilized by friends, relatives, or the impaired person if that is possible. One of the papers has to do with screen magnification for the visually impaired. You have no reason to feel alone with your visual problem.

Nerve Disease, or Neuropathy

The third major organ system of the body that is attacked by poorly controlled diabetes is the nervous system. Sixty percent of people with diabetes are shown to have some abnormality of the nervous system. These patients usually don't realize it because the disease does not have any early symptoms. These patients usually have poor glucose control, smoke, and are over age 40. Nerve disease is found most often in the people who have diabetes the longest. The major problem with respect to diabetic neuropathy is the high frequency of foot infections, foot ulcerations, and amputation — complications that are all entirely preventable. (See the section on "Diabetic Foot Disease," later in this chapter.)

How the high glucose damages nerves remains uncertain. What is found is that the part of the nerve, called the *axon*, that connects to other nerves or to muscle becomes degenerated. It is believed that the damage is due to a cut off of blood to the nerve (vascular) in some cases and to chemical toxins produced by the metabolism of too much glucose (metabolic) in others.

Diabetic neuropathy occurs in any situation where the blood glucose is abnormally elevated for ten years or more. It is therefore not limited to type 1 or type 2 diabetes, although these are the most common diseases where it is found. When the elevated blood glucose is brought down to normal, the signs and symptoms improve. In some cases, the neuropathy disappears.

The fact that intensive control of the blood glucose improves the neuropathy suggests that it is a consequence of abnormal metabolism that damages the nerves.

Diagnosing neuropathy

The speed with which a nervous impulse travels down a nerve fiber is called the *nerve conduction velocity.* In diabetic neuropathy, the nerve conduction velocity (NCV) is slowed. This slowing may not be accompanied by any symptoms at first, providing a way of diagnosing neuropathy in people without symptoms. If patients have very mild symptoms, the improvement that follows medication may be hard to detect except by doing a nerve conduction velocity study. A medication that helps the neuropathy would be expected to speed up the NCV.

In addition to a persistently high blood glucose, neuropathy is made worse by the following conditions:

- ✔ The **age** of the patient is important because neuropathy is most common over the age of 40.
- ✔ The **height** of the patient is a consideration. Neuropathy is more common in taller individuals, who have longer nerve fibers to damage.
- ✔ **Alcohol consumption** is especially important because even small quantities of alcohol can make neuropathy worse.

Doctors can test nerve function in a variety of ways because different nerve fibers seem to be responsible for different kinds of sensation, such as light touch, vibration, and temperature. The connection between the kind of test and the fiber it tests for is as follows:

- ✔ **Vibration testing,** using a tuning fork, for example, can bring out abnormalities of large nerve fibers.
- ✔ **Temperature testing,** using a warm or cold item, tests for damage to small fibers, which are very important in diabetes. When small fibers are damaged, the patient can lose the ability to feel that he is entering a burning hot bath.

✔ **Light touch testing,** perhaps the most important test that is done, reflects the large fibers, which sense anything touching our skin. This test is done using a filament that looks like a hair. The thickness of the filament determines how much force is needed to bend the filament so that it is felt. For example, a filament that bends with 1 gram of force can be felt by normal feet. If a patient can feel a filament that bends with 10 grams of force, it is unlikely that this person will suffer damage to the foot without feeling it. If the patient cannot feel any sensation with a filament that requires 75 grams of force to bend, that area is considered to have lost all sensation.

The 10-gram filament can be used by you or your doctor to discover whether you are at risk for damage to your feet because you cannot feel the pain. This test takes a minute to do and can save your feet from amputation. (See the section about the diabetic foot, later in this chapter.)

Symptoms of neuropathy

The various disorders of the nervous system are broken down into the following categories:

✔ **Disorders associated with loss of sensation,** where the sensory nerves are damaged

✔ **Disorders due to loss of motor nerves,** which carry the impulses to muscles to make them move

✔ **Disorders due to loss of automatic (known as *autonomic*) nerves,** which control muscles we do not have to think about, such as the heart muscles, the intestinal muscles, and the bladder muscles.

The following sections describe the various conditions associated with these disorders.

Disorders of sensation

Disorders of sensation are the most common and bothersome disorders of nerves in diabetes. There are a number of different conditions, which break down into diffuse neuropathies involving many nerves and focal neuropathies involving one or several nerves. This section is about the diffuse neuropathies affecting sensation.

Distal polyneuropathy

Distal polyneuropathy is the most frequent form of diabetic neuropathy. *Distal* means far away from the center of the body — in other words, the feet and hands. *Poly* means many, and *neuropathy* is disease in nerves. So this is a disease of many nerves, which is noticed in the feet and hands. Physicians believe that distal polyneuropathy is a metabolic disease (too much glucose in the blood, specifically) because other diseases where there is a general abnormality of metabolism, such as kidney failure or vitamin deficiency, present with a distal polyneuropathy as well.

The signs and symptoms of distal polyneuropathy are:

- ✔ Diminished ability to feel light touch or feel the position of a foot, whether bent back or forward, resulting from the loss of the large fibers
- ✔ Diminished ability to feel pain and temperature from loss of small fibers
- ✔ Insignificant weakness
- ✔ Tingling and burning
- ✔ Extreme sensitivity to touch
- ✔ Loss of balance or coordination
- ✔ Worsening of symptoms at night

The danger of this kind of neuropathy is that the patient doesn't know, without looking, whether he has trauma to his feet, such as a burn or stepping on a tack. When the small fibers are lost, the symptoms are uncomfortable but not as serious. The patient may feel pain when the night covers are on the feet or other uncomfortable sensations. The majority of patients with this condition are unaware of the loss of nerve fibers, and the disease is picked up by nerve conduction studies.

The complications of this loss of sensation are preventable. If you cannot feel your feet, you must look at them. In the section on the feet, later in this chapter, I offer specific techniques to preserve your feel when neuropathy is present.

The most serious complication of loss of sensation in the feet is the neuropathic foot ulcer. As pressure mounts on an area of the foot, it is felt because of pain. However, in diabetic neuropathy, this pressure is not felt. A callus forms and, with continued pressure, the callus softens and liquifies, finally falling off to leave an ulcer. This ulcer becomes infected. If it isn't promptly treated, it spreads, and amputation may be the only way of saving the patient. In this situation, loss of blood supply to the feet is not an important contributing factor to the ulceration, and, in fact, the blood supply may be very good.

A less common complication in distal polyneuopathy is *neuroarthropathy,* or Charcot's Joint. In this condition, trauma, which isn't felt, occurs to the joints of the foot or ankle. The bones in the foot get out of line, and many painless fractures may occur. The patient has redness and painless swelling of the foot and ankle. The foot becomes unusable and is described as a bag of bones.

Treatment of distal polyneuropathy starts with the best glucose control possible and extremely good foot care.

Your doctor should look at your feet each visit, particularly if you have any evidence of loss of feeling.

Some drugs, such as the nonsteroidal anti-inflammatory agents ibuprofen and salindac, can reduce the inflammation. Other drugs, such as the antidepressants amitriptylene or imipramine, reduce the pain and other discomfort. A drug called capsacin, which is applied to the skin, reduces pain as well. The results of these treatments are variable and seem to work about 60 percent of the time. However, the longer the pain has been present and the worse the pain, the less likely that these drugs will work.

A new drug called gabapentin has been found to work more often than many of the older drugs, but it causes dizziness and sleepiness, which may make treatment more complicated.

Radiculopathy-nerve root involvement

Sometimes a severe pain in a particular distribution suggests that the root of the nerve, as it leaves the spinal column, is damaged. The clinical picture is pain distributed in a horizontal line around one side of the chest or abdomen. The pain can be so severe that it is mistaken for an internal abdominal emergency. Fortunately, the pain goes away after a variable period of time — anywhere from six to 24 months.

Polyradiculopathy-diabetic amyotrophy

Polyradiculopathy-diabetic amyotrophy is a mixture of pain and loss of muscle strength in the muscles of the upper leg so that the patient cannot straighten the knee. Pain extends down from the hip to the thigh. It is second in occurrence after distal polyneuropathy. Polyradiculopathy-diabetic amyotrophy generally has a short course but may continue for years and doesn't particularly improve with better diabetic control.

Disorders of movement

Neuropathy can affect nerves to various muscles. The result is a sudden inability to move or use those muscles. It is thought that these disorders originate as a result of sudden closing of a blood vessel supplying the nerve. The clinical picture depends on which nerve or nerves are affected. If one of the nerves to the eyeball is damaged, the patient cannot turn his eye to the side that nerve is on. If the nerve to the face is affected, the eyelid may droop or the smile on one side of the face may be flat. The patient can have trouble with vision or problems with hearing. Focusing the eye may not be possible. No treatment really exists, but fortunately the disorder goes away on its own after several months.

Disorders of automatic (autonomic) nerves

Many movements of muscles are going on all of the time, but you're unaware of them. The heart muscle is squeezing down and relaxing. The diaphragm is rising up to empty the lungs of air and relaxing to draw air in. The esophagus is carrying food down to the stomach from the mouth where, in turn, the stomach pushes it into the small intestine, which pushes it into the large intestine. All these functions of muscles are under the control of nerves from the brain, and diabetic neuropathy can affect all of them. These automatic functions are called the autonomic nerves. When sensitive tests are done, as many as 40 percent of people with diabetes can be found to have some form of autonomic neuropathy. The clinical presentation of the neuropathy depends upon the involved nerve. Some of the clinical pictures are

- **Bladder abnormalities starting with a loss of the sensation of bladder fullness.** The urine is not eliminated, and urinary tract infections result. After a while, loss of bladder contraction occurs, and the patient has to strain to urinate or loses urine by dribbling. The doctor can easily diagnose this abnormality by finding out how much urine is left in the bladder after urinating. The treatment is to remember to urinate every four hours or take a drug that increases the force of bladder contraction.

- **Sexual dysfunction in 50 percent of males with diabetes and 30 percent of females with diabetes.** Males cannot sustain an erection, and females have trouble lubricating the vagina for intercourse (see Chapter 6 for more information on these problems).

- **Intestinal abnormalities of various kinds.** The most common abnormality is constipation. If nerves to the stomach are involved, the stomach does not empty on time. This can lead to "brittle" diabetes because the insulin is active when there is no food. Fortunately, a drug called metocloprimide helps to empty the stomach.

- **Involvement of the gall bladder leads to gallstones because it does not empty.** Normally, the gall bladder empties each time you eat, especially if you eat a fatty meal because the substances in the bile (within the gall bladder) help to break down fat. If disease of the nerve to the gall bladder prevents it from emptying, these same substances will form stones.

- **Involvement of the large intestine that can result in diabetic diarrhea with as many as ten or more bowel movements in a day.** Accidental loss of bowel contents can occur, and bacteria can grow abnormally in the intestine. This problem responds to antibiotic treatment. Diarrhea is treated with one of several drugs, which quiets the large intestine.

- **Heart abnormalities from loss of nerves to the heart.** The heart may not respond to exercise by speeding up as it should. The force of the heart may not increase when the patient stands, and the patient then becomes lightheaded. A fast fixed heart rate also may occur, and the rhythm of the heart may not be normal. Such patients are at risk for sudden death.

✔ **Sweating problems, especially in the feet.** The body may try to compensate for the lack of sweating in the feet by sweating excessively on the face or trunk. Heavy sweating can occur when certain foods, such as cheese, are eaten.

✔ **Abnormalities of the pupil of the eye.** The pupil determines the amount of light that is let in. As a result of the neuropathy, the pupil is small and does not open up in a dark room.

You can see that you can run into all kinds of problems if you develop diabetic neuropathy. None of them need ever bother you, though, if you follow the recommendations in Part III — and the closest you will ever get to a nerve problem will be when you try to get a date with that cute neighbor.

Heart Disease

In the last three decades, the number of deaths due to heart disease has fallen dramatically, thanks to all kinds of new treatments as well as improved diets. The tremendous increase in the number of type 2 patients predicted for the next few decades may reverse this trend. In this section, you find out about the special problems that diabetes brings to the heart.

Coronary artery disease is the term for the progressive closure of the arteries, which supply blood to the heart muscle. When one or more of your arteries closes completely, the result is a heart attack (myocardial infarction). In diabetes, the incidence of coronary artery disease (CAD) is increased even in the young type 1 patient. It is the duration of time with the diabetes that promotes CAD in type 1 patients. There is no difference in the way CAD affects males or females.

Type 2 diabetes is different. CAD is the most common reason for death in type 2 patients. Women are at increased risk for CAD compared to men. Many other risk factors promote CAD in the type 2 patient. Among them are

✔ **Increased production of insulin** because of the insulin resistance

✔ **Obesity**

✔ **Central adiposity,** which refers to the distribution of fat particularly in the waist area

✔ **Hypertension (high blood pressure)**

✔ **Abnormal blood fats,** especially reduced HDL and increased triglyceride. The abnormal fats may persist even when the glucose is controlled. People without diabetes but with impaired glucose tolerance may show the same abnormalities.

People with diabetes have more CAD than people without diabetes. When x-ray studies of the heart blood vessels are compared, people with diabetes have more arteries involved than nondiabetics.

If a heart attack occurs, the risk of death is much greater for the person with diabetes. Twenty percent of all people with diabetes die of heart attacks. If nondiabetics have a heart attack, they die 15 percent of the time, but people with diabetes die 40 percent of the time. The death rate is worse for the person with diabetes who was in poor glucose control before the heart attack. That same poorly controlled person has more complications, such as shock and heart failure, from a heart attack than the person without diabetes. Once a heart attack occurs, the outlook is much worse for the person with diabetes. A second heart attack occurs in 50 percent (25 percent without diabetes), and the death rate in five years is much worse (80 percent versus 25 percent).

The picture is not a pretty one for the person with diabetes who has coronary artery disease. At least the treatment is the same for the person with diabetes. Therapy to dissolve the clot of blood that is obstructing the coronary artery can be used, but people with diabetes do not do as well with *angioplasty*, the technique by which a tube is placed into the artery to clean it out and open it up.

People with diabetes do as well with surgery to bypass the obstruction (called bypass surgery) as do nondiabetics, but the long-term prognosis for keeping the graft open is not as good.

I want to tell you about three special complications of the heart in diabetes.

Insulin resistance syndrome

The earliest abnormality in type 2 diabetes is insulin resistance, which is found in people even before diabetes can be diagnosed. Those with impaired glucose tolerance and even 25 percent of the population with normal glucose tolerance have evidence of insulin resistance. Several features, all associated with an increased incidence of coronary artery disease, accompany insulin resistance:

✔ **Hypertension:** This problem may be a consequence of the increased insulin required to keep the glucose normal when there is insulin resistance. When people are given insulin to control the glucose, a rise in blood pressure often occurs.

✔ **Abnormalities of blood fats:** The level of triglycerides is elevated as is the amount of small, dense *LDL (low density lipoprotein)*, a particle in the blood that carries cholesterol called "bad cholesterol." At the same time, you see a decline in the amount of *HDL (high density lipoprotein)*, the "good" cholesterol particle that helps to clean out the arteries.

✓ **Increased plasminogen activator inhibitor-1:** This chemical, which blocks the activity of plasminogen activator, prevents the breakdown of blood clots that form in the arteries of the heart and other areas.

✓ **Increased abdominal visceral fat:** You can lose a lot of this fat, which is found at the waistline, by dieting and losing 5 to 10 percent of your body weight.

✓ **Obesity:** This is often present in the insulin resistance syndrome but doesn't need to be there to make the diagnosis.

✓ **Sedentary lifestyle:** This is also often found, but an active lifestyle does not preclude the insulin resistance syndrome.

The preceding features, plus other features that I do not list, are found in people who have an increased tendency to have coronary artery disease and heart attacks. Keep in mind that the condition is present even when diabetes is not. The condition is probably a primary abnormality and not a consequence of an elevated blood glucose over time. When insulin resistance is present in diabetes, the lowering of the blood glucose may decrease the complications of a heart attack, which are related to the high blood glucose, but not the increased tendency to have a heart attack in the first place, which is not dependent on a high blood glucose.

A number of treatments are available for the insulin resistance syndrome. If you are obese and have a sedentary lifestyle, you should correct these problems. It does not take a lot of weight loss or exercise to make a major contribution toward decreasing the risk of a heart attack.

You can treat the elevated triglyceride and the reduced HDL with drugs such as the statins. The *thiazolidendione drugs* (*glitazones*) — a new class of drugs of which rosiglitazone and pioglitazone are the only ones currently available (see Chapter 10) — directly attack the insulin resistance. People with diabetes and the nondiabetics with the features of the insulin resistance syndrome may find these drugs useful in the future.

Cardiac autonomic neuropathy

I discuss cardiac autonomic neuropathy briefly in the section on neuropathy, earlier in this chapter. Basically, the heart is under the control of nerves, and high glucose levels can damage these nerves. There are a number of ways to test for this:

✓ **Measure the resting heart rate.** It may be abnormally high (greater than 100).

✓ **Measure the standing blood pressure.** It may fall abnormally low (a decrease of 20 mm sustained for 3 minutes).

✔ **Measure the variation in heart rate** when the patient breathes in compared to breathing out. It may be abnormally low (under 10).

The presence of cardiac autonomic neuropathy results in a diminished survival even when there is no coronary artery disease.

Cardiomyopathy

Cardiomyopathy refers to an enlarged heart and scarring of the heart muscle in the absense of coronary artery disease. The heart does not pump enough blood with each stroke. The patient may be able to compensate by a more rapid heart rate, but if hypertension is present, a stable condition can deteriorate.

The key treatment in this condition is control of the blood pressure as well as control of the blood glucose. Studies in animals in which diabetic cardiomyopathy is induced have shown healing with control of the blood glucose.

Diabetic Blood Vessel Disease Away from the Heart

The same processes that affect the coronary arteries can affect the arteries to the brain, producing cerebrovascular disease, and the arteries to the rest of the body, producing peripheral vascular disease.

Peripheral vascular disease

Peripheral vascular disease (PVD) occurs much earlier in the person with diabetes than the nondiabetic and proceeds more rapidly. The clogging of the arteries results in loss of pulses in the feet so that after ten years of diabetes, a third of men and women no longer feel a pulse in their feet. People with PVD also have a reduction in life expectancy. When PVD occurs, it is much worse in people with diabetes who have much greater involvement of arteries, just as in the heart. Many risk factors increase the severity of PVD. The following risk factors are unavoidable:

✔ **Genetic factors,** because PVD is more common in some families and certain ethnic groups.

✔ **Age,** because the risk of PVD increases as you age.

✔ **Diabetes,** which certainly makes PVD much worse.

Smoking and diabetes

Smoking has a number of effects on people without diabetes, but the effects have been found to be even worse in people with diabetes. Among other things, smoking:

- Reduces blood flow in arteries and blocks increased flow when it is needed

- Increases pain in the legs in people with PVD and in the heart in people with coronary artery disease

- Increases atheromatous plaques, the changes in arteries in the heart and other areas like the brain and the legs that precede closing of the blood vessels

- Increases clustering of platelets, the blood elements that form a plug or clot that blocks the artery

- Increases blood pressure, which also worsens atheromatous plaques

These problems don't even take into account the effects of smoking on the lungs, the bladder, and the rest of the body.

You can address the following risk factors with some success:

- **Smoking,** which clearly promotes early amputation.
- **Hypercholesterolemia (high cholesterol),** which makes PVD worse.
- **High glucose,** which you can control.
- **Hypertension,** which you can control with pills if necessary.
- **Obesity,** which you can control.

Besides controlling the preceding factors as much as possible, some drugs help prevent closure of the artery and loss of blood supply. Aspirin, which inhibits clotting, is among the most useful. Trental improves the circulation of cells in the blood. In addition, exercise improves blood flow and promotes the development of blood vessels around an obstruction.

Cerebrovascular disease

Cerebrovascular disease (CVD) is disease of the arteries that supply the brain with oxygen and nutrients. What I say about peripheral vascular disease in the preceding section also covers cerebrovascular disease with some exceptions. The risk factors and the approach to treatment are similar. However, the symptoms are very different because the clogged arteries in CVD supply the brain. If a temporary reduction in blood supply to the brain occurs, the person suffers from a *transient ischemic attack,* or TIA. This temporary loss of brain function may present itself as slurring of speech, weakness on one side of the body, or numbness. TIA may disappear after a few minutes, but it comes back again some hours to days later. If a major artery to the brain completely closes, the person suffers a stroke. Fortunately, stroke victims who are seen soon enough after the stroke can take advantage of clot-dissolving materials.

People with diabetes are at increased risk for CVD just as they are for PVD. Their disease tends to be worse than the nondiabetic, and they can have blockage in many small blood vessels in the brain with loss of intellectual function, which is similar to Alzheimer's disease.

The treatable risk factors for CVD are the same as those for PVD (see the preceding section). You should make attempts to improve them.

Diabetic Foot Disease

If I ever have an opportunity to save people from the consequences of diabetes, it's in this section of the book. About 70,000 amputations occur in the United States each year, and more than half of them are done on people with diabetes. Despite the wonderful surgery to bring more blood into the feet, the number of amputations is actually rising. Ironically enough, good medical care can prevent amputations.

Your doctor should look at your feet as routinely as he or she measures your weight.

In the section on neuropathy, earlier in this chapter, I point out that a filament that requires a pressure of 10 grams to be felt can differentiate the patient who will not suffer damage to the feet under normal walking conditions from the patient who will. All doctors who have diabetic patients should have this filament to test the feet at least annually. Even better, you, the patient, should have your own filament and test yourself any time you feel like it. If you can't feel the filament, you had better start looking at your feet every day. See Chapter 7 for where to obtain a filament.

If your feet are dry, you may have loss of sweating. Loss of sweating is usually accompanied by loss of touch sensation and development of ulcers. You need to moisturize your feet, first by soaking them in water, which you test with your hand for its temperature, and then by drying them with a towel and applying a moisturizer.

Ulcers of the foot can develop in a number of ways:

- Constant pressure
- Sudden higher pressure
- Constantly repeated moderate pressure

It takes very little pressure constantly applied to damage the skin. If you have diminished sensation, some of the following ideas may save your feet:

- Change your shoes about every five hours.
- If you have new shoes, you can change them every two hours at first. Your shoes should not be too tight or too loose.
- Never walk barefoot.
- Shake out your shoes before you put them on.
- Inspect your feet daily.
- Do not use a heating pad on your feet.
- Stop smoking. This is like asking for an amputation.

If you do develop an ulcer, the treatment is to take pressure off the site by resting the foot and elevating it. Once the infection is localized in a foot with adequate blood supply, a plaster cast is applied to overcome the natural tendency of everyone to stand or do some other walking. The cast protects the ulcer from the slight trauma necessary to prevent healing.

There is a product that has been shown to speed the healing of deep diabetic foot ulcers when it is combined with good wound care, which means careful removal of dead tissue and keeping your weight off the ulcer, along with treating any infection and controlling the blood glucose. The product, called Regranex Gel, is distributed by Ortho-McNeil and is applied to a clean wound bed once daily. There should be significant reduction in the size of the ulcer within ten weeks and complete healing by 20 weeks. The long duration for healing is the problem because Regranex Gel is very expensive. However, a typical deep diabetic ulcer is very expensive to treat in any case and if this speeds up healing, it may be very worthwhile.

It does not hurt to reiterate that ulcers of the foot, which lead to amputation in people with diabetes, are entirely preventable. The foot without sensation must be examined at every visit by the doctor and daily by the patient. At the first sign of a problem, appropriate action must be taken.

Skin Disease in Diabetes

Many conditions involve the skin and are unique to the person with diabetes because of the treatment and complications of the disease. The most common and important complications include the following:

- Bruises due to cutting of blood vessels by the insulin needle.
- *Vitiligo* (loss of skin pigmentation) is part of the autoimmune aspect of type 1 diabetes and cannot be prevented.

- In *necrobiosis lipoidica,* which also affects people without diabetes, you have patches of reddish-brown skin on the shins or ankles, and the skin becomes thin and can ulcerate. Females tend to have this condition more often than males. Steroid injections are used, and the areas eventually become depressed and brown.

- *Xanthelasma,* which are small yellow flat areas called plaques on the eyelids, occur even when cholesterol is not elevated.

- For unknown reasons, *alopecia,* or loss of hair, occurs in type 1 diabetes.

- *Insulin hypertrophy* is the accumulation of fatty tissue where insulin is injected. This normal action of insulin is prevented by moving the injection site around.

- *Insulin lipoatrophy* is loss of fat where the insulin is injected. Although the cause is unknown, the condition is rarely seen now that human insulin has replaced beef and pork insulin.

- Dry skin, which is a consequence of diabetic neuropathy, leading to a lack of sweating.

- Fungal infections occur under the nails or between the toes. Fungus likes moisture and elevated glucose. Lowering the glucose and keeping the toes dry prevents these infections. Medications may cure this problem, but it recurs if glucose and moisture are not managed.

- *Acanthosis nigricans,* a velvety-feeling increase in pigmentation on the back of the neck and the armpits, causes no problems and needs no treatment. It is usually found when hyperinsulinemia and insulin resistance exist. It is seen in children with type 2 diabetes.

- Diabetic thick skin, which is thicker than normal skin, occurs in diabetics of more than ten years.

Gum Disease in Diabetes

The major problem that people with diabetes may have in their teeth is gum disease. This develops because the higher concentration of glucose in the mouth promotes the growth of germs, which mix with food and saliva to form plaques on your gums. If you do not brush your teeth twice a day and floss your teeth once a day, the plaque may harden into tarter, which is very hard for you to remove. The gums may become brittle and bleed easily, and then you have gingivitis. Eventually the gums may become so weakened that they cannot support your teeth, not to mention the pain and bad breath that precedes that situation.

Controlling the blood glucose is a key step in prevention of gum disease. Visits to your dentist for routine cleaning of your teeth twice a year is another important way to keep your gums healthy. Interestingly, people with diabetes do not seem to develop cavities more often than people who do not have the disease.

Chapter 6

Diabetes, Sexual Function, and Pregnancy

• •

In This Chapter

▶ Treating impotency

▶ Dealing with female sexual problems

▶ Coping with diabetes in pregnancy

• •

*N*othing is quite so pleasant as walking into the hospital room of a mother with diabetes holding her healthy newborn. Perhaps even slightly more pleasant is the knowledge that you have contributed in some way to this outcome. Pregnancy associated with diabetes used to be a disaster for the baby and the mother. No longer. With the proper precautions, the diabetic pregnancy can proceed like a pregnancy without diabetes. This chapter describes everything you need to know to enjoy a healthy pregnancy and deliver a healthy baby.

And, of course, sexual intercourse remains the starting point for most babies. People with diabetes — both male and female — have some problems with this part of the experience of having a baby. I also cover this subject in this chapter.

When the Male Can't Get an Erection

If carefully questioned, up to 50 percent of all males with diabetes will admit to difficulty with sexual function. This difficulty usually takes the form of *erectile dysfunction,* the inability to have or sustain an erection sufficient for intercourse. Many reasons besides diabetes cause this problem, and you should rule them out before blaming diabetes. Some other possibilities include the following:

✔ Trauma to the penis

✔ Medications such as certain antihypertensives and antidepressants

✔ Hormonal abnormalities such as insufficient production of the male hormone testosterone or overproduction of a hormone from the brain, called *prolactin*

✔ Poor blood supply to the penis due to blockage of the artery by peripheral vascular disease (see Chapter 5), which can be treated very effectively by microvascular surgery

✔ *Psychogenic impotence,* an inability to have an erection for psychological rather than physical reasons (see the sidebar "Psychogenic versus physical impotence")

After you eliminate all the possibilities for erectile dysfunction, then diabetes is considered to be the source of the problem. In order to understand how diabetes affects an erection, a brief understanding of the normal production of an erection is necessary.

The erection process

As a result of some form of stimulation, whether by touch, sight, sound, or something else, the brain activates nerves in the parasympathetic nervous system, part of the autonomic nervous system. These nerves cause muscles to relax so that blood flow into the penis greatly increases. As blood flow increases, the veins through which blood leaves the penis compress, and the penis becomes erect. When the penis is erect, it contains about 11 times as much blood as when it's flaccid. With sufficient stimulation, muscles contract, propelling semen through the *urethra*, the tube in the penis that normally carries urine from the bladder, to the outside of the body. The pleasant sensation that occurs along with the muscle contractions (*ejaculation*) is called orgasm.

Orgasm and ejaculation are the result of stimulation by the other side of the autonomic nervous system, the sympathetic nervous system. As the stimulation causes contraction of the muscles, it closes the muscle over the bladder so that urine does not normally accompany expulsion of semen and the semen does not go back into the bladder.

Diabetes can damage the parasympathetic nervous system so that the male cannot get an erection sufficient for sexual intercourse. The sympathetic nervous system is spared, so that ejaculation and orgasm can occur. Of course, intercourse may be unpleasant for the partners because you have a psychological consequence to the inability of the male to provide a firm erection.

The onset of failure of erection is determined by the following factors:

Psychogenic versus physical impotence

Anxiety, stress, depression, and conflict with your significant other can all cause psychogenic impotence. This type of impotence differs from organic (physical) impotence in a number of ways. Psychogenic impotence is often specific to a particular sexual partner and comes on very suddenly. Erections occur during sleep and in the morning, but not when sexual intercourse with that partner is attempted.

Differentiating physical from psychological impotence may require a few nights in a sleep lab, where a device that detects erections during sleep is placed around the penis. Men without physical impotence normally have three or more erections during sleep, while their eyes are going through a state of rapid eye movement

(REM). (Who knows what they are looking at?) Doctors can measure both the erections and REM. If erections occur at various times of day or night, the impotence is psychological and not physical.

(Some doctors have even suggested using postage stamps around the penis at night. If the stamps break, then an erection has occurred. However, this method is associated with problems such as the stickiness of the stamps and the tendency of a male to try to remove a foreign body on the penis.)

Psychological impotence is very responsive to therapy, especially if done together with the female partner with whom the problem occurs.

- **Degree of control of the blood glucose:** Better control is associated with fewer problems.
- **Duration of the diabetes:** The longer you have diabetes, the more likely you will be unable to have an erection.
- **Interaction with the partner:** A positive relationship is important.
- **Use of drugs or alcohol:** Both may prevent erection.
- **State of mind:** A positive frame of mind is associated with more successful erections.

Treatment

Fortunately for the diabetic male with erectile dysfunction, numerous approaches to treatment exist, beginning with drugs, continuing with external devices to create an erection, and ending with implantable devices that provide a very satisfactory erection. Treatment is successful in 90 percent or more of men, but only 5 percent ever discuss the problem with their doctor. Following are treatment options:

✔ **Viagra:** This pill, also called sildenafil, has been specifically studied in diabetic males and is successful in 70 percent of the patients compared to 10 percent of the men who received a pill that contained no active ingredient. (For information on how Viagra works, see the sidebar "How Viagra works.")

However, Viagra is not free of side effects. Some men experience headaches, facial flushing, or indigestion, which generally decline with continued use of the drug. Viagra does not seem to affect diabetic control. It has also been found to cause a temporary color tinge to a man's vision as well as increased sensitivity to light and blurred vision. These side effects do decline with continued use of Viagra.

One important group of men must not take Viagra. Men who have chest pain often take nitrate drugs, the most common of which is nitroglycerine. The combination of Viagra and nitrates may cause a significant and possibly fatal drop in blood pressure.

✔ **Injection into the penis:** The patient himself can use two different kinds of injections to create an erection. The first one, a mixture of drugs called papaverine and phentolamine, has now been replaced for the most part by alprostadil (Caverject or Edex), which is another chemical that relaxes the blood vessels in the penis to allow more flow. The drug is injected about 30 minutes before intercourse and no more than once in 24 hours and three times per week. An injection of either preparation gives a full erection lasting about an hour in 85 to 95 percent of men, except for those who have the most severe loss of blood flow to the penis. Complications of injections are rare but include bruising, pain, and the formation of nodules at the injection site. A very rare complication is *priapism,* where the penis maintains its erection for many hours. If the erection lasts more than four hours, the patient must see his doctor to get an injection of a *vasoconstrictor,* a drug that squeezes down the arteries into the penis so that blood flow is interrupted. Alprostadil does not require sexual stimulation in order to work.

How Viagra works

Certain muscles need to relax for blood to flow into the penis (see the section "The erection process," earlier in this chapter). A certain chemical in the penis permits this to happen. Another chemical breaks down the first one so that the erection ends. Viagra blocks the action of this second chemical so that the erection can continue. Therefore, Viagra depends on some stimulation to get the first chemical flowing and will not work in the absence of stimulation.

Viagra is taken once a day about one hour before sexual intercourse. The dose is usually 50 mg but may be increased to 100 mg if necessary. Viagra is recommended for use no more than once a day. It may accumulate in the body if liver or severe kidney disease exists or certain drugs, especially erythromycin, are used. In those cases, the starting dose is 25 mg.

✔ **Suppository in the penis:** Alprostadil (see the preceding bullet) also comes in a suppository form. The patient inserts a tube containing this small pill into the opening of the penis after urination. Once the tube is fully in the opening, the top is squeezed so that the pill exits from the tube. This preparation, called MUSE, comes in several different strengths so that patients can use a higher dose if the lower dose does not result in a satisfactory erection. It may safely be used twice in 24 hours. It is also associated with some pain in a few men. Again, sexual stimulation is unnecessary.

✔ **Vacuum constriction devices:** These tubes, which fit over the penis, create a closed space when pressed against the patient's body. A pump draws out the air in the tube, and blood rushes into the penis to replace the air. Once the penis is erect, a rubber band is placed around the base of the penis to keep the blood inside it. Sometimes pain and numbness of the penis occur. Because a rubber band is constricting the penis, semen does not get through, so conception does not take place. The rubber band may be kept on for up to 30 minutes.

✔ **Implanted penile prostheses:** If the patient doesn't like the idea of injecting himself in his penis or using a vacuum device and Viagra does not work, a *prosthesis* (an artificial substitute) can be implanted in the penis to give a very satisfactory erection. These come in several varieties. A semi-rigid type produces a permanent erection, but some men do not like the inconvenience of a permanent erection. An inflatable prosthesis involves a pump in the scrotal sac that contains fluid. The pump can be squeezed to transfer the fluid into balloons in the penis to stiffen it. When not pumped up, the penis appears normally soft. In the past few years, the surgery to insert these prostheses has become very satisfactory.

Female Sexual Problems

Because the female does not have a penis that must enlarge during sex, this complication of diabetes is not as visually obvious. However, the problem can be just as difficult for the woman. Several of these problems are also seen in menopause, particularly the dry vagina and irregular menstrual function so that must be ruled out. The following problems are associated with diabetes:

✔ You may have a dry mouth and dry vagina because of the high blood glucose.

✔ Your menstrual function may be irregular when your diabetes is out of control.

✔ You may develop yeast infections of the vagina that make intercourse unpleasant.

- ✔ Because type 2 diabetes is usually associated with obesity, you may feel fat and unattractive.

- ✔ You may feel uncomfortable discussing the problem with your partner or your physician.

- ✔ You may have loss of bladder control due to a neurogenic bladder (see Chapter 5).

- ✔ Your increasing age may predispose to a reduction in estrogen secretion and the vaginal thinning and dryness associated with that.

The female with long-standing diabetes may have several other problems that are specific to her sexual organs. These problems include

- ✔ **Reduced lubrication because of parasympathetic nerve involvement:** Lubrication serves to permit easier entry of the penis, but it also increases the sensitivity of the vagina to touch, thus increasing pleasant sensations.

- ✔ **Reduced blood flow because of diabetic blood vessel disease:** Some of the lubrication comes from fluid within the blood vessels.

- ✔ **Loss of skin sensation around the vaginal area:** This reduces pleasure.

Most women who have problems with lubrication medicate themselves with over-the-counter preparations. These preparations fall into three categories:

- ✔ Water-based lubricants, like K-Y jelly and In Pursuit of Passion

- ✔ Oil-based lubricants, like vegetable oils

- ✔ Petroleum-based lubricants, but these are not recommended for the woman because of the possibility of bacterial infection

Their use is a matter of choice, although water-based products are probably the easiest to use and clean up.

Estrogen, which can be taken by mouth or placed in the dry vagina in suppository form, also may be useful for the menopausal woman.

When psychological or interpersonal issues exist, a discussion with a therapist, the use of antidepressant medications (some of which can dry the vagina, by the way), and sex therapy with your partner are important steps to take to improve sexual pleasure.

As with all of the diabetic problems you read about in this book, maximum control of the blood glucose prevents or slows down a lot of these complications.

Pregnancy and Diabetes

Pregnancy in a diabetic mother is definitely more complicated than in a non-diabetic mother. For this reason, centers around the country employ the latest techniques and equipment, and knowledgeable health care workers are available.

If you have diabetes and want to become pregnant, you need to confer with an expert in pregnancy and diabetes before you conceive.

About 0.4 percent of pregnancies occur in women with preexisting diabetes, called *pregestational diabetes,* and an additional 2 to 4 percent occur in women who develop diabetes some time in the second half of the pregnancy, called *gestational diabetes.* Three million births occur in the United States annually, and diabetes affects about 100,000 or more births each year.

Preventing pregnancy problems when you have pregestational diabetes

In a nondiabetic pregnancy, the body makes enough insulin to overcome the effect of pregnancy hormones (which block insulin action), and the blood glucose stays normal. A woman with type 1 diabetes can't make more insulin and needs two or three times the usual dose. The increasing need for insulin usually stabilizes in the last several weeks of the pregnancy and by the last one or two weeks, you may begin to have hypoglycemia. Once the baby is delivered with the placenta, your insulin needs plummet immediately.

The woman with type 1 diabetes may have some retinopathy (see Chapter 5) before she is pregnant. If it is severe, the eyes may deteriorate during the pregnancy. This is probably the result of rapid improvement of the blood glucose in a woman who has been poorly controlled previously. Once the pregnancy is completed, the eyes will return to their previous state.

Eye disease must be stabilized before pregnancy is attempted.

Nephropathy (see Chapter 5) increases the risk of pregnancy for both the mother and baby. Severe, permanent worsening of the nephropathy is unusual, but a temporary decline in kidney function may occur.

You must take action in advance to avoid the problems of pregnancy by controlling your glucose before conception. (See Part III for more on how to manage your diabetes.) In addition, you need to monitor your diet after you become pregnant. (See the section on "Treating diabetes in pregnancy," later in this chapter, for more information.)

The woman with type 2 diabetes can certainly become pregnant. The precaution about good control at conception holds as well. If you are on oral agents to lower glucose, you need to stop them and use insulin to control the glucose. In addition, obesity, a frequent finding in type 2 diabetes, puts the patient at greater risk for hypertension during the pregnancy. Evaluation of the type 2 patient is similar to the type 1. Most of these pregnancies can be allowed to go to term at 39 weeks, but if hypertension or a previous history of delivery that was not normal is present, earlier delivery is usually done.

Diagnosing diabetes

Experts disagree as to whether all pregnant women who don't already have diabetes need to be checked for it. Some advocate selective screening, suggesting that a thin pregnant woman with no family history of diabetes who is physically active is an unlikely candidate for diabetes. However, the current consensus is to screen all women because a small but significant number of patients with gestational diabetes will be missed if all women are not screened. Everyone agrees that if the glucose tolerance is normal in weeks 27 to 31 of the pregnancy, you don't need to do more screening. (If gestational diabetes was present in a previous pregnancy, the screening test is done as early as the 13th week.)

The screening test is done between weeks 24 and 28 of the pregnancy. No preparation is necessary. You eat 50 grams of glucose, and a blood glucose level is obtained from a vein at one hour. If the glucose level is less than 140, it is considered normal. If it's greater than 140, a further test is done to make a diagnosis of gestational diabetes because many women who have a value greater than 140 will not necessarily have diabetes. The definitive test is done as follows:

✔ The woman prepares by eating at least 150 grams of carbohydrate daily for three days and fasting for at least eight hours before the test.

✔ The woman eats 100 grams of glucose.

✔ Blood glucose is measured before the glucose meal and at one hour, two hours, and three hours.

✔ A diagnosis of gestational diabetes is made if two or more of the samples exceed the levels in Table 6-1.

Table 6-1 Excessive Glucose Levels That Signal Gestational Diabetes			
Before	*1 Hour*	*2 Hours*	*3 Hours*
105 mg/dl	165mg/dl	190 mg/dl	145 mg/dl

Coping with diabetes and pregnancy

If a woman is found to have gestational diabetes or already has pregestational diabetes, a whole new group of considerations arises in order to deliver a healthy baby while maintaining the health of the mother.

A high blood glucose left untreated has major consequences for mother and fetus. If present early in the pregnancy, the result may be *congenital malformations* (physical abnormalities that may be life threatening) in the fetus. In the third trimester, the growing fetus may exhibit *macrosomia* (abnormal largeness) that can lead to a too early delivery or damage to the baby or mother during delivery of the very large baby.

Newborns where only the father has diabetes develop normally. The environment in which the fetus is developing is responsible for the potential abnormalities. Elevated blood glucose, along with abnormalities of proteins and fats that result from the elevated glucose, and the loss of sensitivity to insulin explain the problems.

Early pregnancy problems

The major concern of the pregestational woman with diabetes is to be under good blood glucose control at the time of conception.

Measuring the risks

The hemoglobin A1c is an excellent measurement of overall glucose control and provides a good indicator for the risk of miscarriage. If it is high, it indicates that the diabetic woman was in poor control at conception, and the likelihood of a miscarriage is greater. If overall glucose control is normal, the baby of the woman with diabetes is no more likely to be miscarried than that of a nondiabetic.

The situation for congenital malformations is a little more complicated. They increase with increasing glucose as well, but also with the level of ketones, the breakdown product of fats, but measuring the ketones will not tell you if malformations will definitely occur.

Why macrosomia occurs

Macrosomia, or abnormal largeness, has to do with the elevated glucose, fat, and amino acid levels in the mother in the second half of pregnancy. If these levels aren't lowered, the fetus is exposed to high levels. This stimulates the fetal pancreas to begin to make insulin earlier and to store these extra nutrients. The fetus becomes large wherever fat is stored, such as the shoulders, chest, abdomen, and arms and legs. Because they are large, these macrosomic babies are delivered early in order to make the delivery easier and avoid birth trauma. However, though they are large, they are not fully mature.

Both miscarriages and congenital malformations are a result of poor glucose control at conception and shortly thereafter. The diabetic woman who wants to become pregnant must be in good control before she attempts to become pregnant. It is not only high blood glucose but low blood glucose as well that can induce malformations. (For more on managing diabetes, see Part III.)

However, a woman in poor control of her diabetes has more trouble conceiving a baby than a well-controlled one, which may be the major reason that more babies aren't born with congenital malformations.

The woman who has gestational diabetes mellitus does not have to worry that her baby will have congenital malformations more frequently than babies whose mothers do not have diabetes will. This is because her blood glucose did not start to rise until halfway through the pregnancy, long after the baby's important body structures were formed.

Late pregnancy problems

Both the pregestational and gestational woman with diabetes need to be concerned about a large baby. This largeness is not proportional. The areas that are most responsive to insulin, where fat is stored in the baby, are the ones that enlarge the most.

A baby is considered large if it weighs more than 4 kilograms or 8.8 pounds at birth. Most large babies are the offspring of nondiabetic mothers. Their growth is proportional throughout the pregnancy so that their shoulders are not out of proportion to their heads, and delivery is not complicated.

Treating diabetes in pregnancy

In addition to controlling your glucose levels before conceiving, the pregestational woman with diabetes needs to do the following:

    ✔ Discontinue prescription drugs that harm a fetus.

    ✔ Have your eyes and kidneys evaluated to establish a baseline for future
      damage control.

    ✔ Stop tobacco and alcohol use.

If you are a pregestational woman with diabetes, you need to achieve a
stricter level of control during pregnancy than when you aren't pregnant.
Your fetus is removing glucose from you at a rapid rate, so your blood glucose level is lower than usual. In addition, your body turns to fat for fuel
much sooner, so you produce ketones earlier. Too many ketones can damage
the fetus as well. The fact that you break down fat so early is termed *accelerated starvation*.

In order to maintain your blood glucose at the proper level, you must measure it more frequently. You should measure it before meals, at bedtime, and
occasionally one hour after eating. Your goal is to achieve the levels of blood
glucose listed in Table 6-2.

Table 6-2	Optimum Levels of Blood Glucose	
Fasting and Premeal	*1 Hour After*	*2 Hours After*
65-85	Less than 140-150	Less than 120-130

Studies have shown recently that the one hour after meal glucose may be the
most important for the pregnant woman with diabetes to keep under control.
Although you can deliver insulin in other ways besides a syringe and needle
(see Chapter 10), several studies indicate that the syringe-and-needle method
is as effective as any other is for the pregnant woman with diabetes.

You also need to check for ketones in the urine before breakfast and before
supper. You can do so by placing a test strip in the stream of urine. The strip
indicates whether ketones are present. If the test strip is positive, it means
that you are not eating enough carbohydrates, and your body is going into
accelerated starvation. Too much of this condition is not good for the growing fetus.

Your appropriate amount of weight gain depends upon your weight at the
time you become pregnant. Your BMI determines your weight gain. You
need to determine your BMI (see Chapter 3 if you're not sure how to do this
calculation). If your BMI is normal, you should gain 25 to 35 pounds during
the pregnancy. However, if you are overweight, then you need to gain less
weight through the pregnancy. If you're obese, you should gain no more than
17 or 18 pounds.

Chapter 8 tells you what you need to know about diet and diabetes, but you, as a pregnant woman with diabetes, have some special requirements:

✔ **Your daily food intake should be 35 to 38 kilocalories (rather than calories, which is an incorrect term) per kilogram of ideal body weight (IBW).** You can use your height to determine your ideal body weight. As a woman, you should weigh 100 pounds if you are 5 feet tall, plus 5 pounds for every inch over 5 feet. For example, a 5-foot, 4-inch woman should weigh 120 pounds, ideally (and approximately because this is really a range, not a single weight). You then change that figure to kilograms by dividing the pounds by 2.2. Then multiply that number by 35 to get the low end of the daily calorie intake and by 38 to get the high end. So if you weigh 120 pounds, you weigh 54.6 kilograms. Your daily food intake should then be between 1,900 and 2,100 kilocalories.

✔ **Your protein intake should be 1.5 to 2 grams per kilogram of IBW.** The woman with the IBW of 54.6 should eat about 110 grams of protein daily. Because each gram of protein contains four kilocalories, protein takes up about 440 of the 2,100 daily kilocalories.

✔ **Your carbohydrate intake should be 50 to 55 percent of the approximately 2,000 daily kilocalories, so about 1,000 kilocalories are carbohydrate.** Because each gram of carbohydrate has 4 kilocalories, just like protein, this amounts to 250 grams of carbohydrate.

✔ **Your fat intake should be less than 30 percent of the total daily 2,000 kilocalories, which amounts to 630 kilocalories of fat.** Because fat contains 9 kilocalories per gram, this equals 70 grams of fat a day.

Translating grams of food into amounts of specific foods would require another whole book. Because an excellent one on the subject has already been written, I refer you to *Nutrition For Dummies* by Carol Ann Rinzler (Hungry Minds, Inc.) to get this information.

✔ **Eat three meals a day plus a bedtime snack.** This helps prevent the accelerated starvation that results from the prolonged fast between supper and breakfast.

✔ **Maintain the fasting and premeal glucose between 65 to 85.** Your glucose should be less than 140 one hour after meals.

In addition, you can use a good multivitamin and mineral preparation. A moderate amount of exercise is also very helpful in controlling the blood glucose and keeping the mother in top shape during the pregnancy.

A blood test called a serum alpha-fetoprotein can be done at 15 weeks of the pregnancy to determine whether neural tube defects exist in the fetus. At 18 weeks, an ultrasound can show any malformations of the growing fetus. An ultrasound, by directing a sound at the fetus and catching it as it bounces back to the machine, produces a picture of the fetus that shows the presence of any abnormalities. This harmless test is not painful for the mother or the fetus.

If you have gestational diabetes, you need not worry about congenital malformations in your baby but need to avoid macrosomia. You need to follow the same dietary prescription as the pregestational woman with diabetes, and you need to use insulin if your fasting blood glucose is greater than 130 mg/dl. You cannot use oral antidiabetic agents because these may damage the growing fetus. Your insulin regimen will probably be simpler than that of the pregestational woman with diabetes because your pancreas can make its own insulin. If you are taking insulin, you will stop it at the time of delivery.

Early ultrasound is not necessary for the woman with gestational diabetes unless your doctor suspects that the diabetes was actually there much earlier. An ultrasound at week 38 can show whether fetal macrosomia exists. If macrosomia is present, then your doctor will probably perform a cesarean section, where the baby is removed through an incision made in the abdominal wall and then the uterus.

It's best to deliver the baby at the end of 39 weeks when it has had a chance to mature completely. If the mother does not go into labor spontaneously, then the physician usually induces labor.

If you have been taking insulin, nurses will monitor your blood glucose every four hours after you deliver. You blood glucose is maintained at 70 to 120 mg/dl with insulin, if necessary. The insulin is given in short-acting form as needed and not in large doses of long-acting insulin, which would be around in the circulation when you no longer need it.

After the pregnancy

If you are breastfeeding, which is always a good idea, you need about 300 extra kilocalories above your usual needs. You cannot take oral agents for diabetes because these pass through the milk into the baby.

The diabetes in the gestational woman with diabetes usually disappears with the end of the pregnancy. However, a woman who develops gestational diabetes during pregnancy is at a much higher risk for later development of diabetes. If your fasting blood glucose is greater than 130 during the pregnancy, the risk is as much as 75 to 90 percent.

You need to have a test for glucose tolerance between 6 and 12 weeks after the pregnancy and annually after that if diabetes is not found.

Several factors predispose the woman with gestational diabetes to develop diabetes later on. Some factors cannot be changed and include

✔ **Ethnic origin:** Certain ethnic groups, such as Hispanic American, Native American, Asian American, and African American, are at a higher risk.

✔ **Prepregnancy weight:** Those with a higher prepregnancy weight are at a higher risk.

✔ **Age:** Pregnancies later in life triple the risk of permanent diabetes.

✔ **Number of pregnancies:** The more pregnancies you have, the higher your risk.

✔ **Family history of diabetes:** If a family history is present, you are at a higher risk.

✔ **Severity of blood glucose during pregnancy:** Higher blood glucose levels mean a higher risk.

On the other hand, you can change or modify several factors:

✔ **Future weight gain:** Gain less weight in future pregnancies.

✔ **Future pregnancies:** Have fewer children.

✔ **Physical activity:** Increase your activity.

✔ **Dietary fat:** Limit the fat in your diet.

✔ **Smoking and certain drugs:** Stop smoking and using drugs.

Women who have had gestational diabetes can use oral contraceptives with low levels of estrogen and progesterone to prevent conception. These drugs, along with hormonal replacement therapy after menopause, do not increase your risk of later diabetes. Women with both type 1 and type 2 diabetes can use the same preparations.

The baby in a diabetic pregnancy

The understanding of diabetes and pregnancy has resulted in a great reduction in malformations in these babies as well as the macrosomia that leads to complications at delivery. Unfortunately, many diabetic women do not have tight control at conception, so an incidence of malformations still occurs. If an obvious malformation is present at birth, it is important to search for other malformations.

Also, keep in mind that the fetus was producing a lot of insulin to handle all the maternal glucose entering through the placenta. Suddenly, maternal glucose is cut off at delivery, but the high levels of fetal insulin continues for a while. The danger of hypoglycemia exists in the first four to six hours after delivery. The baby may be sweaty and appear nervous or even have a seizure. It is necessary to do a blood glucose test on the baby hourly until it is stable and at intervals for the first 24 hours.

Besides hypoglycemia, the baby may have several other complications right after birth:

- **Respiratory distress syndrome:** This breathing problem occurs when the baby is delivered early, but it responds to treatment. It's rare with good prenatal care.

- **Low calcium with jitteriness and possibly seizures:** Calcium needs to be given to the baby until its own body can take over. It is usually a result of prematurity.

- **Low magnesium:** This presents itself like low calcium and is also a result of prematurity.

- **Polycythemia:** This condition, where too many red blood cells exist, occurs for unknown reasons. Blood is removed from the baby. The amount is determined by how much extra blood is present.

- **Hyperbilirubinemia:** This condition is the product of too much breakdown of red blood cells. It is treated with light.

- **Lazy left colon:** Occurring for unknown reasons, this condition presents itself like an obstruction of the bowel but clears up on its own.

If the baby was exposed to high glucose and ketones during the pregnancy, it may show diminished intelligence. This is not obvious at birth but is discovered when the baby is expected to learn something.

The large baby of the poorly controlled diabetic mother usually loses its fat by age 1. Starting at ages 6 to 8, however, the child has a greater tendency to be obese. Controlling the blood glucose in the mother may prevent later obesity and even diabetes in the offspring.

Part III

Managing Diabetes: The "Thriving with Diabetes" Lifestyle Plan

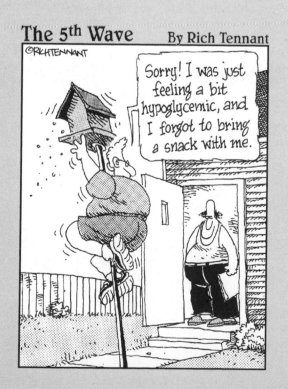

The 5th Wave   By Rich Tennant

©RICHTENNANT

Sorry! I was just feeling a bit hypoglycemic, and I forgot to bring a snack with me.

In this part . . .

Is it possible that you could be healthier with diabetes than your friends who do not have diabetes? This part shows that the answer to that question is yes. While others continue their bad habits leading to illness and perhaps premature death, you can find out exactly what you have to do not just to live with diabetes but to thrive with diabetes. The steps you need to take are simple and basic. You will probably tell yourself many times: "Why didn't I think of that?"

Another function of this part is to show you that lots of people — some of whom you may not have thought of — are out there to provide the information that you need to know.

Chapter 7

Glucose Monitoring and Other Tests

*N*ow the fun begins. If you read Part II, you have gotten through all the bad things that will never happen to you because you're going to practice all the important recommendations in this and the next five chapters. Sure, it's a bit of a bother and will cost a few dollars, but you're worth it.

Not only that, but you're among the most fortunate people with diabetes who have ever lived. Most of the products and treatments I cover in this part were not available just 20 years ago. And the new products coming along will knock your socks off (but put them back on because you should not go barefoot).

How can I get you to make use of these great advances? In the *2,000 Year Old Man* album, Carl Reiner asks Mel Brooks: "Tell me sir, what was the means of locomotion 2,000 years ago?" Brooks says: "What d'ya mean, locomotion?" Reiner asks: "What was it that got you to move quickly from one place to another?" Brooks answers: "Fear."

I did not write Part II with the intention of frightening you, but, whatever works. In this chapter, you discover all you need to know to put your diabetes in its proper place. You find out how well you're currently controlling your blood glucose, whether complications are beginning to show up, and what changes you need to make in your therapy to reverse or slow the progression of these complications.

Testing, Testing: Tests You Need to Stay Healthy

The following procedures should be done by your doctor (and you, if feasible) on at least four visits a year if you take insulin and at least two visits if you do not.

- Evaluate your blood glucose measurements each visit. (See the section "Monitoring Your Blood Glucose: It's a Must," later in this chapter.)

- Obtain hemoglobin A1c four times a year. (See the section "Tracking Your Glucose over Time with the Hemoglobin A1c," later in this chapter.)

- Check for microalbuminuria once a year. (See the section "Testing for Kidney Damage: Microalbuminuria," later in this chapter.)

- Have a dilated eye examination by an ophthalmologist once a year. (See the section "Checking for Eye Problems," later in this chapter.)

- Examine the bare feet at each visit. (See the section "Examining Your Feet," later in this chapter.)

- Obtain a lipid panel once a year. (See the section "Tracking Cholesterol and Other Fats," later in this chapter.)

- Measure blood pressure at each visit. (See the section "Measuring Blood Pressure," later in this chapter.)

- Measure weight at each visit. (See the section "Checking Your Weight," later in this chapter.)

These tests are the minimum standards for proper care of diabetes. Once an abnormality is found, the frequency of testing increases to check on the response to treatment.

How are doctors actually doing in medical care for a person with diabetes? A recent study was an eye-opener. The study looked at five of the standard tests: Patient self-testing of blood glucose, hemoglobin A1c testing, at least four visits to the doctor a year if on insulin and two if not, an annual dilated eye examination, and examination of the feet at each visit.

The results were (sadly) as follows:

- Three percent of insulin users and 1 percent of noninsulin users met all five standards.

- ✔ One of five people with diabetes does no self-testing of blood glucose.
- ✔ Three of four people with diabetes have never heard of the hemoglobin A1c.
- ✔ One of four people with diabetes does not even make an annual visit to the doctor.
- ✔ Two of five have never had their feet examined or had a dilated eye examination.

Another study published in the journal *Ophthalmalogy* in March 2001 looked specifically at annual dilated eye examinations. Of 2,308 people interviewed, 813 (35 percent) did not follow the vision care guidelines of a dilated eye exam in the last year.

In the journal *Stroke* in February 2000, an article stated that although patients' blood pressure commonly exceeded the recommended guidelines after a stroke, blood pressure was especially high among patients with diabetes

There is much to be done. And that's what this chapter is all about.

Monitoring Your Blood Glucose: It's a Must

Insulin was extracted and used for the first time over 75 years ago. Since then, nothing has improved the life of the person with diabetes as much as the ability to measure your own blood glucose with a drop of blood. Prior to blood glucose self-monitoring, testing the urine for glucose was the only way to determine whether your blood glucose was high, but urine testing could not tell at all whether the glucose was low. The urine test for glucose is worthless for controlling blood glucose, actually providing misinformation. All the thousands of research papers in the medical literature before 1980, which used urine testing for glucose, are of no value and should be burned. Testing the urine for other things such as ketones and protein can be of value.

Basically two kinds of test strips are in use today. Both require that glucose in a drop of your blood reacts with an enzyme. In one strip, the reaction produces a color. A meter then reads the amount of color to give a glucose reading. In the other strip, the reaction produces electrons, and a meter then converts the amount of electrons into a glucose reading.

One of the first things that was learned when frequent testing of blood glucose became feasible is that in a person with diabetes, even a fairly stable one, tremendous variation in the glucose occurs in a relatively short time, especially in association with food, but even in the fasting state before breakfast. This is why multiple tests are needed.

How often should you test?

How often you test is determined by the kind of diabetes you have, the kind of treatment you're using, and the level of stability of your blood glucose.

- ✔ **If you have type 1 diabetes or type 2 diabetes and you're taking insulin, you need to test before each meal and at bedtime.** The reason is that you're constantly using this information to make adjustments in your insulin dose. No matter how good you think your control, you cannot feel the level of the blood glucose without testing unless you're hypoglycemic. I have had my patients try this out on numerous occasions. I ask them to guess their blood glucose and then test it. They are close less than 50 percent of the time. That degree of accuracy is not sufficient for good glucose control. Occasionally, people with type 1 diabetes should test one hour after a meal and in the middle of the night to see just how high the glucose goes after eating and whether it's going too low in the middle of the night. These results guide you and your physician to make the changes you need.

- ✔ **If you have type 2 diabetes and you're on pills or just diet and exercise, then testing twice a day before breakfast and dinner gives you the information needed to measure the effect of the treatment.** I'm assuming that you're fairly stable as shown by mostly good blood glucose tests (in the area of 80 to 120 mg/dl) and by the hemoglobin A1c (see the section later in this chapter). I even have some of my most stable patients testing once a day, alternating a prebreakfast test with a presupper test on consecutive days. Any less testing than that is not enough to keep you aware of the state of your control.

- ✔ **If you're pregnant, see the testing guidelines I outline in Chapter 6.** I would guess that you're probably willing to test numerous times in a day to keep your developing fetus as healthy as possible.

The blood glucose test can be useful many other times of day. If you eat something off your diet and want to test its effect on your glucose, do a test. If you're about to exercise, a blood glucose test can tell you whether you need to eat before starting the exercise or can use the exercise to bring your glucose down. If your diabetes is temporarily unstable and you're about to drive, you may want to test before getting into the car to make sure that you're not on the verge of hypoglycemia.

A key point is that you're not being graded on your glucose test results. The human body has too much variation in it to expect that each time you take the same medication, do the same exercise, eat the same way, and feel the same emotionally, you will necessarily get the same test result. If the person who reviews your results with you sees your abnormal results as bad, he or she does not understand this point. You may want to consider finding someone who does.

Another key point is that the occasional blood glucose done in your doctor's office is of little or no value in understanding the big picture of your glucose control. It is exactly like trying to visualize an entire painting by Seurat, who painted with dots, by looking at one dot on the canvas.

Using a lancet

To get the drop of blood, you have to use a spring-loaded device that contains a sharp lancet. You push the button of the device and the lancet springs out and pokes your finger.

One lancet device that seems less painful than the others is the Softclix Lancet Device. It allows you to select one of ten depth settings so that you can penetrate your finger no deeper than necessary. It uses its own type of lancet that is a little more expensive. Becton Dickinson makes another lancet, called BDGenie Lancet, that works like a lancet and lancing device all in one. It is less painful and a little less expensive.

When you go to your doctor's office, the doctor often uses a lancet to stick your finger for blood. A new device, called the Lasette, is now available for personal use (with a doctor's prescription), for doctor's offices, and for laboratories (see the figure in this sidebar). It penetrates the finger painlessly and without the use of sharp items. It's available from Cell Robotics, Inc., in Albuquerque, New Mexico (800-846-0590). Until someone makes a laser lancet that is affordable to patients, though, you still have to use the needle lancet. Although you do not have to use alcohol on your fingers, they should be reasonably clean. (After millions of finger sticks, I know of no problems with infections of the fingers.) Use the side of your finger to avoid the more sensitive tips that you don't want to hurt, especially if you type. Change fingers often so that no finger becomes very sensitive.

Remember never to use a used lancet on someone else. They last for a few pokes and should then be discarded in a special sharps container so that they do not poke someone else accidentally. Sharps containers are available in drugstores.

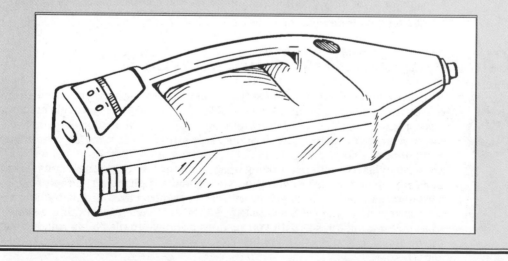

How do you perform the test?

If you don't already have a meter, be sure to check out the following section. All meters require a drop of blood, usually from the finger. You place the blood on a specific part of a test strip and allow enough time, sometimes 20 seconds to one minute, for a reaction to occur. Some strips allow you to add more blood within 30 seconds if the quantity is insufficient. In less than a minute, the meter reads the product of that reaction, which is determined by the amount of glucose in the original blood sample.

Keep the following tips in mind when you're testing your glucose:

- ✔ **If you have trouble getting blood, you can use a rubberband at the point where your finger joins your hand.** You will be amazed at the flow of blood. Take off the rubberband before a major hemorrhage (just joking).

- ✔ **Keep in mind that some meters use whole blood and some use the liquid part of the blood, called the *plasma*.** A lab glucose tests the plasma. The blood value is about 12 percent less than the plasma value, so it is important to know which you're measuring. The various recommendations for appropriate levels of glucose are plasma values.

- ✔ **Studies have shown that the qualities of test strips, which are loose in a vial, deteriorate rapidly if the vial is left open.** Be sure to cap the vial. Two hours of exposure to air may ruin the strips. Strips that are individually foil-wrapped do not have this problem.

- ✔ **Do not let others use your meter.** Their test result will be mixed in with your tests when they are downloaded into a computer. In addition, a meter invariably gets a little blood on it and can be a source of infection.

Choosing a Blood Glucose Meter

So many meters are on the market that you may be confused about which one to use. One consideration that should play no part in your decision is the cost of the meter. Most manufacturers are happy to practically give you the meter so that you're forced to buy their test strips. Each manufacturer makes a different test strip, and they're not interchangeable in other machines. Some even make a different strip for each different machine that they make. Because the meters are so cheap and the science is changing so rapidly, it is a good idea to get a new meter every year or two to make sure that you have the latest state of the art. The cost of test strips is generally about the same from meter to meter, so cost of strips does not have to play a big role in your meter decision, either.

A second nonconsideration is the accuracy of the various machines. All are accurate to a degree acceptable for managing your diabetes. Keep in mind, though, that they do not have the accuracy of a laboratory. They are probably about plus or minus 10 percent compared to the lab.

Questions you should answer before buying your meter

Your doctor may have a meter that he or she prefers to work with because a computer program can download the test results from the meter and display them in a certain way. This analysis can be enormously helpful in deciding how to alter your therapy for the best control of your glucose.

Any meter you buy should have a memory that records the time and date so that you can read that information along with the glucose result. The memory should be at least 100 glucose values if you test four times a day; 100 values represents 25 days at this testing frequency, and your visits with your doctor will usually occur once a month.

Do not buy a meter without the capability to download the results to a data management system in a computer. Bring your meter with you to your monthly appointments so that your doctor, or one of his or her assistants, can download your glucose test results and evaluate them with the aid of a data management system. Evaluating pages of glucose readings in a log book is virtually impossible.

Your insurance company also may mandate a certain meter, and then you have no choice.

You should ask yourself the following questions when choosing a meter:

- ✔ If a small child is to use it, can the child easily use the meter and strips?
- ✔ Are the batteries common ones, or hard to get and expensive?
- ✔ Does the meter have a memory that you and your doctor can check?
- ✔ Is the meter downloadable to a computer program that can manipulate the data?
- ✔ Are the test strips reasonable in cost?

Profiles of the different meters

There are really four major players in the meter game and a few minor ones. Among them, they produce more than 25 machines. Like everything in business, mergers and acquisitions have and will occur so that the field will narrow. It is probably wise to stick with one of the four major companies, which I describe in the following sections, unless a minor company comes out with irresistible features. Their strips will be available anywhere and they tend to have excellent service should you have a problem with their meter.

You want to know what I use in my practice? All of my patients use the Accu-Chek Advantage meter or one of the other Roche meters that utilizes the same data management system. They bring the meter to every visit, and I download their test results.

Abbott Laboratories

Abbott Laboratories purchased the MediSense Company, which first made and sold these meters. The company has one of the longest warranties (four years) on its meters. The company is speedy about taking care of problems that arise. The batteries are permanent, unless otherwise noted, and good for 4,000 tests. When the batteries die, the company replaces the meter.

- **ExacTech:** It requires 30 seconds to do a test, is accurate, and recalls the last reading. I do not recommend this meter because it lacks the ability to download the results to a data management system on a computer.

- **ExacTechRSG:** This meter is the same as the Exactech but requires no calibration. I do not recommend it because it also lacks the ability to download the results to a data management system.

- **Precision QID:** It's very small, requires little blood, and allows the addition of blood within 30 seconds if necessary. This meter works with diabetes management software (DMS) through a data port and can hold 125 results. You cannot see the date and time for the results, but they appear when the data is downloaded.

- **Precision QID pen sensor:** This meter is basically the same as the Precision QID, but it's shaped like a pen, making it smaller and easier to carry, and it is no more expensive.

- **PrecisionXtra:** It is similar to the Precision QID but holds 450 results. It does averaging of the blood glucose levels. You can also test for ketones with this machine. You can use it in one of five languages, and you can change the batteries.

- **Optium:** This meter is the same as the PrecisionXtra, but you cannot check ketones.

- **Sof*Tact:** This meter allows you to test the blood glucose at alternate sites away from the fingers. It does averaging of the blood glucose levels and is otherwise similar to the Optium.

Bayer Corporation

Bayer Corporation sells these meters in the United States. It is a branch of Bayer Group, a German company. The meters are accurate and carry the longest warranty (five years) in the industry. You can replace the batteries at home. The meters are descendants of some of the first meters available.

- ✔ **Glucometer Elite:** This meter uses strips that require little blood and draw the blood up instead of placing the drop on top of the strip, making it easier for you to use with small children. Children, though, will probably have trouble with the foil-wrapped test strips. This meter does not have a data port for DMS, and I do not recommend it for this reason

- ✔ **Glucometer Elite XL:** This meter remembers 120 tests and does have a data port for DMS, but it's otherwise similar to the preceding meter.

- ✔ **Glucometer DEX:** This meter provides a 10-test cartridge that replaces the test strips. The cartridge calibrates the meter. It has a 100 test memory and can do averaging. The tests can be downloaded to a DMS. This meter draws the blood in by capillary action like the Elite.

Roche Group

Roche Group, which did not sell meters originally, merged with Boehringer Mannheim and now sells their meters. The batteries in their meters are replaceable at home.

- ✔ **Accu-Chek Complete:** This meter works with a DMS. It has a very large memory, storing up to 1,000 blood glucose values, and can also record other information such as insulin dosages and carbohydrate intake. It requires a tiny sample of blood and can produce on-screen graphs and statistics.

- ✔ **Accu-Chek Advantage:** It also has a DMS but stores only 100 blood glucose values. It uses a test strip that takes 40 seconds but does not require cleaning or wiping, and it draws the blood up by capillary action.

- ✔ **Accu-Chek Compact:** This new meter uses a 17-test drum with no test strip handling or calibration. The results are displayed in 15 seconds, and it has a 100 test value memory that is downloadable to a DMS.

- ✔ **Accu-Chek Active:** This meter uses a tiny sample of blood and gives a result in five seconds. It has a 200 value memory that is downloadable to a DMS.

- ✔ **Accu-Chek Voicemate:** This meter is for the visually impaired. It identifies the type of insulin used, and audibly takes the user through the glucose test and gives the reading. It also uses the Comfort Curve test strips that draw the blood in by capillary action, and is downloadable to a DMS.

Roche also makes a software program for people with diabetes called Accu-Chek Compass. It helps patients to better manage their diabetes by providing reports and summaries of the glucose tests.

LifeScan

Johnson & Johnson purchased LifeScan, which has a number of meters in competition with one another. The company is very reliable, taking care of problems within 24 hours. You can replace the batteries in LifeScan meters at home.

- **FastTake Compact Blood Glucose Monitoring System:** This meter has a data port and a DMS for its 150 blood glucose memory. It has a fast test time of 15 seconds. It can give a 14-day average of its readings.

- **SureStep Meter:** The meter has a 150 test memory with averaging and a data port for DMS. This meter is useful for the visually impaired because the blood can be smeared onto the strip.

- **One Touch Profile:** This meter has a DMS and the test takes 45 seconds. The meter remembers the last 250 blood glucose readings and can give a 14- and 30-day test average. The display can appear in English, Spanish, or 17 other languages.

- **One Touch Basic:** This meter has a 75 test memory with a data port. It does not average blood glucoses, and can be used in 17 languages.

- **One Touch Ultra:** This new system allows alternate site testing away from the fingers. It uses a tiny sample and therefore can work with Lifescan's ultrafine lancets. The result is displayed in five seconds, and the blood is drawn up by capillary action. The meter has a 150 test memory that allows averaging on the screen and connects to a data port.

How I use my patients' test results

I encourage my patients to keep their own written records so that they can see for themselves how they are doing. I have several years of records and can compare and contrast each patient. I use the software to generate pictures of their diabetic control. The figures in this sidebar show you a typical patient before starting therapy and after insulin treatment had time to work. It is easy to see how helpful the graphic information can be.

The first figure shows the patient's blood glucose levels in three different formats. The top, called the Trendgraph, shows the blood glucoses each day, in this case, between 6/11 and 7/1. The shaded area represents the blood glucoses from 80 to 180 mg/dl. The line below the shaded area is the 50 mg/dl line. Each X represents a distinct blood glucose test. You can see that the glucose is often high, going up to 300, and sometimes low, going down to 50 with large excursions. This graph also shows that the mean of the tests is 159 and that 5 percent of the time, the patient is less than 80; 63.4 percent of the time, she is between 80 and 180; and 31.7 percent of the time, she is above 180. The next level, called the Standard Day, puts all those glucose levels in a 24-hour day so that tests taken between certain hours, regardless of the day, appear close to one another. This grouping allows me to see whether the patient has a tendency to be high or low at a given time each day. The software averages out the blood glucose at different times, providing a number to compare to other time periods. This information permits me to adjust her insulin to correct for that particular time.

The bottom level, called the Pie Chart, clearly shows how much of the time she is high, how much of the time she is within the target of 80–180, and how much of the time she is below 80.

These three figures provide an excellent picture of the patient's diabetic control and permit me to easily compare it to the result of treatment.

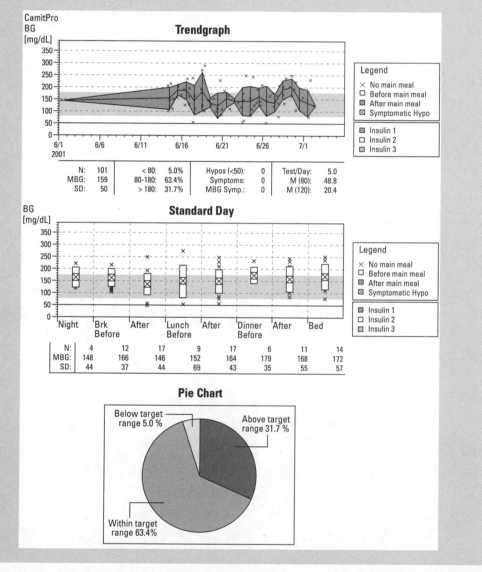

(continued)

(continued)

The second figure is after treatment with a new form of insulin, Lantus, for one week. The results are dramatic. Now almost all the glucoses are in the shaded area, and there is little excursion of the tests. A few X's fall above 180 and a few fall below 80. The Standard Day now shows fairly low averages throughout, except perhaps after lunch. The Pie Chart shows much more in the target range and far fewer above the target range. Comparing the two graphs, the above target range figure has dropped from 31.7 percent to 6.5 percent.

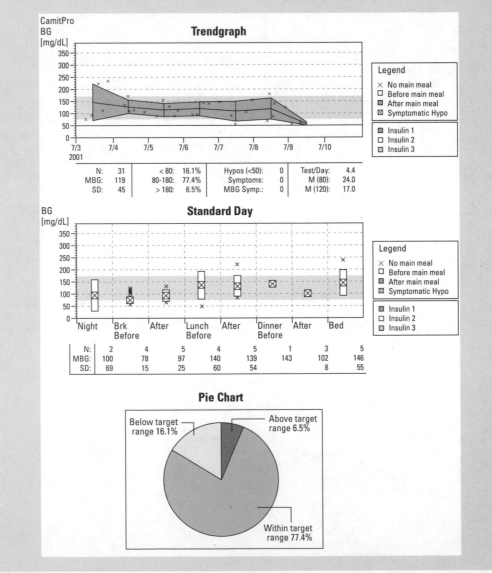

CamitPro
BG [mg/dL]

Trendgraph

Legend
- × No main meal
- ☐ Before main meal
- ▨ After main meal
- ⊠ Symptomatic Hypo

- ▨ Insulin 1
- ☐ Insulin 2
- ▨ Insulin 3

N:	31	< 80:	16.1%	Hypos (<50):	0	Test/Day:	4.4
MBG:	119	80-180:	77.4%	Symptoms:	0	M (80):	24.0
SD:	45	> 180:	6.5%	MBG Symp.:	0	M (120):	17.0

BG [mg/dL]

Standard Day

Legend
- × No main meal
- ☐ Before main meal
- ▨ After main meal
- ⊠ Symptomatic Hypo

- ▨ Insulin 1
- ☐ Insulin 2
- ▨ Insulin 3

	Night	Brk Before	After	Lunch Before	After	Dinner Before	After	Bed
N:	2	4	5	4	5	1	3	5
MBG:	100	78	97	140	139	143	102	146
SD:	69	15	25	60	54		8	55

Pie Chart

Below target range 16.1%

Above target range 6.5%

Within target range 77.4%

I can print all these graphs and charts. In later visits, I can compare the current control with the way the patient was doing before. When patients can see so clearly how they're improving from time to time, it keeps them motivated to take their medicine and follow their diet and exercise plan.

A non-invasive meter

MiniMed has a "Continuous Glucose Monitoring System." This consists of a sensor implanted under the skin of the abdomen and left in place for three days. It takes glucose readings every five minutes and stores them in the meter to which it is attached. The meter is then downloaded into a computer to provide 24-hour analysis of glucose levels. The glucose levels are not measured in blood but in the fluid found around tissues called *interstitial fluid.* This correlates very well with blood glucose levels. Such a system can be used to design a very accurate program for giving insulin. In the future, it could be hooked up to an insulin delivery device and provide instant responses to changes in blood glucose. It does not give immediate readings, but this feature is planned for the future as well. It must be calibrated by taking blood glucose measurements three times a day and entering them in the meter.

Tracking Your Glucose over Time with the Hemoglobin A1c

Individual blood glucose tests are great for deciding how you're doing at that moment and what to do to make it better, but they do not give the big picture. They are just a moment in time. Glucose can change a great deal even in an hour. What is needed is a test that gives an integrated picture of many days or weeks or even months of blood glucose levels. The test that accomplished this important task is called the *hemoglobin A1c.*

With this test, you can look back and say that you were or were not in control of the blood glucose for whatever period of time the test looks back at. This is a perfect test, for example, for the diabetic woman who wants to get pregnant. She can know whether her blood glucose has been well controlled before she tries to conceive. If it has not, then she can wait until the test shows good control and then get pregnant. In this way, she avoids the possibility of fetal malformations (see Chapter 6 for more on pregnancy and diabetes). It's also a great way to follow the effects of treatment. If treatment is working, this test should show improvement.

Unfortunately, all labs do not do the hemoglobin A1c test the same way. Some labs report both the hemoglobin A1c and the total glycohemoglobin. As a result, there are different normal levels depending on how the test was done. You need to know the normal value in the lab where you did the test. Fortunately, each lab usually has a column on its result form showing the normal values for each test. Still, it makes for a lot of confusion.

My medical building has two different labs, each reporting the results differently. As a result of insurance requirements, I have to send patients to one or the other. When I get back the result, I have to be sure I know which lab did it. The standard method should be the way it was done in the Diabetes Control and Complications Trial, the study that showed that controlling the blood glucose prevents complications in type 1 diabetes. In that study, a normal level was about 6.05 percent. Figure 7-1 shows you the correlation between the hemoglobin A1c and the blood glucose when this method is the one that is used.

Blood Glucose Control Chart

Hemoglobin A1c (%)

| 5 | 6 | 7 | 8 | 9 | 10 | 11 | 12 | 13 | 14 |

| Normal | Good | Fair | Poor |

| 90 | 120 | 150 | 180 | 210 | 240 | 270 | 300 | 330 | 360 |

Average Bood Glucose (mg/dL)

Figure 7-1: Comparison between hemoglobin A1c and blood glucose.

As you can see in the figure, a normal hemoglobin A1c of less than 6 percent corresponds to a blood glucose of less than 120, while a fair hemoglobin A1c of 7 percent reflects an average blood glucose of 150.

Large-scale studies have shown that the average hemoglobin A1c in the United States for type 2 diabetes is around 9.4 percent, which means the average blood glucose is 220. The American Diabetes Association recommends taking action to control the blood glucose if the hemoglobin A1c is 8 percent or greater with the goal being less than 7 percent.

How hemoglobin A1c works

Hemoglobin is a protein that carries oxygen around the body and drops it off wherever it's needed to help in all the chemical reactions that are constantly taking place. The hemoglobin is packaged within red blood cells that live in the bloodstream for 60 to 90 days. As the blood circulates, glucose in the blood attaches to the hemoglobin and stays attached. It attaches in several different ways to the hemoglobin and the total of all the hemoglobin attached to glucose is called *glycohemoglobin.* Glycohemoglobin normally makes up about 6 percent of the hemoglobin in the blood. The largest fraction, two-thirds of the glycohemoglobin, is in the form called hemoglobin A1c, making it easiest to measure. The rest of the hemoglobin is made up of hemoglobin A1a and A1b. The more glucose in the blood, the more glycohemoglobins form. Because glycohemoglobin remains in the blood for two to three months, it is a reflection of the glucose control over the entire time period and not just the second that a single glucose test reflects.

Your physician should be testing for hemoglobin A1c as follows:

- ✔ If you have type 1 diabetes or type 2 and you're on insulin, you should be tested four times a year.

- ✔ If you have type 2 diabetes and you're not on insulin, you should be tested two times a year.

In my own practice, I test all patients every three months. A good hemoglobin A1c is highly motivating to keep up good self-care, while a poor result gives immediate feedback as to the need for tighter control.

Currently, the National Glycohemoglobin Standardization Program, created by the American Association for Clinical Chemistry, is working to get the hemoglobin A1c test standardized so that a 6 percent result will mean the same for every patient. The program might start by doing only one test, the hemoglobin A1c, and calling it by only one name.

A company called Metrika, Inc., has come up with a clever home version of the hemoglobin A1c, called A1c Now. You do a finger stick to produce a large drop of blood. The blood is mixed with a solution that is provided, and a sample of that mixture is placed in the testing device. Eight minutes later, the hemoglobin A1c appears in the device window. The device is then discarded. The device appears to be highly accurate and may save the trouble of going to a lab for this test. Because it's so quick, your doctor can have the test results while you're at his office and can act on them immediately, instead of waiting for a lab to return the test results at a later time.

Another test similar to the hemoglobin A1c is the *fructosamine*. This test, which measures the glucose combined with protein in the blood, reflects the level of blood glucose for the past three weeks. Fructosamine is a relatively new test that has not seen a lot of use, so its place in diabetes care has not been established. The test should prove very useful for the pregnant woman with diabetes, for example, where you need to know the effect of a treatment change very rapidly. As doctors become more familiar with its use, more fructosamine tests will be ordered.

The Food and Drug Administration has approved a home-testing device called the Duet Glucose Control Monitoring System, which can measure both the blood glucose and the fructosamine. The machine costs around $300, and the test strips are $64 for eight. How useful it will be is yet to be determined.

Testing for Kidney Damage: Microalbuminuria

The finding of very small but abnormal amounts of protein in the urine, called *microalbuminuria,* is the earliest sign that high glucose may be damaging the kidneys (see Chapter 5 for more on nephropathy). When microalbuminuria is found, it is still early enough to reverse any damage.

When the diagnosis of type 2 diabetes is made and within the fifth year after the diagnosis of type 1 diabetes, your doctor must order a urine test for microalbuminuria. If the test is negative, it must be repeated annually. If it is positive, the test is done a second time to verify the result. If the test is positive again, your doctor should

- ✔ **Put you on a drug called an ACE inhibitor.** After you have been on this drug for some months, the test can be repeated to see whether it has turned negative. The ACE inhibitor can be stopped and restarted later if microalbuminuria appears again.

- ✔ **Bring your blood glucose under the tightest control possible.** This helps to reverse the damaging process as well.

- ✔ **Normalize your body fats so that your cholesterol and triglycerides (see "Tracking Cholesterol and Other Fats," later in this chapter) are made normal.** Elevated cholesterol and triglycerides have been found to damage the kidneys.

Doing this simple little test can protect your kidneys from damage. Ask your doctor about it if you think it has never been done. Show him or her this page if the doctor is unclear as to why it is performed.

Checking for Eye Problems

All people with diabetes need to have a dilated eye exam done annually by an ophthalmologist or optometrist. No other physician, including the endocrinologist (yours truly excepted, of course), can do the exam properly.

For this exam, the doctor instills drops into your eyes and uses various instruments to examine the pressure, the appearance of your lens, and, most importantly, the retina of your eye.

All kinds of things can be done if abnormalities are found, but they must be discovered first. (See Chapter 5 for more information on eye problems.)

This test is something you must demand. Your doctor must refer you to an ophthalmologist or optometrist every year. Better yet, set up the appointment yourself with the eye doctor's nurse at the end of your first visit so that you are reminded about it each year.

Examining Your Feet

Unfortunately, foot problems often end in an amputation. An amputation is really evidence of inadequate care. (For more on foot problems, see Chapter 5.) The doctor is not necessarily at fault here. The doctor sees you once in a while. You're with yourself much more often.

If you have any problem sensing touch with your feet, you need to take the following precautions:

- ✔ You must use your eyes to examine your feet every day.
- ✔ You must use your hand to test hot water before you step into it so that you do not get burned.
- ✔ You must shake out your shoes before you step into them to make sure no stone or other object is inside them.
- ✔ You must not go barefoot.
- ✔ You must keep the skin of your feet moist by soaking them in water, drying them, and applying a moistening lotion.

Your doctor can test your ability to feel an injury by using a ten gram filament, but, again, that is done only when you have an appointment. You can obtain one of these filaments for yourself. Call the National Institutes of Health at 800-438-5383 and ask for the "Feet Can Last a Lifetime" package.

If you have any suggestion of a loss of sensation, at each visit to the doctor who takes care of your diabetes, you should take off your shoes and socks and have your feet inspected by the doctor.

Tracking Cholesterol and Other Fats

Most people these days know the level of their cholesterol. What they actually know is the level of their *total* cholesterol. Cholesterol circulates in the blood in small packages called *lipoproteins*. These tiny round particles contain fat (*lipo,* as in liposuction) and protein. Because cholesterol does not dissolve in water, it would separate from the blood if it were not surrounded by the protein, just like oil separates from water in salad dressing. (That's why you have to shake the salad dressing each time you use it.)

A second kind of fat found in the lipoproteins is *triglyceride.* Triglyceride actually represents the form of most of the fat you eat each day. Although you eat only a gram or less of cholesterol (an egg yolk is one-third of a gram of cholesterol), you eat up to 100 grams of triglyceride a day. (For more on the place of fats in your diet, see Chapter 8.) The fat in animal meats is mostly triglycerides.

As you might imagine, we need to know which particle the cholesterol comes from in order to understand whether you have too much bad cholesterol (LDL) or a satisfactory level of good cholesterol (HDL).

You do not have to fast to do a test for total cholesterol and HDL cholesterol. However, you do need to fast for eight hours to find out your LDL cholesterol, because the blood has to be cleared of chylomicrons, which rise greatly when you eat.

You should have a fasting lipid panel at least once each year.

Table 7-1 lists the current recommendations for the levels of these fats in terms of the risk for coronary artery disease.

Table 7-1	Levels of Fat and the Risk for Coronary Artery Disease		
Risk	*LDL Cholesterol*	*HDL Cholesterol*	*Triglycerides*
Higher	Greater than 130	Less than 35	Greater than 400
Borderline	100 to 129	35 to 45	200 to 399
Lower	Less than 100	Greater than 45	Less than 200

Types of fat particles

✔ **Chylomicrons,** the largest particles, which contain the fat that is absorbed from the intestine after a meal. They are usually cleared from the blood rapidly. Ordinarily, chylomicrons are not a concern with respect to causing *arteriosclerosis* (hardening of the arteries).

✔ **Very Low Density Lipoprotein (VLDL) particles,** which contain mostly triglyceride as the fat. These are smaller than chylomicrons.

✔ **High Density Lipoprotein (HDL),** known as "good" cholesterol, the next smallest in size. This particle functions to clean the arteries, helping to prevent coronary artery disease, peripheral vascular disease, and strokes.

✔ **Low Density Lipoprotein (LDL),** known as "bad" cholesterol. This particle seems to be the one that carries cholesterol to the arteries where it's deposited and causes hardening of the arteries.

You can see from Table 7-1 that the risk goes up as the LDL cholesterol goes up and the HDL cholesterol goes down. A huge study of thousands of citizens of Framingham, Massachusetts, shows that you can get a good picture of the risk by dividing the total cholesterol by the HDL cholesterol. If this result is less than 4.5, the risk is lower. If it's greater than 4.5, you're at higher risk for coronary artery disease. The higher it is, the worse the risk.

With diabetes, it gets a little more complicated because of insulin resistance syndrome (see Chapter 5). In insulin resistance syndrome, the total cholesterol may not be very high, but the HDL cholesterol is low and the triglycerides are elevated. These patients also have a lot of a dangerous form of LDL cholesterol, so they are also at higher risk for coronary artery disease. This increased risk must be taken into account in considering treatment for the fats.

In deciding whether and how to treat the fats, you have to consider other risk factors. You're at:

✔ Highest risk if you already have coronary artery disease, stroke, or peripheral vascular disease.

✔ High risk if you

- Are a male over 45.

- Are a female over 55.

- Smoke cigarettes.

- Have high blood pressure.

- Have HDL cholesterol less than 35.

- Have a father or brother with a heart attack before age 55.

- Have a mother or sister with a heart attack before age 65.
- Have a body mass index greater than 30.

✔ Low risk if you have none of the preceding risk factors.

The treatment then depends on your risk category and level of LDL cholesterol (see Table 7-2).

Table 7-2	Your Treatment Based on Risk Category	
Risk	*Dietary Treatment if LDL Greater Than*	*Diet and Drug Treatment if LDL Greater Than*
Low	160	190
High	130	160
Very high	100	100

All these decisions depend on obtaining a lipid (fat) panel.

Measuring Blood Pressure

The United States is experiencing an epidemic of high blood pressure (*hypertension*) similar to the epidemic of diabetes. The reasons are the same:

✔ Americans are getting fatter.

✔ Americans are storing fat in the center of our body, the so-called *abdominal visceral fat.*

✔ Americans are getting older as a population. The fastest growing segment of the population is over 75 years of age. Of people with diabetes age 50 to 55, 50 percent have high blood pressure. Of people with diabetes older than 75, 75 percent have high blood pressure.

✔ Americans are more sedentary than before.

People with diabetes have high blood pressure more often than the nondiabetic population for a lot of other reasons besides the preceding ones:

✔ People with diabetes get kidney disease.

✔ People with diabetes have increased sensitivity to salt that raises blood pressure.

✔ People with diabetes lack the nighttime fall in blood pressure that normally occurs in people without diabetes.

The meaning of your blood pressure

What does the blood pressure measurement mean, and what is high blood pressure? When you get a reading, it usually looks something like 120/70, an upper reading and a lower reading.

✔ The upper reading, called the *systolic pressure,* is the amount of force exerted by the heart when it contracts to push blood around the body. A cuff around your arm connects to a column of mercury. You, your doctor, or a machine listens for the first sound you hear on the side of the cuff away from your heart. That is the sound of blood finally able to overcome the pressure in the cuff and get through to the other side. The systolic blood pressure is the height of the column of mercury, read in millimeters, just

as the blood comes through. Sometimes the cuff is not connected to a column of mercury but to a gauge that is calibrated so the reading on the gauge is in millimeters of mercury even though no mercury is present. In this case, the systolic blood pressure reading is 120 mm of mercury.

✔ The lower reading, called the *diastolic blood pressure,* is the pressure in the artery when the heart is at rest. A valve in the heart keeps the blood from flowing backwards so that the pressure does not fall to zero (you hope). When the sound stops, the height of the mercury column gives the diastolic blood pressure, in this case 70 mm of mercury.

It is generally agreed that a normal blood pressure is less than 140/90. For years, the diastolic blood pressure was considered more damaging, and an elevation in that pressure was treated with greater importance than an elevation in the systolic blood pressure. Recent studies have shown that it is the systolic blood pressure, not the diastolic blood pressure that may be more important.

All of the complications of diabetes are made worse by an elevation in blood pressure, especially diabetic kidney disease but also eye disease, heart disease, nerve disease, peripheral vascular disease, and cerebral arterial disease (see Chapter 5).

The most recent evidence of the importance of controlling blood pressure in diabetes comes from the United Kingdom Prospective Diabetes Study, published in late 1998. This study found that a lowering of blood pressure by 10 mm systolic and 5 mm diastolic resulted in a 24 percent reduction in any diabetic complication and a 32 percent reduction in death related to diabetes.

Controlling the blood pressure is absolutely essential in diabetes. The goal in diabetes is an even lower blood pressure than in the nondiabetic because studies have shown that lower normal blood pressures result in less diabetic damage than higher normal blood pressures. Your blood pressure should be no higher than 130/85, and 130/80 is even better.

How well are doctors doing at controlling blood pressure in people with diabetes? A study has shown that only 15 percent of people with diabetes with hypertension have a blood pressure as low as 140/90, and only 5 percent have a blood pressure down to 130/85.

Your doctor should measure blood pressure at every visit. Better yet, get a blood pressure device and measure it yourself. If you detect an elevation, bring it to the attention of your doctor.

Checking Your Weight

To give you a general idea of how much you ought to weigh, you can use the following formula:

- If you're a woman, give yourself 100 pounds for being 5 feet tall and add 5 pounds for each inch over 5 feet. For example, if you're 5 feet 3 inches, your appropriate weight is 115 pounds.

- If you're a man, give yourself 106 pounds for being 5 feet tall and add 6 pounds for each inch over 5 feet. A 5 foot 6 inch male should weigh 142 pounds.

Body Mass Index (BMI) relates the weight to the height so that a tall person will have a lower BMI than a short person of the same weight (see Chapter 3 for more on BMI). A person with a BMI under 20 is considered slim. A person with a BMI from 20 to 25 is normal. A person with a BMI from 25 to 29.9 is overweight, and a person with a BMI over 30 is obese. By this definition, more than half the people in the United States are overweight or obese.

You cannot step on a scale and get a reading of the BMI, but you can get your weight. This is one of the easiest measurements in medicine.

Your doctor should measure your weight at every visit.

To save you some time in figuring out your BMI, Table 7-3 shows your height in inches and meters and your weight in pounds. If you know your weight in kilograms, convert it to pounds by multiplying by 2.2. Find your height in the left-hand column. Move your finger across that row until you come to your weight in pounds. Look at the top of that column to find your BMI. For example, if your height is 66 inches and your weight is 161 pounds, your BMI is 26 kilograms per meter squared. Alternately, you can calculate your BMI as shown in Chapter 3.

Table 7-3					Body Mass Index Chart									
	Body Mass Index (kg/m²)													
	19	20	21	22	23	24	25	26	27	28	29	30	35	40
Height (inches/ meters)	Body Weight (pounds)													
58/1.47	91	96	100	105	110	115	119	124	129	134	138	143	167	191
59/1.50	94	99	104	109	114	119	124	128	133	138	143	148	173	198
60/1.52	97	102	107	112	118	123	128	133	138	143	148	15	179	204
61/1.55	100	106	111	116	122	127	132	137	143	148	153	158	185	211
62/1.57	104	109	115	120	126	131	136	142	147	153	158	164	191	218
63/1.60	107	113	118	124	130	135	141	146	152	158	163	169	197	225
64/1.63	110	116	122	128	134	140	145	151	157	163	169	174	204	232
65/1.65	114	120	126	132	138	144	150	156	162	168	174	180	210	240
66/1.68	118	124	130	136	142	148	155	161	167	173	179	186	216	247
67/1.70	121	127	134	140	146	153	159	166	172	178	185	191	233	255
68/1.73	125	131	138	144	151	158	164	171	177	184	190	197	230	262
69/1.75	128	135	142	149	155	162	169	176	182	189	196	203	236	270
70/1.78	132	139	146	153	160	167	174	181	188	195	202	207	243	278
71/1.80	136	143	150	157	165	172	179	186	193	200	208	215	250	286
72/1.83	140	147	154	162	169	177	184	191	199	206	213	221	258	294
73/1.85	144	151	159	166	174	182	189	197	204	212	219	227	265	302
74/1.88	148	155	163	171	179	186	194	202	210	218	225	233	272	311
75/1.90	152	160	168	176	184	192	200	208	216	224	232	240	279	319
76/1.93	156	164	172	180	189	197	205	213	221	230	238	246	287	328

Maintaining a BMI in the normal range makes controlling your diabetes and blood pressure easier.

You need to eliminate obesity as a risk factor for coronary artery disease.

Testing for Ketones

When your blood glucose rises above 250 mg/dl (13.9 mmol/L) or if you are pregnant with diabetes and your blood glucose is below 60 mg/dl (3.3 mmol/L), it is a good idea to check for ketones. Finding ketones means that your body has turned to fat for energy. With a high glucose, it may mean you need more insulin. With a low glucose in pregnancy, it may mean the need for more carbohydrates in your diet.

Testing for ketones is done by inserting a test strip into your urine and observing a purple color. The deeper the color, the greater the ketone level. If you find a large amount of ketones, you should contact your physician.

Chapter 8

Diabetes Diet Plan

· ·

In This Chapter

▶ Concentrating on diet-total calories

▶ Checking carbohydrates, glycemic index, and fiber

▶ Picking proteins

▶ Choosing fat in your diet

▶ Understanding vitamins, minerals, and water

▶ Adding alcohol

▶ Substituting sweeteners — caloric and artificial

▶ Considering dietary needs of type 1 diabetes

▶ Focusing on diet for type 2 diabetes

▶ Accomplishing weight reduction

▶ Coping with eating disorders and diabetes

· ·

*A*re you watching your weight go higher and higher? Do you think that low calorie means the food on the bottom shelf of the supermarket? Language specialists claim that the five sweetest phrases in the English language are

✔ I love you.

✔ Dinner is served.

✔ All is forgiven.

✔ Sleep until noon.

✔ Keep the change.

To that, most people would certainly add, "You've lost weight."

For the diabetic population, most of whom are overweight, appropriate nutrition and weight loss are not an option but a necessity. The Diabetes Control and Complications Trial clearly demonstrates that a person with diabetes who follows a careful nutrition program can reduce his or her hemoglobin A1c (see Chapter 7) by as much as 1 percent compared to the person with diabetes who is careless about diet. The consequence of that lowering is a very significant reduction in both short- and long-term complications of diabetes. In this chapter, you find out all you need to know to make your diet work for you, not only to improve your diabetes and control your blood glucose, but to generally feel that you have an improved quality of life.

Consider Total Calories First

Wanda B. Thinner, age 46, was a new type 2 diabetic patient who came to me because of high blood glucose levels, some blurring of her vision, and some numbness in her toes. She was 5 feet 5 inches tall and weighed 165 pounds. She was taking pills for the diabetes, but they were not helping. Her doctor had told her she needed to lose weight, but gave no further instructions. I started her on a diet based on the principles in this chapter. She was willing to follow the diet and lost 20 pounds, which she has kept off. Her blood glucose is now in the range of 110 most of the time. She no longer has blurring of vision, and her toes are beginning to improve. She is not taking the diabetes medication and feels much better.

No matter how you slice it, your weight is determined by the number of calories you take in, minus the number of calories you use up by exercise or loss of calories in the urine or bowel movement. If you have an excess of calories in and have insulin with which to store them, you will gain weight. If you have fewer calories in than out, you will lose weight. (See Chapter 7 if you're not sure how much you should weigh.) If you are overweight, you will benefit from even a small weight loss:

- Weight loss markedly reduces the risk of developing type 2 diabetes.

- Weight loss prevents the progression of impaired glucose tolerance to type 2 diabetes.

- Weight loss can reverse the failure to respond to drugs for diabetes that develops after responding at first (see Chapter 10).

- Weight loss reduces the risk of death from diabetes.

- Weight loss increases life expectancy in patients with type 2 diabetes.

- Weight loss has beneficial effects on high blood pressure and abnormal fats.

To have an approximate idea of how many kilocalories (actually not calories, which are much smaller) you need each day, you need to figure your desirable weight. Using the method I describe in Chapter 7, a 5 foot 6 inch male with a moderate frame should weigh around 142 pounds. To find the number of kcalories needed without taking exercise into consideration, you multiply your weight times 10, which, in this example, gives a value of about 1,400 kcalories. Then you add kcalories for the level of exercise. A sedentary male adds 10 percent of the basal kcalories, a moderately active male adds 20 percent, and a very active male adds 40 percent or more, depending on the length of exercise and the degree of exercise. These formulas are true for women as well, but women usually require fewer calories to maintain the same weight as men. Be aware that this is an approximation that differs not only for different people but even the same person on different days.

In the preceding example, the male, who is moderately active, needs 1,400 kcalories plus 1,400 times 20 percent (or about 300 more) for a total of 1,700 kcalories. You then try a diet based on your rough estimate of caloric needs, modifying the diet if you don't have enough energy and aren't maintaining your desired weight. Especially when a person is very physically active, the extra caloric needs may be very large and will quickly be noticed because the person will lose weight.

Caloric needs are different for different ages, different sexes, and different levels of activity. If a woman is pregnant or breastfeeding, she obviously needs more kcalories. If a person is trying to lose weight, then reducing the total kcalories per day can help to accomplish this. I say a lot more about this in the section on weight reduction in this chapter.

Once you determine the total kcalories, the question becomes how to divide the calories among the various foods. There are basically three foods that contain calories: Carbohydrates, proteins, and fats. Within these foods, you have many variables, which I explain in each section.

Carbohydrates

If there were a more controversial area in nutrition for the diabetic person than carbohydrates, I would like to know about it. For years, the American Diabetes Association told people with diabetes that they should be eating 55 to 60 percent of their calories as carbohydrate. Other experts said that that amount was too much. Some even said that that amount was too little. The ADA has now modified its recommendation so that it says in the Clinical Practice Recommendations for 2001: "The percent of calories from carbohydrate will vary and is individualized based on the individual's eating habits and glucose and lipid (fat) goals." In this section, I give you my suggestions for carbohydrate in your diet based on my reading of the medical literature and my clinical experience. You are free to disagree with me and use whatever level of carbohydrate you like as long as it helps to promote a lower blood glucose without increasing blood fats or weight.

Carbohydrates are the source of energy that starts with glucose, the sugar in your bloodstream that is one sugar molecule, and includes substances containing many sugar molecules called complex carbohydrates, starches, cellulose, and gums. Some of the common sources of carbohydrate are bread, potatoes, grains, cereals, and rice.

Physicians know a lot of information about carbohydrate in the body:

- ✔ Carbohydrate is the primary source of energy for muscles.
- ✔ Glucose is the carbohydrate that causes the pancreas to release insulin.
- ✔ Carbohydrate causes the triglyceride (fat) level to rise in the blood.
- ✔ When insulin is not present or is ineffective, more carbohydrate raises the blood glucose higher.
- ✔ If simple sugars are in the diet in increased amounts, they are not harmful as long as the total calorie count is satisfactory. (The major reason to reduce simple sugars in the diet is the harmful effect on dental cavities. Cavities are no more severe or common in people with diabetes than in people without diabetes.)

Although the fat intake of the American population has declined because of the fear of coronary artery disease caused by cholesterol, Americans are getting fatter. In fact, 55 percent of Americans are considered overweight or obese. Because Americans are not eating more protein, the culprit is most probably excess carbohydrate, such as that found in concentrated sweets like pastry and candy as well as the more complex carbohydrate found in bread. Within the body, carbohydrate can be turned into fat and stored. This function was great when everyone lived in caves and got little food for prolonged periods of time, but it doesn't fit today's lifestyle, consisting as it does of abundant food (and minimal foraging for it in the supermarket).

Because carbohydrate is the food that raises the blood glucose, which is responsible for the complications of diabetes, it seems right to recommend a diet that is lower in carbohydrate than previously suggested. Furthermore, a major source of coronary artery disease in diabetes is the insulin resistance syndrome (see Chapter 5). Because increased carbohydrate triggers increased triglyceride, which is the beginning of a number of abnormalities that lead to increased coronary artery disease, recommending less carbohydrate on this basis as well seems prudent.

My experience has been that a diet of 40 percent carbohydrate makes controlling my patients' blood glucose much easier. It also leads to weight loss because you don't tend to substitute protein or fat for the reduced amount of carbohydrate in the diet. My patients on lower carbohydrate diets are able to reduce the amounts of drugs such as insulin, which can cause weight gain and complicate controlling their diabetes. They also have a better fat profile.

Therefore, a man on a diet of 1,700 kcalories should eat about 680 kcalories as carbohydrate. Because each gram of carbohydrate is 4 kcalories, he eats about 170 grams of carbohydrate a day. Translating this into the foods you know and love, this is the same as 11 slices of white bread a day or 6 cups of cereal a day or 4 cups of rice a day.

Glycemic index

All carbohydrates are not alike in the degree to which they raise the blood glucose. This fact was recognized some years ago, and a measurement called the *glycemic index* was created to quantify it. The *glycemic index* (GI) uses white bread as the indicator food and assigns it a value of 100. Another carbohydrate of equal calories is compared to white bread in its ability to raise the blood glucose and assigned a value in comparison to white bread. A food that raises glucose half as much as white bread has a GI of 50, while a food that raises glucose 1½ times as much has a GI of 150. The point is to select carbohydrates with low GI levels to try to keep the glucose response as low as possible.

GI has problems that have caused it to be underutilized:

- ✔ The GI of a carbohydrate may be different when it is eaten alone or as part of a mixed meal.
- ✔ The GI of a food may differ if it's processed and prepared differently.
- ✔ Some low GI foods, like chocolate, contain a lot of fat.
- ✔ Diabetes educators have been reluctant to teach the concept of the glycemic index because they believe it is hard to understand and will create confusion.

However, good clinical studies have shown that knowledge of the glycemic index of food sources can be very valuable. Evaluation of the diet of people who develop diabetes compared with those who don't shows that, all other things being equal, the people with the highest GI diet most often developed diabetes. Once diabetes is present, those who eat the lowest GI carbohydrates have the lowest levels of blood glucose. Patients in these studies have not had great difficulty changing to a low GI diet. The other thing that happens when low GI food is incorporated into a diet is that the levels of triglycerides and LDL (or "bad" cholesterol) fall in both type 1 and type 2 diabetes.

I believe that switching to low GI carbohydrates can be very beneficial for controlling the glucose. You can easily make some simple substitutions in your diet, as shown in Table 8-1.

Table 8-1	Simple Diet Substitutions
High-GI Food	*Low-GI Food*
Bread (whole meal or white)	Whole grain bread
Processed breakfast cereal	Unrefined cereals like oats or processed low GI cereals
Plain cookies and crackers	Cookies made with dried fruits or whole grains like oats
Cakes and muffins	Cakes and muffins made with fruit, oats, and whole grains
Tropical fruits like bananas	Temperate climate fruits like apples and plums
Potatoes	Pasta or legumes
Rice	Basmati or other low GI rice

Because bread and breakfast cereal are major daily sources of carbohydrates, these simple changes can make a major difference in lowering your glycemic index. Foods that are excellent sources of carbohydrate but have a low GI include legumes such as peas or beans, pasta, grains like barley, parboiled rice and bulgar, and whole grain breads.

Even though a food has a low GI, it may not be appropriate because it is too high in fat. You need to evaluate each food's fat content before assuming that all low GI foods are good for a person with diabetes.

If you want to go into this in deeper detail, you can find a listing of many foods by category of food and by level of GI on the Web at www.mendosa.com/gilists.htm.

Fiber

Fiber is the part of the carbohydrate that is not digestible and therefore adds no calories. Fiber is found in most fruits, grains, and vegetables. Fiber comes in two forms:

- **Soluble fiber:** This form of fiber can dissolve in water and has a lowering effect on blood glucose and fat levels, particularly cholesterol.

- **Insoluble fiber:** This form of fiber cannot dissolve in water and remains in the intestine. It absorbs water and stimulates movement in the intestine. Insoluble fiber also helps prevent constipation and possibly colon cancer. This is the fiber called bulk or roughage.

Before the current trend to refine foods, people ate many sources of carbohydrate that were high in fiber. These were all in plant foods, such as fruits, vegetables, and grains. Animal foods contain no fiber.

Protein chemistry

Just as most carbohydrate contains no protein, most protein contains no carbohydrate. Therefore, protein does not raise blood glucose levels significantly under normal circumstances.

When the protein enters the small intestine, it is broken down into the smaller molecules of amino acids of which it is made. The amino acids are absorbed into the bloodstream and head for the liver where some are converted into glucose. So dietary protein can raise glucose, but this takes place slowly and is not a major contributor to the blood glucose. Some of the amino acids are used to build new protein.

Because too much fiber causes diarrhea and gas, you need to increase the fiber level in your diet fairly slowly. The recommendation for daily fiber is 20 to 30 grams. Most Americans eat only about 15 grams daily.

Many of the foods listed as having a low glycemic index contain a lot of fiber and that helps to reduce the blood glucose.

The way to eat the right amount of carbohydrate without increasing your blood glucose or triglycerides is to make it a low-glycemic, high-fiber carbohydrate.

Proteins

Unless you are a vegetarian, protein in your diet is actually the muscle of other animals, such as chicken, turkey, beef, or lamb. For this reason, it was thought that you could build your own muscle by eating lots of another animal's muscle (but you can build up the muscle only by exercising or weightlifting). You need little protein to maintain your current level of muscle.

Your choice of protein is very important because some is very high in fat while some is relatively fat free. The following lists can give you an idea of the fat content of various sources of protein. (In the next section, I explain how to integrate fat into your diet.)

One ounce of **very lean** meat, fish, or substitutes has 7 grams of protein and 1 gram of fat. Examples are

- ✔ Skinless white meat chicken or turkey
- ✔ Flounder, halibut, or tuna canned in water
- ✔ Lobster, shrimp, or clams
- ✔ Fat free cheese

An ounce of **lean** meat, fish, or substitutes has 7 grams of protein and 3 grams of fat. For example:

- Lean beef, lean pork, lamb, or veal
- Dark meat chicken without skin or white meat chicken with skin
- Sardines, salmon, or tuna canned in oil
- Other meats or cheeses with 3 grams of fat per ounce

An ounce of **medium-fat** meat, fish, or substitutes has 7 grams of protein plus 5 grams of fat. Examples include

- Most beef products
- Regular fat pork, lamb, or veal
- Dark meat chicken with skin or fried chicken
- Fried fish
- Cheeses with 5 grams of fat per ounce such as feta and mozzarella

High fat meat, fish, or substitutes contains 8 grams of fat and 7 grams of protein per ounce. Examples of this category are

- Pork spareribs or pork sausage
- Bacon
- Regular cheeses like cheddar and Monterey Jack
- Processed sandwich meats

You can see that there is a huge difference in kcalories between low-fat sources of protein and high fat sources. An ounce of skinless white meat chicken contains about 40 kcalories, while an ounce of pork spareribs has 100 kcalories. Because most people eat a minimum of four ounces of meat at a meal, they're eating from 160 to 400 kcalories depending upon the source.

My recommendation is that 30 percent of your kcalories come from protein. This would be about 500 of the kcalories of the gentleman who weighs 142 pounds and needs 1,700 kcalories each day. Because a gram of protein is 4 kcalories, he can eat 125 grams of protein. Translating that into ounces of meat, because there are 7 grams of protein in each ounce, he can eat 18 ounces of meat daily. Using the preceding lists, he can eat 8 ounces of flounder at one meal and 8 ounces of dark meat chicken at another with 2 glasses of milk providing the rest.

A lot of controversy exists with regard to how much protein should be in the diet. Many authorities call for less than 30 percent, usually preferring a diet that has 20 percent of calories as protein. One reason has to do with the large fat content of some protein sources. However, if you select protein with less fat, you can solve that problem.

A second reason cited for less protein is the suggestion that protein has a damaging effect on the kidneys. Several studies have shown this to be the case, but a very large study in the *New England Journal of Medicine* (volume 330, page 877 in 1994) a few years ago came to a different conclusion. It showed that low-protein diets did not preserve kidney function any better than a high-protein diet. The jury remains out on this question of lower versus higher protein diets.

Fat

The amount of fat you need is a lot less controversial than the carbohydrate and protein in your diet. Everyone agrees that you should eat no more than 30 percent of your diet as fats. (Currently, the American population eats 36 percent of its diet as fats.)

Keep in mind that some fats are more dangerous in their tendency to promote coronary artery disease than others. These fats should make up less of the dietary fat than the safer fats.

Cholesterol is the fat everyone knows. It has been shown to be the culprit in the development of coronary artery disease as well as peripheral vascular disease and cerebrovascular disease (see Chapter 5). The recommendation is that no more than 300 milligrams a day of fat come from cholesterol. One egg can take care of that prescription. Most other foods that you eat regularly do not contain a lot of cholesterol, but whole milk and hard cheeses like Jack and cheddar contain saturated fat, which raises the cholesterol in the body.

The other kind of fat is triglyceride, which comes in several forms:

- ✔ **Saturated fat** is the kind of fat that comes from animal sources. The streaks of fat in a steak are saturated fat. Butter is made up of saturated fat. Bacon, cream, and cream cheese are other examples.

  Eating a lot of saturated fat increases the blood cholesterol level.

- ✔ **Unsaturated fat** comes from vegetable sources like olive oil, canola oil, and margarine. It comes in several forms:

  - **Monounsaturated fat** does not raise cholesterol. Avocado, olive oil, and canola oil are examples. The oil in nuts like almonds and peanuts is monounsaturated.

  - **Polyunsaturated fat** also does not raise cholesterol but causes a reduction in the good or HDL cholesterol. Examples of polyunsaturated fats are soft fats and oils such as corn oil, mayonnaise, and margarine.

Eskimos eat a lot of fat (more than is recommended) and yet they have a low incidence of coronary artery disease. It has been shown that their protection comes from essential fatty acids. These acids are found in fish oils, which the Eskimos consume to a great extent. Essential fatty acids reduce triglycerides, reduce blood pressure, and increase the time that it takes for blood to clot, which protects against a blood clot in the heart. You can have the benefits of fish oil by substituting fish for meat two or three times a week in your diet. Pills containing fish oil have not been shown to provide the same benefit. If you don't like fish (which means you have probably never tasted salmon cooked on a barbecue), you can't get this benefit.

Keeping in mind that 30 percent of total daily calories should come from fat, it is recommended that less than a third of that amount come from saturated fats. You should also keep dietary cholesterol under 300 milligrams per day.

For the gentleman who weighs 142 pounds and needs 1,700 kcalories, slowly starving waiting for us to figure out how much to feed him, his final 500 kcalories come from fat. Fat has 9 kcalories per gram, so he can eat about 56 grams of fat daily.

Remember that he has already taken in 40 grams of fat with his flounder and chicken, so he is only left with 16 grams, 8 of which come with his milk. That leaves about a teaspoon of butter from the fat sources.

Getting Enough Vitamins, Minerals, and Water

Your diet must contain sufficient vitamins and minerals, but the amount you need may be less than you think. If you eat a balanced diet that comes from the various food groups, you generally get enough vitamins for your daily needs. Table 8-2 lists the vitamins and their food sources.

Table 8-2	Vitamins You Need	
Vitamin	*Function*	*Food Source*
Vitamin A	Needed for healthy skin and bones	Milk and green vegetables
Vitamin B1 (thiamin)	Converts carbohydrates into energy	Meat and whole grain cereals

Vitamin	Function	Food Source
Vitamin B2 (riboflavin)	Needed to use food properly	Milk, cheese, fish, and green vegetables
Vitamin B6 (pyridoxine), pantothenic acid, and biotin	All needed for growth	Liver, yeast, and many, other foods
Vitamin B12	Keeps the red blood cells and the nervous system healthy	Animal foods (for example, meat)
Folic acid	Keeps the red blood cells and the nervous system healthy	Green vegetables
Niacin	Helps release energy	Lean meat, fish, nuts, and legumes
Vitamin C	Helps maintain supportive tissues	Fruit and potatoes
Vitamin D	Helps with absorption of calcium	Dairy products and is made in the skin when exposed to sunlight
Vitamin E	Helps maintain cells	Vegetable oils and whole grain cereals.
Vitamin K	Needed for proper clotting of the blood	Leafy vegetables and is made by bacteria in your intestine

As you look through the vitamins in Table 8-2, you can see that most of them are easily available in the foods you eat every day. In certain situations, such as the pregnant woman, you need to be sure that you are getting enough every day so you take a vitamin supplement. Some evidence also suggests that extra vitamin C protects against colds.

As far as the other vitamins, the proof just does not exist that large amounts of the vitamins are beneficial, and in some cases, they may be harmful. I do not recommend that you take megadoses of these vitamins.

Minerals are also key ingredients of a healthy diet. Most are needed in tiny amounts, which are easily consumed from a balanced diet with a few exceptions:

- **Calcium, phosphorus, and magnesium build bones and teeth.** Milk and other diary products provide plenty of these minerals, but evidence suggests that people are not getting enough calcium. It is recommended that adults get 1,000 milligrams of calcium every day and 1,500 milligrams if you are growing up (adolescents) or out (pregnant women). Older people must be sure to eat 1,500 milligrams a day.

- **Iron is essential for red blood cells and is gotten from meat.** However, a menstruating woman tends to lose iron and may need to supplement her food with a pill.

- **Sodium regulates body water.** You need only about 220 milligrams a day but take in 20 to 40 times that much, which probably explains a lot of the high blood pressure in the United States. Don't add salt to your food because it already has plenty in it and you will enjoy the taste a lot more without it.

- **Chromium is needed in tiny amounts.** No scientific evidence shows that chromium is especially helpful to the person with diabetes in controlling the blood glucose despite reams of articles in health food magazines to the contrary.

- **Iodine is essential for production of thyroid hormones.** It is added to salt in order to assure that people get enough of it. In many areas of the world where iodine is not found in the soil, people suffer from very large thyroid glands known as *goiters*.

- **Various other minerals, like chlorine, cobalt, tin, and zinc are found in many foods.** These minerals are rarely lacking in the human diet.

Water is the last important nutrient I discuss in this section, but it is by no means the least important. Your body is made up of 60 percent or more water. All the nutrients in the body are dissolved in water. You can live without food for some time, but you will not last long without water. Water can help to give a feeling of fullness that reduces appetite. In general, people do not drink enough water.

You need to drink a minimum of ten cups, or 2½ quarts, of water a day.

Adding Alcohol

Alcohol is a chemical that has calories but no particular nutritional value, although it has been shown that a moderate amount (a glass or two of wine a day) may reduce the risk of a heart attack. You notice that I call alcohol a chemical. That's because alcohol is often taken to excess and does major damage to the body. It wrecks the liver and can lead to bleeding and death.

This book is not the place for a discussion of the social issues that surround the use of alcohol. Suffice it to say that excess alcohol destroys lives and families. In this section, I want to explain the part that alcohol plays in the life of the person with diabetes.

Because alcohol has calories, if you drink some, you must account for it in your diet. The proof of the alcohol is the percentage of alcohol in an ounce of the drink multiplied by 2. Wine that is 12.5 percent alcohol is 25 proof. Beer is 12 proof most of the time. Liquor is often 80 proof. To determine the calories, you use the following formula:

Calories = 0.8 x proof of the drink x number of ounces

So, for example, for a 12-ounce can of beer, you use the formula 0.8 x 12 x 12 for a total of 115 kilocalories.

For a couple of 6-ounce glasses of wine, you use the formula 0.8 x 25 x 12 to come up with 240 kilocalories.

You can see that the alcohol calories add up pretty quickly. You might even wonder why alcoholics are not often overweight. The answer is that alcohol becomes their primary source of nutrition, and they develop wasting diseases associated with inadequate intake of protein, carbohydrate, fat, vitamins, and minerals.

In addition to the calories, alcohol plays other roles in diabetes. If alcohol is taken without food, it can cause low blood glucose by increasing the activity of insulin without food to compensate for it. Some alcoholics, even without diabetes, go to bed with several drinks and are unconscious the next morning because of a very low blood glucose. They can have brain damage unless their body is able to manufacture enough glucose to wake them up.

If you're having a couple of glasses of wine or other alcohol, make sure that you eat some food along with it.

Substituting Sweeteners (Caloric and Artificial)

Fear of the "danger" of sugar in the diet has led to a vast effort to produce a compound that could add the pleasurable sweetness without the liabilities of sugar. Interestingly enough, despite the availability of a number of excellent sweeteners, some containing no calories at all, the incidence of diabetes continues to rise. Still, if you can reduce your caloric intake or your glucose response by using a sweetener, it will have an advantage. Sweeteners are divided into those that contain calories and those that do not.

Among the calorie-containing sweeteners are

- **Fructose found in fruits and berries:** Fructose is actually sweeter than table sugar *(sucrose)*. It is absorbed more slowly from the intestine than glucose, so it raises the blood glucose more slowly. It is taken up by the liver and converted to glucose or triglycerides.

- **Xylitol, found in strawberries and raspberries:** Xylitol is about like fructose in terms of sweetness. It is taken up slowly from the intestine so that it causes little change in blood glucose. Xylitol does not cause cavities of the teeth as often as the other nutritive sweeteners, so it is used in chewing gum.

- **Sorbitol and mannitol, sugar alcohols occurring in plants:** Sorbitol and mannitol are half as sweet as table sugar and have little effect on blood glucose. They change to fructose in the body. (If you read Chapter 5, you may remember sorbitol. When taken as a food, sorbitol does not accumulate and damage tissues.)

The non-nutritive or artificial sweeteners are often much more sweet than table sugar. Therefore, much less of them are required to accomplish the same level of sweetness as sugar. The current artificial sweeteners include

- **Saccharin:** This sweetener is 300 to 400 times sweeter than sucrose. It is rapidly excreted unchanged in the urine.

- **Aspartame:** This sweetener is more expensive than saccharin, but people seem to prefer its taste. It's 150 to 200 times sweeter than sucrose.

- **Cyclamate:** Because it has been associated with cancer when given in huge doses, cyclamate is banned in the United States. It is 30 times as sweet as sucrose.

The use of sugar in the diet of the person with diabetes has been changed so that some sugar is permitted. The point is to count the calories eaten as sugar and subtract that from your permissible intake. If you do this, you'll have little use for either the nutritive or the non-nutritive sweeteners.

Special Nutritional Considerations for People with Type 1 Diabetes

A person with type 1 diabetes takes insulin (see Chapter 10) to control the blood glucose. At this time, doctors and their patients cannot match the human pancreas in the way that it releases insulin just when the food is entering the bloodstream so that the glucose remains between 80 and 120 mg/dl. Therefore, the diabetic patient needs to make sure that his or her food enters as close to the expected activity of the insulin as possible.

Most people with type 1 diabetes are taking two different types of insulin, one that acts soon after the injection and has a brief period of activity and a second kind of insulin that acts more slowly and lasts longer. The rapid-acting insulin is meant to cover the food eaten at meals, while the slower acting insulin covers the rest of the time, particularly overnight when a lot of circumstances tend to raise the blood glucose.

Fortunately, you can take a new type of insulin when you start to eat or even in the middle or at the end of the meal (see Chapter 10 for more information on this insulin). This insulin overcomes the problem that has always existed — that the shot had to be taken 30 minutes before eating to give it time to be active. A person with diabetes who had a meal delayed for any reason often became hypoglycemic using the old preparation.

The person with type 1 diabetes needs to be more careful in drinking alcohol. Alcohol increases the activity of insulin and can bring the blood glucose way down if food is not taken with it. (See the section on "Adding Alcohol," earlier in this chapter.)

Because the person with type 1 diabetes always has some insulin circulating whether food is available or not, this patient should not miss a meal. A mid-morning snack, a midafternoon snack, and even a bedtime snack, if necessary, are particularly good ideas.

The person with type 1 diabetes needs to be willing to test the blood glucose frequently. That way, he or she can identify problems in advance. If, for example, blood glucose is low before exercise (see Chapter 9), you can take some nutrition to avoid hypoglycemia.

Special Nutritional Considerations for People with Type 2 Diabetes

Because most people with type 2 diabetes are overweight, weight control and reduction should be the major consideration. (See the next section for specific techniques to lose weight.)

The benefits of weight loss are rapidly seen, even when relatively little has been lost. There is a rapid fall in blood glucose. The blood pressure declines. The cholesterol falls. The triglycerides drop and the good cholesterol (HDL) rises. As I point out in Chapter 5, even a modest reduction of 10 percent of body weight has a significant positive effect on coronary artery disease.

The person with type 2 diabetes has to be very aware of the fats in his or her diet. The insulin resistance syndrome (see Chapter 5) is commonly found in this type of diabetes. You must pay attention to foods that increase triglycerides, which lead to production of small, dense LDL particles that are connected to coronary artery disease.

Because hypertension is so prevalent in both types of diabetes and it makes diabetic complications occur earlier, reduction of salt intake is an important consideration.

Reducing Your Weight

Weight reduction is difficult for many reasons. In my experience, most patients do very well initially but tend to return to old habits. There is evidence that this tendency to regain weight is built into the human brain. When fat tissue is decreased or even increased, a central control system in the brain acts to restore the fat to the previous level. If liposuction is done, for example, the remaining cells swell up to hold more fat.

Still, losing weight and keeping it off is possible. At one time, it was calculated that only one out of 20 people who lost weight would keep it off. Now the figure is closer to one out of five.

In the next chapter, I cover the value of exercise in a weight loss program. At this point, you need to realize that successful maintenance of weight loss practically requires a willingness to make exercise a part of your daily life. If, for some reason, you cannot move your legs to exercise, you can get a satisfactory workout using your upper body alone. A recent study showed that 92 percent of the people who maintained weight loss were exercising regularly, while only 34 percent of those who regained their weight continued to exercise.

Mathematics of weight loss

A pound of fat contains 3,500 kcalories. In order to lose a pound of fat, therefore, you must eat 3,500 kcalories less than you need. You can do this by a daily reduction of 500 kcalories or by doing 200 kcalories extra of exercise daily and reducing the diet by only 300 kcalories per day. Using the first method, a man eating 1,700 kcalories per day needs to decrease his diet to 1,200.

Types of diets

The numerous methods that are available for weight loss certainly suggest that no one method is especially better than all of the rest. Some are fairly drastic in the degree to which they cut calories, and weight loss is fairly rapid. But these methods are particularly prone to result in restoration of the original weight. Among the many more drastic diets are the following:

- ✔ **Very low calorie diets:** These diets provide 400 to 800 kcalories daily of protein and carbohydrate with supplemental vitamins and minerals. They are safe when supervised by a physician and are used when you need rapid weight loss — for example, for a heart condition. They result in rapid initial weight loss with a fall in the need for medications. Weight restoration commonly occurs, however.

- ✔ **Animal protein diets like the Atkins diet:** Food is limited to animal protein sources in an effort to maintain body protein, along with vitamins and minerals. Patients often complain of hair loss. Weight is rapidly regained when the diet is discontinued. This is not a balanced diet and is not recommended by me for more than a few weeks.

- ✔ **Fasts:** A *fast* means giving up all food for a period of time and taking only water and vitamins and minerals. A fast is such a drastic change from normal eating habits that patients do not remain on the fast for very long, and weight is regained.

Several diets are associated with large organizations in the community and may require that you purchase only their foods. The support given by these organizations seems to be extremely helpful in weight-loss maintenance. In addition, the slower loss of weight and the connection to more normal eating seems to result in a greater tendency to stay with the program and keep the weight off. The leading contenders for this type of diet are

- ✔ **Jenny Craig:** This organization provides the food that you eat, which you must pay for. It offers some information on behavior modification. They also have special diets for people with diabetes. In May 1997, the government required Jenny Craig to tell its customers that the weight-loss methods may only be temporary because customers had no way to judge from their advertising that many people regain their weight.

✔ **Weight Watchers:** This organization emphasizes slow weight loss, exercise, and behavior modification. It charges for weekly attendance at its meetings, which are held all over the world. It does not require that you purchase any products. Foods are available for purchase. Its point program for increasing fiber in your diet may be especially helpful to the person with diabetes.

Surgery for weight loss

I want to say a word about surgery for weight reduction. Surgery is used in the most severe and resistant cases of obesity. It has impressive effects such as correction of high glucose and reduction or discontinuation of glucose-lowering drugs. Results are so successful in some patients that some surgeons consider type 2 diabetes to be a surgical disease. That, I believe, is a little extreme. Some of the reasons for bypass surgery include

✔ You have a body mass index that is greater than 40.

✔ You have an obesity-related physical problem such as inability to walk.

✔ You have a high-risk obesity-related health problem like heart disease.

The best surgical treatment for obesity is the *gastric bypass operation* where the stomach is stapled to create a small pouch. A section of the small intestine is attached to the pouch so food passes through very little of the small intestine, reducing calorie and nutrient absorption. Because the pouch is small, you tend to eat less. The usual loss of weight is two-thirds of the excess in two years. Some of the problems of gastric bypass include

✔ The pouch may stretch.

✔ The staple line can break down.

✔ Malabsorption of iron and calcium may occur.

✔ Anemia may occur from lack of vitamin B12.

✔ The dumping syndrome may occur. In this condition, stomach contents move too fast into the small intestine, provoking a lot of insulin with resultant hypoglycemia.

When you have bypass surgery for obesity, you must be willing to be committed to lifelong medical follow-up. You must be willing to give up large meals and be determined to lose weight.

Behavior modification

Years of working with obese patients have shown that diet and exercise must be accompanied by changes in behavior with respect to food. The first behavior changes are diet and exercise. After that, you can change eating behavior to make the diet easier to follow. Some of the best techniques include the following:

- Eat according to a schedule to avoid unscheduled eating.
- Find a single place to eat all food.
- Slow down your eating to make the meal last.
- Put high calorie foods away. Remove serving dishes and bread from the table.
- Don't dispense food to others to avoid exposure for yourself.
- Do not clean your plate.
- Set realistic goals for weight loss.
- When eating out, be careful of salad dressing, alcohol, and bread.
- Get a 10-pound weight and carry it around for a while to appreciate the importance of a loss of even that little.
- At the market, buy from a list, carry only enough money for the food on that list, and avoid aisles containing loose foods, other than fruits and vegetables, like loose candy.

You can incorporate one technique into your life each week (or even longer) until you feel you have mastered it and have added it to your eating style. Then go on and take up another technique.

As you go about this difficult task of losing weight and keeping it off, remember to seek the help of those around you. A loving partner provides great help through the roughest days.

Coping with Eating Disorders and Diabetes

You can't be too rich or too thin. How much damage has this statement done to society, especially the thin part? Young people, particularly girls, are preoccupied with their body weight. When this preoccupation becomes too great, it can result in an eating disorder. The young girl (and young boys about a tenth as often) will either starve herself and exercise excessively or eat a great deal and then induce vomiting and/or take laxatives and water pills. The one who starves herself has *anorexia nervosa,* while the one who binges and purges has *bulimia nervosa.* By themselves, these conditions can result in severe illness and even death when carried to extremes. When combined with diabetes, there is very great danger to the health of the young girl.

Anorexia is usually found in middle- and upper-class girls. They have a distorted body image and are fearful of weight gain. The prevalence may be as high as one in 200 in these girls. Their parents are usually very concerned with slimness. The girls may appear unusually thin and do not menstruate. Their malnutrition may be so severe that they die from it. These girls are in a constant state of starvation. When they have diabetes, their condition is just like that of people with type 1 diabetes before the availability of insulin. They have very low blood glucose levels, so little or no insulin is required (see Chapter 10). They develop problems with their hearts and have low blood pressure and low body temperature. They lose a lot of body musculature once the fat is gone.

If you think you know someone with this disorder, here are some of the clues to look for:

- ✔ She eats more rapidly than others do.
- ✔ She eats until uncomfortably full.
- ✔ She eats large amounts of food even when she is not hungry.
- ✔ She eats by herself because she is embarrassed.
- ✔ She feels guilty or disgusted after overeating.

Management of diabetes requires a certain amount of routine from day to day. There is no way to achieve such systematization when the amount of food coming into the body is so uncertain. The girl with severe anorexia may require intravenous feeding until she is stabilized a little bit. This will sometimes lead to very high blood glucose levels necessitating the use of insulin. Once the life-threatening starvation is under control, it is possible to achieve good blood glucose control with help from the patient and a therapist who can help her to understand her distorted body image. If there is clinical depression, antidepressant medication may be necessary.

Bulimia involves eating large quantities of easily digested food and then purging it by vomiting and taking laxatives or water pills. These patients are not as severely thin as those are with anorexia. Their background is similar to the anorexia patients. They may represent up to 40 percent of college-age female students. Because their weight is closer to normal, they usually will menstruate normally.

Girls with bulimia are more likely to go on to adult obesity and are harder to treat. They actually do not do as well with therapy as those with anorexia. They end up with more psychiatric problems later in life.

Their food intake is extremely variable but less severe than that of the anorexics. Therefore, their diabetes is a little easier to treat.

If you would like to know more about anorexia and bulimia, you can obtain a publication from the National Institutes of Health called "Binge Eating Disorders." It is NIH Publication No. 94-3589 and is available from the Weight-Control Information Network at 1 Win Way, Bethesda, MD 20892-3665 or call 800-946-8098. This publication also contains a list of treatment programs throughout the United States for this eating disorder.

Another source of useful information is the National Eating Disorders Organization, which publishes the "Overview of Eating Disorders: Anorexia Nervosa, Bulimia Nervosa and Related Disorders" available at 445 E. Granville Road, Worthington, OH 43085 or call 614-436-1112.

Both of these conditions make it impossible to control blood glucose but one other activity makes diabetic control difficult. Some women and men skip insulin shots in order to lose weight. Weight will be lost as the body turns to fat for fuel because glucose can't be used (see Chapter 2). Again, there is loss of muscle mass and the blood glucose rises very high. This is not a way of avoiding complications of diabetes.

Chapter 9

Keeping It Moving: Exercise Plan

• •

• •

More than 60 years ago, the great leaders in diabetes care declared that proper management has three major aspects:

✔ Proper diet

✔ Appropriate medication

✔ Sufficient exercise

Since then, millions of dollars and man (and woman) hours have been spent to define the proper diet and the right medication, but exercise has rarely received its proper place in the triad of care. I am writing this chapter to correct that omission.

Getting Off the Couch: Why Exercise Is Important

When they wrote their recommendations, the experts were really talking about type 1 diabetes just after the isolation and administration of insulin. In fact, many studies have shown that exercise doesn't normalize the blood glucose or reduce the hemoglobin A1c (see Chapter 7) in type 1 diabetes. Many other studies have shown that exercise does normalize blood glucose and reduce hemoglobin A1c in type 2 diabetes.

Exercise your way to health

John Plant is a 46-year-old male who has had type 1 diabetes for 23 years. He takes insulin shots four times daily and measures his blood glucose multiple times a day. He follows a careful diet.

Prior to developing diabetes, he was a very active person, participating in vigorous sports and doing major hiking and mountain climbing. At the time, his doctor warned him that he would have to give up many of the most strenuous activities because he would never know his blood glucose level and it might drop precipitously during his heavy exercise. He ignored this advice and continued his active way of life. He found that he could do with much less insulin than his doctor prescribed and rarely became hypoglycemic. He has been able to continue these activities without limitation. His blood glucose level is generally between 75 and 140. His last hemoglobin A1c was slightly elevated at 5.7. A recent eye examination showed no diabetic retinopathy. He has no significant microalbuminuria in his urine and no tingling in his feet.

Is John lucky? You bet he is. But it is like most "luck." It is based on a self-realization that the human body is made up of both a mind and a body. If humans were meant to spend their lives munching potato chips in front of a TV set, why do they have all these muscles?

When a new diabetic patient enters my office, I give him a bottle of 50 pills. I instruct him not to swallow the pills but to drop them on the floor three times daily and pick them up one at a time. The condition a person is in can be judged by what he or she takes two at a time, pills or stairs.

The major benefit of exercise for both types of diabetes is to prevent macrovascular disease (see Chapter 5), which affects the entire population of nondiabetics and people with diabetes alike but is particularly severe in people with diabetes. Exercise does prevent macrovascular disease in numerous ways:

- ✔ Exercise helps with weight loss in type 2 diabetes.
- ✔ Exercise lowers bad cholesterol and triglycerides, and raises good cholesterol.
- ✔ Exercise lowers blood pressure.
- ✔ Exercise lowers stress levels.
- ✔ Exercise reduces the need for insulin or drugs.

The feeling of fatigue that occurs with exercise is probably due to the loss of stored muscle glucose. (See the sidebar "How exercise works its magic" for more detail.)

With exercise, insulin levels in nondiabetics and people with type 2 diabetes decline because insulin acts to store and not release glucose and fat. Levels of glucagon, epinephrine, cortisol, and growth hormone increase to provide more glucose. Studies show that glucagon is responsible for 60 percent of the glucose, and epinephrine and cortisol are responsible for the other 40 percent. If insulin did not fall, glucagon could not stimulate the liver to make glucose.

You might wonder how insulin can open the cell to the entry of glucose when insulin levels are falling. In fact, two things are at work here. Glucose is getting into muscle cells without the need for insulin and the rapid circulation that comes with exercise is delivering the smaller amount of insulin more frequently to the muscle. The muscle seems to be more sensitive to the insulin as well. This is exactly what the person with type 2 diabetes hopes to accomplish when insulin resistance is the major block to insulin action.

One way to preserve glucose stores is to provide calories from an external source. Any marathoner knows that additional calories can delay the feeling of exhaustion. The timing is important. If the glucose is given an hour before exercise, it will be metabolized during the exercise and increase endurance. However, if it's given 30 minutes before exercise, it may decrease stamina by stimulating insulin, which blocks liver production of glucose. (See the sidebar "How exercise works its magic" for more information.)

How exercise works its magic

In order to understand how exercise reduces the blood glucose in type 2 diabetes and helps prevent macrovascular disease in both types, you need to have some understanding of the dynamics of metabolism during exercise.

As exercise begins, the demand for both glucose and fat for energy is increased. Glucose and fat leave the sites where they are stored and enter the bloodstream, heading for muscles. At first, glycogen, the storage form of glucose in the liver, begins to break down and release glucose. With continued exercise, glycogen is used up, and the liver begins to make large amounts of glucose from other substances to continue to provide energy.

With steady, moderate exercise, the body eventually turns to fat as the glucose production begins to diminish. This is a wonderful situation, especially because most people with type 2 diabetes have plenty of fat to offer. On the other hand, if the exercise is very vigorous, the liver actually makes more glucose than the muscles can use immediately, and the blood glucose begins to rise. This explains some of the instances where the glucose is higher after exercise than it is before exercise. The reason the liver makes so much glucose is that very vigorous exercise depletes the stores of glucose in the muscle very rapidly. Vigorous exercise will not be continued for very long, and the extra glucose will be there to replenish the muscle tissue, once exercise ends.

Glucose is a better source of energy when the exercise is very vigorous because it is converted to energy much faster than fat. For less intense exercise, fat is preferred because it provides more energy than an equal amount of glucose.

Fructose can replenish you when you're doing prolonged exercise. This sweetener can replace glucose because it is sweeter but is absorbed more slowly and does not provoke the insulin secretion that glucose provokes. Fructose is rapidly converted into glucose inside the body. (See Chapter 8 for more on fructose.)

Exercising When You Have Diabetes

Prior to beginning a new exercise program, a person with diabetes who has not exercised previously should check with a doctor, especially if over the age of 35 or if diabetes has been present for ten years or longer. You should check with a doctor if you have any of the following risk factors:

- The presence of any diabetic complications like retinopathy, nephropathy, or neuropathy (see Chapter 5)
- Obesity
- A physical limitation
- A history of coronary artery disease or elevated blood pressure
- Use of medications

You need to discuss any of these problems with your doctor in order to choose the appropriate exercises. I say more about the choice of exercise in the section "Is Golf a Sport? Choosing Your Activity," later in this chapter.

Once exercise is begun, the person with type 1 diabetes as well as the person with type 2 diabetes can do a lot to make it safe and healthful. Some important steps to take include

- Wearing an ID bracelet
- Testing the blood glucose very often
- Choosing proper socks and shoes
- Drinking plenty of water
- Carrying treatment for hypoglycemia
- Exercising with a friend

If you have diabetes, you don't need to do the following things to exercise:

- You don't need to buy special clothing other than the right shoes and socks (and possibly soft pants for the cyclist).
- Don't expect to lose certain "spots" by repetitively exercising them.

> ✔ Don't exercise to the point of pain.
>
> ✔ You don't need to use exercise gadgets like belts or other objects that do not require you to move.

Exercise for the person with type 1 diabetes

The person with type 1 diabetes depends on insulin injections to manage the blood glucose. He or she does not have the luxury of a "thermostat" that automatically shuts off during exercise and turns back on when exercise is finished. Once an insulin shot is taken, it is active until it is used up.

The person with type 1 diabetes has to avoid overdosing on insulin before exercise, which can lead to hypoglycemia, or underdosing, which can lead to hyperglycemia. If the body does not have enough insulin, it turns to fat for energy. Glucose rises because it is not being metabolized, but its production is continuing. If exercise is particularly vigorous in a situation of not enough insulin, the blood glucose can rise extremely high.

Reduction of the insulin dosage prior to exercise helps prevent hypoglycemia. In one study, an 80 percent reduction of the dose allowed the person with diabetes to exercise for 3 hours, while a 50 percent reduction forced the person with diabetes to stop after 90 minutes due to hypoglycemia. Each person with diabetes varies, and you must determine for yourself how much to reduce insulin by measuring the blood glucose before, during, and after exercise.

Another way to prevent hypoglycemia, of course, is to eat some carbohydrate. You need to have some carbohydrate (which quickly raises blood glucose) available during exercise.

In addition, the site of the insulin injection is important because this determines how fast the insulin becomes active. If you are running and inject insulin into your leg, it will be taken up more quickly than an injection into the arm.

You can exercise whenever you will do it faithfully. If you like to sleep late and schedule your exercise at 5:30 a.m., you probably won't consistently do it. Your best time is probably about 60 to 90 minutes after eating because this is when the glucose is peaking, providing the calories you need, avoiding the usual post-eating high in your blood glucose, and burning up those food calories.

Exercise for the person with type 2 diabetes

Even though you have type 2 diabetes, many of the suggestions for the type 1, other than the insulin discussion, apply to you, too. If you haven't already, read the section "Exercising When You Have Diabetes," earlier in this chapter.

With sufficient exercise and diet, some people with type 2 diabetes can revert to a nondiabetic state. This does not mean that they no longer have diabetes, but it certainly means that they will not develop the long-term complications that can make life so miserable later in life (see Chapter 5).

Determining How Much Exercise You Can and Should Do

Unless you have a physical abnormality, there is no limitation on what you can do. You need to select an activity that you enjoy and will continue to perform.

In the recent past, exercise physiologists said that you needed to make sure that you monitored your exercise intensity by periodically checking your heart rate. Your exercise heart rate was supposed to be based on your age. The usual formula to figure this out is to take the number 220, subtract your age, and multiply that number by 60 to 75 percent to get the recommended exercise heart rate for aerobic exercise. (See the sidebar "What are aerobic and anaerobic exercise?" if you're not sure what aerobic exercise is.)

Now studies have shown that people can sustain aerobic exercise at higher heart rates. Perhaps the best way to know whether you're meeting your exercise goals is to use the "Perceived Exertion Scale" described in the nearby sidebar, "Checking the value of your exercise."

What are aerobic and anaerobic exercise?

Aerobic exercise is exercise that can be sustained for more than a few minutes, uses major groups of muscles, and gets your heart to pump faster during the exercise, thus training the heart. I give you many examples of aerobic exercise throughout this chapter.

Anaerobic exercise, on the other hand, is brief (sometimes a few seconds) and intense and usually cannot be sustained. Lifting large weights is an example of an anaerobic exercise. A 100-yard dash is another example.

Checking the value of your exercise

Measuring your pulse during exercise (or even at rest) may be hard for you. Instead, you can use the Perceived Exertion Scale. Exercise is given a descriptive value from very, very light to very, very hard with very light, fairly light, somewhat hard, and very hard in between. You want to exercise to a level of somewhat hard and you will be at your target heart rate in most cases.

As you get into shape, the amount of exertion that corresponds to somewhat hard will increase.

Do not continue exercising if you have tightness in your chest, chest pain, severe shortness of breath, or dizziness.

The younger you are, the faster your exercise heart rate may be. Like everything in this book, your exercise heart rate is an individual number. If you are a world-class athlete training for your ninth marathon, your exercise heart rate may be higher. If you have some heart disease, your exercise heart rate may be significantly lower.

Once you know your maximal exercise heart rate, you can choose your activity and use the "Perceived Exertion Scale" to be sure that you achieve that level during exercise. The best choice for you is an exercise you enjoy and will continue to perform. The choices are really limitless. The number of kcalories you use for any exercise is determined by your weight, the strenuousness of the activity, and the time you spend actually doing it. In order to have a positive effect on your heart, you need to do a moderate level of exercise for 20 to 45 minutes at least three times a week.

Although you only need to do aerobic exercise three or four times a week to have an effect on your heart fitness, a daily program of aerobic exercise has a major impact on your diabetes. Twenty to 30 minutes of moderate aerobic exercise every day provides enormous physical, mental, and emotional benefits.

You need to warm up and cool down for about five minutes before and after you exercise. You can warm up by stretching or just standing in one place and hitting the ball before starting to run around.

I am not spending a lot of time on stretching because the place of stretching for the healthy exerciser is not clear. One study showed that a group of runners who did not stretch did better than a group who did. Most doctors agree that stretching after an injury is appropriate but whether all the advice about stretching before exercise for an uninjured person is much ado about nothing is yet to be determined. If you do stretch, do not stretch to the point that it hurts. This is where muscle tears occur. See the excellent book *Fitness For Dummies,* 2nd Edition, by Suzanne Schlosberg and Liz Neporent, M.A. (Hungry Minds, Inc.) for more about stretching.

When you need support

The Diabetes Exercise and Sports Association is an organization that you can turn to for help, instruction, and friendship as you add exercise to your good diabetes care. You can reach this organization by writing P.O. Box 1935, Litchfield Park, AZ 85340, or by calling 800-898-4322. They know all about diabetes and sports and are eager to share the information with you. See the Web site at http://www.diabetes-exercise.org/index.html.

Moderate exercise is a moving definition. If you're out of shape, moderate exercise for you may be slow walking. If you're in good shape, moderate exercise may be jogging or cross-country skiing. Moderate exercise is simply something you can do and not get out of breath. For ideas on the types of exercise you can do, see the following section.

How long can you stop exercise before you start to decondition? It takes only about two to three weeks to lose some of the fitness your exercise has provided. Then it takes up to six weeks to get back to your current level, assuming that your holiday from exercise does not go on too long.

Is Golf a Sport? Choosing Your Activity

The following factors can help you determine your choice of activity:

- Do you like to exercise alone or with company? Pick a competitive or team sport if you prefer company.

- Do you like to compete against others or just yourself? Running or walking are sports you can do alone.

- Do you prefer vigorous or less vigorous activity? Less vigorous activity over a longer period is just as effective as more vigorous activity.

- Do you live where you can do activities outside year-round, or do you need to go inside a lot of the year? Find a sports club if weather prevents year-round outside activity.

- Do you need special equipment or just a pair of running shoes? Special equipment is very helpful when it's needed.

- What benefits are you looking for in your exercise: Cardiovascular, strength, endurance, flexibility, or body fat control? You should probably look for all these benefits, but you may have to combine activities to get them all in.

Fore!

You are probably wondering why I chose to title this section "Is Golf a Sport? Choosing Your Activity." I have to say that some of my best friends are golfers. Golf is currently the favorite sport of executives throughout the United States, so if you're planning to reach the executive level, you'd better take it up. My objection to golf has to do with the requirement that golfers use carts to get from hole to hole. This virtually eliminates the exercise associated with it. If you enjoy golf, by all means continue to play it as often as you like but add some other activity to provide the fitness that will not only help your diabetes but your golf game as well.

Perhaps a good starting point in your activity selection is to focus on the benefits. Table 9-1 gives you some ideas.

Table 9-1	Match Your Activity to the Results You Want
If You Want to . . .	**Then Consider . . .**
Build up cardiovascular condition	Vigorous basketball, racquetball, squash, cross-country skiing, handball
Strengthen body	Low-size, high repetition weight lifting, gymnastics, mountain climbing, cross-country skiing
Build up muscular endurance	Gymnastics, rowing, cross-country skiing, vigorous basketball
Increase flexibility	Gymnastics, judo and karate, soccer, surfing
Control body fat	Handball, racquetball, squash, cross-country skiing, vigorous basketball, singles tennis

You can tell from Table 9-1 that living in the mountains where you have plenty of snow is helpful because cross-country skiing is in practically every list. On the other hand, so is vigorous basketball, so you don't have to give up exercise if you live in a warm climate like Florida.

The special needs of many of these sports may turn you off to exercise. The curious thing is that the best exercise that you can sustain for life is right at your feet. A brisk daily walk improves heart function, adds to muscular endurance, and helps control body fat. So many people drive their cars to the gym and try to park as close as possible so that they can get to the building with as little effort as possible. Seems a little strange, doesn't it?

Of course, the social benefits of exercise are very important. You are together with people who are concerned with health and appearance. These people usually share many of your interests. The person who likes to jog often likes to hike and climb and camp out. Many lifetime partnerships begin on one side of a tennis court (and some end there as well).

Cross-training, where you do several different activities throughout the week, is a good idea. Cross-training reduces the boredom that may accompany one thing done day after day. It also permits you to exercise regardless of the weather because you can do some things indoors and some outside.

Table 9-2 lists a variety of exercises that you can try. I also include the amount of kcalories that you burn in 20 minutes.

Table 9-2	Exercise and the Amount of Calories You Burn in 20 Minutes at Different Body Weights	
Activity	*Kcalories Burned (125 pounds)*	*Kcalories Burned (175 pounds)*
Standing	24	32
Walking, 4 mph	104	144
Running, 7 mph	236	328
Gardening	60	84
Writing	30	42
Typing	38	54
Carpentry	64	88
House painting	58	80
Baseball	78	108
Dancing	70	96
Football	138	192
Golfing	66	96
Swimming	80	112
Skiing, downhill	160	224
Skiing, cross-country	196	276
Tennis	112	160

Everything you do burns calories. Even sleeping and watching television use 20 kcalories in 20 minutes if you weigh 125 pounds.

Your choice of an activity must take into account your physical condition. If you have diabetic neuropathy (see Chapter 5) and cannot feel your feet, you do not want to do pounding exercises that may damage them without your awareness. You can swim, bike, row, or do armchair exercises where you move your upper body vigorously.

If you have diabetic retinopathy (see Chapter 5), you won't want to do exercises that raise your blood pressure (like weight lifting), cause jerky motions in your eyes (like bouncing on a trampoline), or change the pressure in your eye significantly (like scuba diving or high mountain climbing). You also should not do exercises that place your eyes below the level of your heart, such as when you touch your toes.

Patients with nephropathy (see Chapter 5) should avoid exercises that raise your blood pressure for prolonged periods. These exercises are extremely intense activities that you do for a long time, like marathon running.

Some people have pain in the legs after they walk a certain distance. This may be due to diminished blood supply to the legs so that the needs of the muscles in the legs cannot be met by the inadequate blood supply. Although you need to discuss this problem with your doctor, you do not need to give up walking. You can determine the distance you can walk up to the point of pain. Then you should walk about three-quarters of that distance and stop to give the circulation a chance to catch up. Once you have rested, you will find that you can go about the same distance again without pain. By stringing several of these walks together, you can get a good, pain-free workout. You may even find that you are able to increase the distance after a while because this kind of training tends to create new blood vessels.

Is there a medical condition that should absolutely prevent you from doing exercise? Short of chest pain at rest, which must be addressed by your doctor, the answer is no. If you cannot figure out an exercise that you can do, get together with an exercise therapist. You will be amazed at how many muscles you can move that you never knew you had.

Benefiting from Training

As your body becomes trained with regular exercise, the benefits for your diabetes are very significant. Your body starts to turn to fat for energy earlier in the course of your exercise. At the same time, the hormones that tend to raise the blood glucose during exercise are not produced at the same high rate because they aren't needed. Because you don't require as much insulin, your insulin doses can be reduced, and it's much easier to avoid hypoglycemia during exercise.

Lifting Weights

Weight lifting is a form of anaerobic exercise. (See the sidebar earlier in this chapter if you're not sure what anaerobic exercise is.) It involves the movement of heavy weights, which can only be moved for brief periods of time. It results in significant muscle strengthening and increased endurance.

Because weight lifting causes a significant rise in blood pressure as it is being done, people with severe diabetic eye disease should not do it.

Weight training, which uses lighter weights, can be a form of aerobic exercise. Because the weights are light, they can be moved for prolonged periods of time. The result is improved cardiovascular fitness along with strengthening of muscles, tendons, ligaments, and bones. Weight training is an excellent way to protect and strengthen a joint that is beginning to develop some discomfort.

Older people in nursing homes who were given weights of just a few pounds have shown excellent return of strength to what appeared to be atrophied muscles. The benefits for you will be that much greater.

Weight training may be good for the days that you do not do your aerobic exercise, or you can add it for a few minutes after you finish your activity. Weight training is also good for working on a particular group of muscles that you feel is weak. Very often, this muscle is the back. Weight-training exercises can isolate and strengthen each muscle.

If you do a lot of aerobic exercise that involves the legs, you may want to use upper body weight training only. I can tell you from personal experience that you not only feel a stronger upper body, but your ability to do your usual exercise is enhanced as well.

Chapter 10

Medications: What You Should Know

*Y*ou don't know how lucky you are. You are the beneficiary of the greatest advances in medications for diabetes in the history of this disease. From 1921, when insulin was isolated and used for the first time, to 1955, when a class of glucose-lowering drugs called sulfonylureas became available, insulin was all there was. For another 40 years, nothing new showed up in the United States until 1995. Now four new classes of drugs, each in its own unique way, lower blood glucose. In Chapter 16, you see that even more drugs are coming, and soon.

In this chapter, you find out all you need to know to use these drugs effectively and safely. (You need to take medication if diet and exercise are not keeping your blood glucose under control; see this part for more information.)

This chapter helps you become an educated consumer. Not only can you find out about the medication you're taking and how it works, but you discover when to take it, how it interacts with other medications, what side effects it may cause, and how to use several of these medications together, if necessary, to normalize your blood glucose. Right now, today, this year, you have all the tools needed to control your diabetes, and there is more to come. In the immortal words of the great entertainer Al Jolson, "You ain't seen nothin' yet."

Taking Drugs by Mouth: Oral Agents

Most people do not care for shots. You may be an exception, but I doubt it. Fortunately, drugs that can be taken by mouth have been available for some time. One thing you should know about these pills: You can take them or leave them, but they work much better if you take them.

Sulfonylureas

Scientists discovered sulfonylureas accidentally when it was noticed that soldiers given certain sulfur-containing antibiotics developed symptoms of low blood glucose. Once scientists began to search for the most potent examples of this effect, they came up with several different versions of this drug. They all have the following characteristics:

- They work by making the pancreas release more insulin.
- They are not effective in type 1 diabetes where the pancreas is not capable of releasing any insulin.
- Sometimes they don't work when first given (primary failure) but almost always they stop working later on (secondary failure).
- They are all capable of causing hypoglycemia.
- When you use any of a class of antibiotics called *sulfonamides,* the glucose-lowering action of the sulfonylureas is prolonged.
- They should not be taken by a pregnant woman or a nursing mother.
- They can be fairly potent when given in combination with one of the other classes of oral agents.

The original sulfonylureas from the 1950s, the first-generation sulfonylureas, are not used as initial treatment as much anymore but are actually just as useful as the newer, second-generation sulfonylureas. The old ones are just as potent, but more milligrams are required for the same effect. All the first-generation drugs are available in a generic form, which makes them less expensive. The first-generation sulfonylureas include

- **Tolbutamide,** brand name Orinase. This is the only short-acting sulfonylurea. Because it is rapidly broken down in the liver, tolbutamide begins to work in one hour and is gone from the body in ten hours. It is available in 250 and 500 milligram strength. Tolbutamide is usually given before each meal, but some patients require only one or two doses a day. Because it lasts for such a short time, tolbutamide is much safer in elderly people. The maximal dose is 3 grams daily (six 500 mg pills).

✔ **Tolazamide,** brand name Tolinase. This agent is absorbed more slowly than other sulfonylureas, so it takes four or more hours to notice its effects and its activity lasts up to 20 hours. Tolazamide is available in 100, 250, and 500 milligrams. When more than 500 mg is needed, the dose is divided. The maximum dose is 1,000 mg. The drug is changed in the liver, but the new products have the ability to lower the blood glucose just like tolazamide. Because the new products are then disposed of in the urine, a person with kidney disease should be careful about taking this medication.

✔ **Acetohexamide,** brand name Dymelor. Acetohexamide begins to work about one hour after it's taken and lasts for 12 hours. It comes in 250 and 500 mg strength. Acetohexamide is given in one or two doses daily, and the maximum useful dose is 1.5 grams (three 500 mg tablets). Acetohexamide is inactivated and excreted just like tolazamide, so it requires the same precautions about kidney problems.

✔ **Chlorpropamide,** brand names Diabinase or Glucamide. Chlorpromamide is the longest acting of the first-generation sulfonylureas and was responsible for many cases of hypoglycemia in the past. It is active for 24 hours or longer. Chlorpropamide causes a very prolonged hypoglycemia that sometimes requires treatment with intravenous glucose for several days. Chlorpropamide comes in 100 and 250 mg sizes. The maximum recommended dose is 750 mg. It is broken down into other chemicals, which are also active and are slowly eliminated in the urine, so any kidney problem will greatly lengthen its time of activity. It is given only once a day because it lasts so long. Chlorpropamide has several unique side effects. It causes water retention that sometimes results in low levels of sodium in the blood. When alcohol is taken by a person on chlorpropamide, the face flushes shortly after taking the alcohol, lasting for ten minutes. Other sulfonylureas do not cause this flushing.

In making a choice among the first-generation drugs, tolbutamide, acetohex-amide, and tolazamide are considered less potent, and chlorpropamide is felt to be the most potent of them. If the first three (of which tolbutamide is the mildest) do not work, then chlorpropamide is tried. If chlorpropamide doesn't lower the blood glucose sufficiently, then the second-generation drugs are used. Doctors, too often, do not try the first-generation drugs today and go right to the second-generation pills. For many people, the second-generation pills are too potent, and hypoglycemia becomes a problem. For others, the second-generation drugs provide no greater benefit than the earlier ones. All these drugs suffer from the fact that, sooner or later, they no longer control the blood glucose.

Three second-generation sulfonylureas now exist:

- Glyburide, brand names Micronase, Diabeta, and Glynase. Among the foreign brand names for glyburide are Antibet, Azuglucon, Betanase, Gliban, Glibil, Gluben, and Orabetic. Pretty confusing, huh? Glyburide comes in 1.25, 2.5, and 5 mg strengths. The usual starting dose is 2.5 to 5 mg with breakfast, and the maintenance dose is 1.25 to 20 mg. Glyburide leaves the body equally in the bowel movement and the urine, so patients with either liver or kidney disease are at greater risk for low blood glucose. Glyburide is carried around the bloodstream bound to proteins, so if other drugs that bind to proteins are taken, such as aspirin, the activity of glyburide may increase. When these drugs are withdrawn, the activity of glyburide may decrease. Other than hypoglycemia, the incidence of negative effects is very low. Glynase is a form of glyburide that is slightly more active, so less is required for the same effect. The starting dose is 1.5 mg, and it's available as 1.5, 3, or 6 mg tablets with a maximum dose of 12 mg. You can take either form once a day in the morning, but sometimes it works better when given twice a day.

- **Glipizide,** brand names Glucotrol, Glucotrol XL. Among the foreign brand names are Digrin, Glibenase, Glican, Glyco, Glynase (same name as glyburide in the USA!), Mindiab, Napizide, and Sucrazide. Glipizide is similar to glyburide but slightly less potent so that it comes as 5 and 10 mg pills. You take it 30 minutes before food. The starting dose is 5 mg. Up to 40 mg can be given daily in several doses. Because it's less potent, glipizide is preferred in the elderly. Glucotrol XL is an extended release form of glipizide that lasts for 24 hours, so it usually is given as 5 or 10 mg once a day.

- **Glimepiride,** brand name Amaryl. This drug also lasts a longer time and is fairly potent, so it is given once a day. It comes in 1, 2, and 4 mg sizes with a maximum daily dose of 8 mg.

Choosing among the second-generation sulfonylureas, I generally select glimepiride because of its long duration of action. However, the other two are available as generic preparations and are, therefore, less expensive.

Metformin

Metformin, brand name Glucophage, is an entirely different kind of glucose-lowering medication. Outside the USA, it's called Benoformin, Dextin, Diabex, Diaformin, Fornidd, Glucoform, Gluformin, Metforal, Metomin, and Orabet.

More than 20 years ago, the United States banned a sister medication called Phenformin because of an association with a fatal complication. Metformin has been used in Europe for years without much trouble and was finally approved in this country in 1995. Metformin is rarely, and perhaps never, associated with the fatal complication lactic acidosis that caused Phenformin to be banned.

Metformin has the following characteristics:

- ✔ It lowers the blood glucose mainly by reducing the production of glucose from the liver (the hepatic glucose output) and by itself (monotherapy) does not cause hypoglycemia.

- ✔ It may increase the sensitivity of the muscle cells to insulin and slow the uptake of glucose from the intestine.

- ✔ It must be taken with food because it causes gastrointestinal irritation, but this side effect declines with time.

- ✔ It's available in 500 mg, 850 mg, and 1,000 mg tablets.

- ✔ The maximum dose is 2,500 mg taken in divided doses with each meal.

- ✔ It does not depend on stimulating insulin to work as do the sulfonylureas.

- ✔ It's often associated with weight loss, possibly from the gastrointestinal irritation or because of a loss of taste for food.

- ✔ It's not recommended when you have significant liver disease, kidney disease, or heart failure.

- ✔ It's usually stopped for a day or two before surgery or an x-ray study using a dye.

- ✔ It's not recommended for use in alcoholics.

- ✔ It's not recommended for use in pregnancy or by a nursing mother.

- ✔ When given in combination with the sulfonylureas, hypoglycemia can occur. If persistent, the dose of sulfonylurea is reduced.

Metformin can be a very useful drug, especially when *fasting hyperglycemia* (high blood glucose upon awakening) is present. Metformin has some positive effects on the blood fats, causing a decrease in triglycerides and LDL cholesterol and an increase in HDL cholesterol. About 10 percent of patients fail to respond to it when it is first used, and the secondary failure rate is 5 to 10 percent a year. It occasionally causes a decrease in the absorption of vitamin B12, a vitamin that is important for the blood and the nervous system.

Bristol-Myers Squibb, the makers of the brand name of metformin, Gluophage, have come up with two new preparations of metformin, which, they believe, have some advantages over the original drug. Because metformin had to be taken at each meal, they have produced a longer-acting preparation called Glucophage XR, which lasts for 24 hours. It comes in a 500 mg strength and helps overcome the problem of patients not taking their medication the required multiple times a day.

Their second new version of metformin is Glucovance. This pill combines glyburide, the sulfonylurea described previously, with metformin at a dose of 250 or 500 mg. The various combinations are 1.25 mg of glyburide with 250 mg metformin, 2.5 mg glyburide with 500 mg metformin, and 5 mg glyburide with 500 mg metformin. The advantage is the convenience of having to take only one pill instead of two. The company also claims that the combination works better than both drugs taken alone, although it is hard to see why this would be true.

Acarbose

Acarbose, brand name Precose, seems to have a lot greater popularity in Europe than it does in the United States. It's the first of a group of drugs called *alpha-glucosidase inhibitors*. These drugs block the action of an enzyme in the intestine that breaks down more complex carbohydrates into smaller molecules like glucose and fructose so that they can be absorbed. The result is that the rate of rise of glucose in the bloodstream is slowed after meals. These carbohydrates are eventually broken down by bacteria lower down in the intestine and produce a lot of gas, abdominal pain, and diarrhea, which are the major drawbacks to this drug.

The main characteristics of acarbose are

- It's supplied in 25, 50, and 100 mg strengths.
- The recommended starting dose is 25 mg at the beginning of each meal. This dose can be increased to 50 or 100 mg three times daily, depending on the blood glucose. The highest dose is not given unless the patient weighs more than 130 pounds.
- It does not cause hypoglycemia when used alone but does in combination with sulfonylureas. If hypoglycemia is persistent, the dose of sulfonylurea is decreased.
- It does not require insulin for its activity.
- Many people do not like it because of the gastrointestinal effects.
- The lowering of glucose and hemoglobin A1c is modest at most.

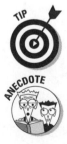

Because its action is to block the breakdown of complex carbohydrates, hypoglycemia occurring with acarbose and sulfonylurea combinations must be treated with a preparation of glucose, not more complex carbohydrates.

In my own practice, I have not found a use for acarbose. I tried it on a number of patients, and even though they started at a low dose and gradually built up to a more effective level, they complained about the gas and abdominal pain and asked me to take them off the drug. Because I was not seeing much change in the blood glucose, I did not object.

Thiazolidinediones (the glitazones)

This is the first group of drugs for diabetes that directly reverses insulin resistance.

Troglitazone

Troglitazone, brand name Rezulin (called Prelay outside the United States), was the first oral agent for type 2 diabetes that actually reversed the basic lesion in this disease, namely the insulin resistance. It does this by causing changes within the muscle and fat cells where the insulin resistance resides. These changes take several weeks to occur, and if troglitazone is stopped, they take several weeks to subside.

In March 2000, because of continuing occurrences of severe liver disease sometimes leading to death in a small number of patients taking troglitazone, the FDA removed troglitazone from the market. The other glitazone drugs currently on the market — rosiglitazone and pioglitazone — have not had this problem, although the FDA requires monitoring the patient's liver function when these drugs are first used.

Rosiglitazone

Rosiglitazone was the second thiazolidinedione to be approved by the FDA. It is marketed by Glaxo SmithKline as Avandia. The characteristics of rosiglitazone are:

- ✔ It's available as 2, 4, and 8 milligram tablets.

- ✔ Tablets are taken with or without food once a day.

- ✔ The recommended starting dose is 4 mg, and 8 mg is the maximum recommended dose. Increases in the dose are made no more often than every two to four weeks. Rosiglitazone may take three months or longer to have its maximum effect.

- ✔ Because it improves insulin resistance, rosiglitazone has its greatest effect on the blood glucose after eating, rather than the first morning glucose.

- ✔ Rosiglitazone is an excellent drug when used together with metformin or a sulfonylurea in a poorly controlled patient. You often need to reduce the dosage of sulfonylurea after a while because of hypoglycemia.

- ✔ If given to a patient on sulfonylurea or metformin, those drugs must not be stopped when the rosiglitazone is started.

- ✔ Rosiglitazone is insulin-sparing, meaning that the body does not have to make as much insulin to control the blood glucose when rosiglitazone is given.

- ✔ By itself, rosiglitazone does not cause hypoglycemia. It results in hypoglycemia only when combined with insulin or sulfonylurea.

Rosiglitazone can be extremely helpful in controlling blood glucose. So far, secondary failure, where this drug works initially but stops working later, does not seem to be a problem. A major advantage is that rosiglitazone needs to be taken only once a day, which greatly helps with one of the major problems in all medicine, namely compliance.

However, rosiglitazone does have some problems:

- ✔ Although rosiglitazone has not been shown to cause severe liver damage, the FDA requires that liver testing be done before starting treatment, every two months for the first year, and periodically thereafter. If the specific liver test called ALT rises more than three times the upper limit of normal, the drug must be stopped. So far, I have had no such problem after treating several hundreds of patients with this drug.

- ✔ It causes water retention and swelling of the ankles, especially in the older population, which some people do not find tolerable. Occasionally the drug is stopped for this reason. This water retention may also be responsible for a mild decrease in red blood cells called anemia.

- ✔ It should not be taken by a pregnant diabetic or a nursing mother.

- ✔ It's eliminated from the body almost entirely through the bowels, so no adjustment of the dose is needed when the kidneys are poorly functioning.

Rosiglitazone has been found to have unexpected effects in women of child-bearing age, specifically, an unintended pregnancy due to improved fertility. Many such women have reduced fertility as a result of insulin resistance. When these women take rosiglitazone, their fertility may improve, and they may become pregnant.

In my practice, I have found rosiglitazone to be an extremely valuable treatment in type 2 diabetes. I now use rosiglitazone as the initial treatment in all people with type 2 diabetes in whom diet and exercise are not successful and the blood glucose is still mildly to moderately elevated. I also add it to the treatment of a patient already on metformin or a sulfonylurea to improve control.

Pioglitazone

Pioglitazone, manufactured by Eli Lilly and Takeda in the U.S., was the third thiazoledinedione to come to market. It is called Actos, and its properties are the same as rosiglizone with the following differences:

- ✔ The initial dose is 15 mg once a day with or without food, but most patients require 30 or even 45 mg. It comes in all three sizes.

- ✔ In addition to restoring fertility in some women who are infertile due to insulin resistance, pioglitazone reduces estrogen levels in women taking estrogen and may result in making hormone-based contraception, such as the Pill or Depo-Provera, less effective.

✔ It is authorized for use alone, with insulin with metformin, or with a sulfonylurea.

Repaglinide

Repaglinide, brand name Prandin, is the last of the current group of new medications for type 2 diabetes. It's the first of a group of drugs called *meglitinides,* which are chemically unrelated to the sulfonylureas but work by squeezing more insulin out of the pancreas just like the sulfonylureas do. Repaglinide, however, is taken just before meals to stimulate insulin for only that meal.

The characteristics of repaglinide include:

✔ It is available as 0.5, 1, and 2 mg tablets taken just before or up to 30 minutes before meals.

✔ The starting dose is 0.5 mg with a mild elevation of blood glucose or 1 or 2 mg if the initial blood glucose is higher. The dose may be doubled once a week to a maximum of 4 mg before meals.

✔ Because it acts through insulin, it can cause hypoglycemia.

✔ It's not recommended in pregnancy or for nursing mothers.

✔ It's not used with the sulfonylureas but can be combined with metformin. Use in combination with rosiglitazone has not been studied.

✔ It lowers the blood glucose and the hemoglobin A1c effectively when used in combination with metformin.

✔ It's mostly broken down in the liver and leaves the body in the bowel movement. Therefore, if liver disease is present, the dose has to be adjusted downward.

✔ Despite the lack of excretion through the kidneys, increases in the dose have to be made more carefully when kidney impairment is present.

Experience with repaglinide has shown that it causes no problems when given with other medications. It's bound to protein in the blood, so other medications like aspirin, which also bind to protein, may, theoretically, increase its activity. I have not seen this as a problem with my patients who are on this medication.

Combining oral agents

As you might expect, taking one oral agent alone often does not control the blood glucose to the point where complications of diabetes are prevented. (This would be a hemoglobin A1c of less than 7 percent.) In this section, I explain to you how you can use several of these drugs together.

No drug should be taken as a convenient way of avoiding the basic diet and exercise that is the key to diabetic control. (See Chapters 8 and 9 for more information on these crucial points.)

I currently start all new type 2 patients who are mildly out of control on rosiglitazone. I give this medication at least eight weeks to work. Many patients need no more treatment than this in addition to their diet and exercise. I usually begin with a 4 mg dose and increase to 8 mg if the blood glucose is still elevated after four weeks. I check liver function before starting this drug and every two months thereafter.

If this dosage does not control the blood glucose, it's often the first morning glucose that is still elevated, the fasting blood glucose. Metformin is an excellent second drug to add at this point, usually at a dose of 500 mg with breakfast and supper, but most patients need 1,000 mg twice daily to achieve sufficient reduction of the glucose. Several articles in the medical literature have shown that rosiglitazone and metformin is a highly effective and safe combination.

When these two drugs still leave some lowering of blood glucose to be accomplished, then I add a sulfonylurea. I like to use a longer acting form such as glimepiride because I always prefer a drug that can be taken only once a day to drugs that require multiple dosing. That's one of the reasons I like rosiglitazone so much in addition to its effectiveness. I have found that 2 to 4 mg of glimepiride with the others is all the treatment needed to achieve the goal.

A few patients will still have elevated blood glucose and hemoglobin A1c levels, even with all the preceding treatments. For them, repaglinide in place of the sulfonylurea usually does the trick. Starting at 1 mg before each meal, this medication has been very helpful for those patients.

If low blood glucose starts to be a problem, then the dose of the sulfonylurea or repaglinide is lowered because the other medications are not responsible for hypoglycemia.

It is generally believed that the pancreas gradually fails to make insulin in type 2 diabetes and that most patients need insulin sooner or later (see the sidebar "Combining insulin and oral agents in type 2 diabetes"). My experience is that this is not necessarily true and that the modern medications, particularly the glitazones and metformin, can delay or eliminate the need for insulin. Certainly, numerous people with diabetes are well controlled with only a small dose of an oral medication. And I have seen many others who used insulin when nothing else was available but have come off insulin and do not appear as though they will ever need it again. Some people need no drugs at all, and some do well on one of the oral agents I discuss in the preceding sections.

Insulin

If you're a person with type 1 diabetes, insulin is your savior. If you have type 2 diabetes, you may need insulin late in the course of your disease. Insulin is a great drug, but it must be taken through a needle at the present time and that is the rub (or the pain). Inventors have come up with many different ways to administer insulin, but most people still use the old technique of a syringe and a needle. I tell you about the newer methods in this section. You may even want to consider switching to one of them because they are easier and possibly more accurate than the old method. However, the new syringes and needles are just about painless.

Until a few years ago, insulin could only be obtained by extracting it from the pancreas of cows, pigs, salmon, and some other animals. This was not entirely satisfactory because those insulins are slightly different from human insulin. Using them resulted in an immune reaction in the blood and certain skin reactions. The preparation was purified but there were always tiny amounts of impurities. In 1978 researchers were able to trick bacteria called E coli into making human insulin. Almost all insulin is now perfectly pure human insulin. In a short while, no insulin besides human insulin will be available.

How I would treat you

If you have had diabetes for a few years, chances are you are already taking a sulfonylurea but you are not well controlled. If you were to come to me, I would add a glitazone to your treatment. You would be amazed and delighted, as I have been, at the improvement that takes place.

Because most of the medications I discuss in this chapter are relatively new, you might come to me on both sulfonylurea and insulin treatment. (For more on insulin, see the section surrounding this sidebar.) As a specialist, I get the patients who are not in good control, so I usually have to adjust the medications. If you're being treated with insulin and sulfonylurea, I would add a glitazone. Within a week or two, your blood glucose levels would drop, and I would probably have to reduce the insulin dose. A few weeks after that, I might have to stop the insulin because the blood glucose levels would be continuing to fall.

Previously insulin came in two different strengths, U40 and U80, which meant 40 units per milliliter or 80 units per milliliter. This measurement was confusing, especially if the wrong syringe was used — you had to use a U40 syringe for U40 insulin. This double standard was eliminated in the United States, and now all insulin is U100 or 100 units per milliliter, and all syringes are U100 syringes. This standardization is not necessarily so in Europe or elsewhere, so check the strength of the insulin and the markings on the syringe.

In the human body, insulin is constantly responding to ups and downs in the blood glucose. No simple device is currently available to measure the blood glucose and give insulin as the pancreas does. In order to avoid having to take many shots a day, forms of insulin were invented to work at different times. These forms of insulin include

- **Rapid-acting lispro insulin:** The newest preparation and the shortest acting, lispro insulin (called Humalog insulin by its manufacturer, Eli Lilly) begins to lower the glucose within five minutes after its administration, peaks at about one hour, and is no longer active by about three hours. Lispro is a great advance because it frees the person with diabetes to take a shot just when he or she eats. With the previous short-acting insulin (regular insulin), a person had to take a shot and eat within 30 minutes or hypoglycemia might occur. Because its activity begins and ends so quickly, lispro does not cause hypoglycemia as often as the older preparations.

- **Short-acting regular insulin:** Regular insulin takes 30 minutes to start to lower the glucose, peaks at three hours, and is gone by six to eight hours. This insulin is the preparation that was used before meals to keep the glucose low until the next meal.

- **Intermediate-acting NPH or Lente insulins:** Both begin to lower the glucose within 2 hours of administration and continue their activity for 10 to 12 hours. They can be active for up to 24 hours. The purpose of this kind of insulin is to provide a smooth level of control over half the day so that a low level of active insulin is always in the body. This attempts to parallel the situation that exists in the human body.

- **Long-acting Ultralente insulin:** This insulin begins to act within 6 hours and provides a low level of insulin activity for up to 26 hours. It was invented to provide a smooth, basal level of control requiring only one shot a day. It can act differently in different people, looking more like intermediate insulin in some patients.

- **Long-acting insulin glargine:** Aventis is selling a new insulin called insulin glargine or Lantus. Studies have shown that insulin glargine has its onset in 1 to 2 hours after injection, and its activity lasts for 24 hours without a specific peak time of activity, which is exactly what is needed to control the blood glucose over an entire day. Insulin glargine is released in a smooth fashion from the site of injection, and it doesn't matter what part of the body is injected. Because of its smooth and predictable activity, insulin glargine does not often cause low blood glucose at night, which often happens with NPH insulin. I have used this insulin in a number of my patients with type 1 diabetes and have been extremely pleased with the results. I am now using it with all new type 1 diabetes patients.

TIP

If you do not have good diabetic control (hemoglobin A1c of 7 percent or less is good control) with NPH insulin, ask your doctor to consider using insulin glargine.

✔ **Premixed insulins:** These contain 70 percent NPH insulin and 30 percent regular or a 50-50 mixture. These insulins are helpful for people who have trouble mixing insulins in one syringe, have poor eyesight, or are stable on a preparation that does not change.

TIP

You need to know a few things that are common to all insulins:

✔ Insulin may be kept at room temperature for four weeks or in the refrigerator until the expiration date printed on the label. After four weeks at room temperature, it should be discarded.

✔ Insulin does not take too well to excessive heat, such as direct sunlight or excessive cold. Protect your insulin against these conditions.

✔ You can safely give an insulin shot through clothing.

✔ If you take less than 50 units in a shot, there are ½ cc syringes that make it easy to measure up to 50 units. The same is true if you take less than 30 units, which would use ³⁄₁₀ cc syringes.

✔ Shorter needles may be more comfortable, especially for children, but the depth of the injection helps to determine how fast the insulin works.

✔ You can reuse disposable syringes a couple of times.

✔ Used syringes and needles must be disposed of in a puncture-proof container that is sealed shut before being placed in the trash.

How to shoot yourself

Whatever the type, drawing up insulin is done in the same way. If you look at the syringe in Figure 10-1, you see that it's lined. Starting at the needle end of the syringe, you can see nine small lines above the needle, followed by a tenth longer line where the number 10 may be found. Each line is one unit of insulin up to ten units. Above the 10 unit line, you see a succession of four small lines followed by a larger line representing 15, 20, 25, and so on.

Combining insulin and oral agents in type 2 diabetes

Sometimes the characteristics of the currently available oral agents do not provide the tight control needed to avoid complications. This is particularly true after many years of type 2 diabetes. Then insulin may be required. Insulin may be added in a number of ways, but often a shot of NPH insulin at bedtime is all that is needed to start the day under control and continue it with oral agents. Rosiglitazone may control the day-time glucoses very well after eating, but the first morning glucose may need the overnight shot of NPH insulin.

As type 2 diabetes progresses, the oral agents may be less effective, and insulin is taken more often. Two shots a day of intermediate and short-acting insulin may do the trick. Usually you take two-thirds of the dose in the morning and one-third before supper because you need short-acting insulin to control the supper car-bohydrates. This is a situation where 75 percent protamine lispro (like NPH) and 25 percent lispro insulin may be useful, allowing the patient to measure from only one bottle. This combination is especially valuable in the older person with diabetes, where the tightest level of control is not being sought because the expected lifespan of the patient is shorter than the time necessary to develop complications. In this patient, doctors want to prevent problems like frequent urination leading to loss of sleep or vaginal infections, so they give enough to treat this but not so much that a frail, elderly patient is having hypoglycemia on a frequent basis.

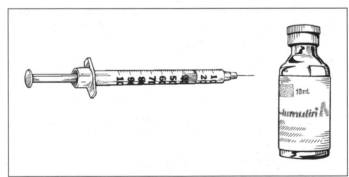

Figure 10-1:
The insulin syringe and bottle.

If the insulin is lispro or regular, it should be clear and you do not have to shake the bottle. The other kinds of insulin are cloudy, and you need to shake the bottle a few times to suspend the tiny particles in the liquid. A new bottle has a cap on the top, which you break off and discard. When you're ready to take insulin, wipe the rubber stopper in the top of the bottle with alcohol.

Pull up the number of units of air that corresponds to the number of units of insulin you need to take. Turn the insulin bottle upside down and penetrate the rubber stopper with the needle of the syringe. Push all the air inside and pull out the insulin dose you need. Because air replaces the insulin, the pressure inside the bottle is unchanged, and no vacuum is created. Check and make sure that you have the right amount of the right insulin and no air bubbles in the syringe.

To give the injection, use alcohol to wipe off an area of skin on the arm, the chest, the stomach, or wherever you're injecting it. Insert the needle at a right angle to the skin and push it in. When the needle has penetrated the skin, push the plunger of the syringe down to zero to administer the insulin.

If you're taking two kinds of insulin at the same time, you can mix them in one syringe, thus avoiding two shots. Here's how you do that:

1. **Wipe both bottles with alcohol.**
2. **Draw up the total units of air corresponding to the total insulin you need.**
3. **Push the units of air into the longer acting insulin bottle that correspond to the number of units of longer acting insulin that you need and withdraw the needle.**
4. **Push the rest of the units of air into the shorter acting insulin bottle and withdraw the correct units of insulin.**
5. **Go back to the longer acting bottle and withdraw the correct units of insulin from there.**

    By doing this, you do not contaminate the shorter acting insulin with the additive in the longer-acting insulin.

Where you inject the insulin helps determine how fast it will work. Insulin injected into the abdomen is most rapidly absorbed, followed by the arms and legs and then the buttocks. You might use these differing rates of uptake of the insulin to get faster action when your blood glucose is high. If the body part that gets the insulin is exercised, the insulin enters more quickly. If you use the same site repeatedly, the absorption rate slows down, so rotate the sites.

When you inject the insulin helps to determine the smoothness of your glucose control. The more regular you are in your injections, your eating, and your exercise, the smoother your glucose level.

Conducting intensive insulin treatment

Intensive insulin treatment is essential in type 1 diabetes if you hope to prevent the complications of the disease. This means measuring your blood glucose at least before each meal and at bedtime and using both short-acting and longer-acting insulin to keep the blood glucose between 80 and 100 before meals and less than 140 after eating. How you do this is the subject of this section.

ANECDOTE

Carbohydrate counting to maximum health

To find out how you can accomplish carbohydrate counting in everyday life, take a typical type 1 patient. Salvatore Law is a 41-year-old who has had type 1 diabetes for 31 years. He has been well controlled because he follows a good diet, does lots of exercise, and takes his insulin appropriately. He takes 30 units of insulin glargine at bedtime. He has a list of dosages of lispro insulin that tell him to take 1 unit of insulin for each 20 grams of carbohydrate. He is about to have breakfast and knows that it will contain 80 grams of carbohydrate. Therefore, he needs four units of lispro insulin. He measures his blood glucose before breakfast and finds that it is 202 mg/dl. His doctor has told him to take an extra unit of lispro insulin for each 50 mg/dl above 100 mg/dl. He adds two more units for a total of six units of insulin taken just before breakfast.

At lunch, his blood glucose measures 58. He is about to have a lunch of 120 grams of carbohydrate, so he needs 6 units for that, but he reduces it by 1 unit for the low measurement that is approximately 50 mg/dl lower than 100 for a final dose of 5 units.

Before supper, Law's blood glucose measures 120. His supper contains only 60 grams of carbohydrate, so he needs 3 units for that. He does not have to adjust the dose because the glucose is close to 100, so he takes only 3 units. When he measures his blood glucose at bedtime, it's 108, so he is doing very well. Unless the blood glucose is 200 or greater, he does not need to take any bedtime lispro because he is taking insulin glargine to control his glucose overnight.

In the human body (except in type 1 diabetes), a small amount of circulating insulin is always present in the bloodstream and, after eating, insulin increases temporarily to control the glucose in the meal. Intensive insulin treatment attempts to mirror the normal human pancreas as much as possible.

In intensive insulin treatment, you usually take a certain amount of longer-acting insulin (I prefer insulin glargine because it produces a smooth basal level of glucose control over 24 hours) at bedtime. In addition, you take a dose of rapid-acting insulin before each meal. I prefer lispro because it is more convenient and less hypoglycemia occurs. The dose of lispro is determined by the expected grams of carbohydrates in the meal about to be taken plus the blood glucose at that moment. Your doctor should provide you with a list of how much insulin to take for a given situation. Each patient is different, and this must be individualized.

When you use the carbohydrates in the meal to determine the insulin dose, it is called *carbohydrate counting*. You can quickly figure out how much carbohydrate is in each meal if you know how large your portion is and how much carbohydrate is in it. This calculation is especially easy for breakfast because most people eat the same things at breakfast time. It gets harder at lunch and supper, when meals tend to be different, but a little practice makes carbohydrate counting not too difficult then either.

Then you need to know how many grams of carbohydrate are controlled by each unit of insulin. For example, one person may need 1 unit to control 20 grams of carbohydrate, while another person needs 1 unit to control 15 grams of carbohydrate. If both of them eat a breakfast of 75 grams of carbohydrate, the first person might take 4 units of lispro, while the second person takes 5 units of lispro. Then additional units are added for the amount that the blood glucose needs to be lowered. A typical schedule is to take 1 unit for every 50 mg/dl that the blood glucose is above 100 mg/dl. Insulin can also be subtracted if the blood glucose is too low. For every 50 mg/dl that the glucose is below 100, subtract 1 unit. (To see how carbohydrate counting works in practice, see the sidebar "Carbohydrate counting to maximum health".)

The key to this system is to know the carbohydrates in your food. Here is where you make use of your friendly dietitian, who can go over your food preferences and show you how many carbohydrates are in them. The dietitian can also show you where to find carbohydrate counts for any other foods that you might eat.

By measuring your blood glucose frequently, you can find out how different carbohydrates affect your blood glucose. By using the carbohydrate sources that have a low glycemic index, you will need to use less insulin to control them. (See Chapter 8 for more on carbohydrates.)

In an attempt to mirror normal insulin and glucose dynamics, you often have to deal with a greater frequency of hypoglycemia. The best way to handle hypoglycemia is by eating slightly smaller meals and using the unused calories as between-meal snacks. This technique smoothes out the ups and downs.

At what point do you adjust your insulin glargine? If you find that several mornings in a row your fasting blood glucose is too high, you might add a unit or two to your bedtime glargine. If it's too low, you might reduce your insulin glargine by a unit or two or try eating a small bedtime snack. A high blood glucose level throughout the day is an indication to raise the glargine. Getting a lot of hypoglycemia at different times of day is a reason to lower the glargine. These adjustments are best done in consultation with your doctor, but sometimes your doctor is not available or you are away. As a knowledgeable person, you can make these adjustments on your own.

Adjusting insulin when you travel

Time changes of under three hours require no modifications, but changes above three hours require progressively more, and you should probably discuss these with your physician before you go.

As you travel through time zones, you lose or gain hours in the day, depending upon the direction. From California to New York, for example, you lose three hours. Say that you're taking the red-eye flight at 10 p.m. from San Francisco, arriving at 6 a.m. at Kennedy Airport. If you are taking insulin glargine, you do not have to change your dose. Just start using lispro at the beginning of your meals, which is earlier than on the West Coast. If you're returning to California, you can add three hours to your day. In this case, you need to make an extra measurement of your blood glucose. If it's around 150, you need do nothing, but if it's 200 or more, you can take a couple of units of lispro insulin to bring it down. If your blood glucose is much below 100, you can take a small snack. Again, you do not have to adjust your insulin glargine.

Delivering insulin with a pen

Several manufacturers, including Eli Lilly, Novo Nordisk, and Becton Dickinson, have sought ways to make delivering insulin easier. The insulin pen, shown in Figure 10-2, is one useful tool. Either the pen comes with the cartridge already inserted or the cartridge is placed inside the pen just like the old ink cartridges used to be put in pens. Each cartridge contains 1.5 or 3.0 milliliters of either NPH, regular, lispro, or a mixture of NPH-like lispro and lispro (such as 75 percent NPH-like lispro and 25 percent lispro). You can then dial the amount of insulin that you need to take. Each unit (sometimes two units) is accompanied by a clicking sound so that the visually impaired can hear the number of units. The units also appear in a window on the pen. If you take too many units, one of the pens forces you to waste the insulin by pushing it out of the needle while the other allows you to reset the pen and start again. Depending on the pen, you can deliver from 30 to 70 units of insulin. You screw on a new needle as needed.

Patients tell me that whether they use the Eli Lilly or the Novo Nordisk pen, the Novo Fine Pen Needles are less painful to use.

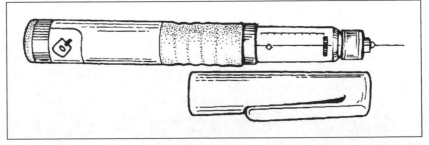

Figure 10-2:
The insulin
pen.

Should you shift from your syringe and needle to a pen? If you're comfortable with the syringe and needle and feel your technique is accurate, you probably have no reason to do so. If you're new to insulin, have some visual impairment, or feel that you're not getting an accurate measurement of the insulin, then a pen may be the solution for you.

Delivering insulin with a jet injection device

Jet injection devices (see Figure 10-3) are for the person who just can't stick a needle into his or her skin. At around $1,000 or more, they're expensive, but they last a long time and replace the syringe and needle. They're made by at least three different manufacturers.

The leading manufacturer is Antares Pharma, formerly Medi-Ject Corporation. They make a device called the Medijector Vision that is easy to dose, has a safety lock on it so the insulin is not delivered until it is fully measured, and uses the newer technology of so-called needle free syringes. This is a advance that allows the patient to see the insulin and does not require washing a stainless-steel nozzle. (The stainless-steel nozzle was a feature of the older jet injection devices that had to be cleaned regularly or else the correct dose of insulin might not be delivered.)

Activa Corporation makes the Advanta Jet injection device. They make the Gentle Jet for children and the Advanta Jet ES for especially tough skin. However they continue to use the old stainless-steel technology, which puts their device at a disadvantage.

Bioject makes devices that are similar to the Medijector. Their current device is the VitaJet 3. It uses the newer technology but may not be as easy to dose as the Medijector.

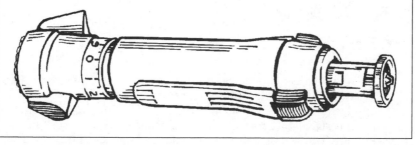

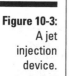

Figure 10-3:
A jet injection device.

A large quantity of insulin is taken into the injection device, enough for multiple treatments. The amount of insulin to be delivered is measured, usually by rotating one part of the device while the number of units to be delivered appears in a window. The device is held against the skin. With the press of a button, a powerful jet of air forces the insulin through the skin into the subcutaneous tissue, usually with no pain perceived by the patient. The devices come in a lower power form for smaller children. These devices can deliver up to 50 units at one time.

Should you try an insulin jet injector? If you have no trouble with the syringe and needle or find the pen to be an easy substitute, you don't need a jet injector. If you hate needles or need to give frequent shots to a small child who is very resistant to them, then a jet injector may solve your problems.

Delivering insulin with an external pump

For some people — and you may be one of them — the external insulin pump (see Figure 10-4) is the answer to their prayers. These devices are as close as you currently can come to the gradual administration of rapid-acting insulin that is normally taking place in the body. They're expensive, costing more than $4,000, but the insulin pump may be the answer for patients who simply cannot achieve good glucose control with syringes, pens, or jet injectors.

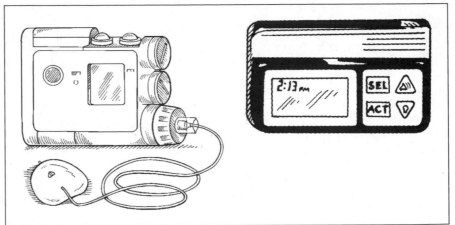

Figure 10-4:
The insulin pump with its infusion set.

Currently, three companies, Animas, MiniMed, and Disetronic Medical Systems sell these pumps, which are the size of a pager. Inside the pump is a motor. A syringe filled with short-acting insulin is placed within the pump, with the plunger against a screw that slowly pushes it down to push insulin out of the syringe. The end of the syringe is attached to a short tube, which ends in a needle pushed into the skin of the abdomen. Insulin is slowly pushed under the skin.

The rate at which insulin slowly enters the abdomen is called the *basal rate*. It can be set, by way of computer chips, to vary as often as every half hour to an hour. For example, from 8 a.m. to 9 a.m., the pump may deliver 0.8 units, while from 9 a.m. to 10 a.m., the pump may deliver 1.0 units, depending upon the needs of the patient. This amount is determined, of course, by measuring the blood glucose with a meter (see Chapter 7).

When a meal is about to be eaten, the patient can push a button to deliver extra insulin, called a *bolus* of insulin. (The amount is determined by carbohydrate counting.) You can get extra insulin if the blood glucose is too high at any time.

Pump usage has its advantages:

- ✔ It's flexible because the bolus is taken just before the meal.

- ✔ It often smoothes out the swings of glucose during the day because the insulin is administered slowly and in small doses.

- ✔ It can be rapidly disconnected and reconnected to take a shower or swim but can take a little getting used to when worn to bed.

- ✔ It's safe from overdosage because it has built-in protective devices to prevent this occurrence.

On the other hand, pump usage has definite disadvantages besides the high cost:

- ✔ Infections of the skin are frequent because the infusion set is left in place for several days. These infections are usually mild, however.

- ✔ Overall diabetic control is not necessarily better with the pump than with other ways of delivering insulin, especially with the new insulin glargine.

- ✔ Because short-acting insulin is the only form the patient receives, if insulin stops entering, ketoacidosis may come on rapidly (see Chapter 4).

- ✔ Some patients are allergic to the tape that holds the infusion set on to the abdomen.

- ✔ Blood glucose must be measured often to adjust the pump for optimal control.

Pump usage is definitely not treatment to be done on your own at the beginning. You need a diabetologist to help with dosages, a dietician to help with amounts of boluses based upon carbohydrate intake, and someone from the manufacturer to teach you how to set the pump and to be there for any malfunctions.

Is an insulin pump for you? If you're willing to invest the time and effort at first, if your schedule is very uncertain particularly with respect to meals, and if your control has not been good with other means, you should look into this option.

My experience with my patients has generally been positive. None of them are willing to give up the pump now that they have it. Occasionally, they disconnect the pump to allow their skin to heal. They have generally shown improved control and a better hemoglobin A1c.

Do I recommend using an insulin pump? With the new form of insulin called insulin glargine, you can accomplish a continuous basal control of the blood glucose much like the pump does. The pump proponents say that you need to be able to alter the basal dose for different conditions throughout the day and you can't do that with a single shot of insulin. Although this is true, I am not sure that it makes a great difference in the course of controlling the blood glucose.

Is one pump better than another? All seem to have excellent mechanical features, and all provide you with the ability to adjust your insulin in numerous ways. They all have alarms for any eventuality like blockage of the tube, an electrical failure, and so forth. They try to differentiate themselves by offering different options for how the insulin is delivered, but you may find that you need the help of a rocket scientist to figure them out.

Aids to insulin delivery

For those of you still using the old needle and syringe method, I want you to be aware of the numerous aids that can make it easier for you to take your insulin:

- **Spring-loaded syringe holders:** You place your syringe in the holder, hold it against the skin, and press a button. The needle enters, and you've administered the insulin.
- **Syringe magnifiers:** These help the visually impaired administer insulin.
- **Syringe-filling devices:** You can feel and hear a click as you take up insulin.
- **Needle guides:** You can use these guides when you can't see the rubber part of the insulin bottle to insert the needle to take up the insulin.

You can call your branch of the American Diabetes Association or look in the back of the ADA's Diabetes Forecast magazine to find sources for these products.

Avoiding Drug Interactions

In some studies, patients are taking as many as four to five drugs, including their diabetes medications. These drugs often interact and end up costing more than $4 billion in drug toxicity costs. Sometimes (believe it or not) even your doctor is not aware of the interactions of common drugs. You need to know the names of all the drugs you take and whether they affect one another.

Many common medications used for the treatment of high blood pressure also raise the blood glucose, sometimes bringing out a diabetic tendency that might otherwise not have been recognized:

- **Thiazide diuretics** often raise the glucose by causing a loss of potassium. Among these drugs are Diuril, hydroDiuril, Oretic, and Zaroxolyn.

- **Beta blockers** reduce the release of insulin and include such drugs as Inderal, Lopressor, and Tenormin.

- **Calcium channel blockers** also reduce insulin secretion and include Adalat, Calan, Cardizem, Isoptin, Norvasc, and Procardia.

- **Minoxidil** can raise blood glucose.

Drugs used for other purposes can also raise blood glucose:

- **Corticosteroids,** even topical use, can raise blood glucose (see Chapter 2 for more on corticosteroids).

- **Cyclosporine,** used to prevent organ rejection, can raise the blood glucose by poisoning the insulin-producing beta cell.

- **Diphenylhydantoin,** known as Dilantin, is a drug for seizures and blocks insulin release.

- **Oral contraceptives** were accused of causing hyperglycemia when the dose of estrogen was very high, but current preparations are not a problem.

- **Nicotinic acid and niacin,** used to lower cholesterol, can bring out a hyperglycemic tendency.

- **Phenothiazines,** such as Compazine, Serentil, Stelazine, and Thorazine, can block insulin secretion and cause hyperglycemia.

- **Thyroid hormone,** in elevated levels, raise the blood glucose by reducing insulin from the pancreas.

Many common medications, either on their own or by doing something to make the oral hypoglycemic agents more potent, also lower the blood glucose. The most important of these include the following:

- **Salicylates and acetaminophen,** known as Aspirin and Tylenol, both can lower the blood glucose, especially when given in large doses.

- **Ethanol,** in any form of alcohol, can lower the blood glucose, particularly when taken without food.

- **Angiotensin converting enzyme inhibitors,** used for high blood pressure, such as Accupril, Captopril, Lotensin, Monopril, Prinivil, Vasotec, and Zestril, can lower the blood glucose, though the mechanism is unclear.

    ✔ **Alpha-blockers,** another group of antihypertensives that includes Prazosin, lower the glucose as well.

    ✔ **Fibric acid derivatives** like Clofibrate, used to treat disorders of fat, cause a lowering of blood glucose.

 If you start a new medication and suddenly find that your blood glucose is significantly higher or lower than usual, ask your doctor to check for the possibility that the new medication has a definite glucose-lowering or glucose-raising effect.

Acquiring Financial Assistance for Medications

Diabetes can be expensive, especially if you need several drugs to control your blood glucose. The pharmaceutical companies understand, and several offer programs to provide medication for a period of time. Table 10-1 tells you what you need to know about these companies.

Table 10-1	How You Can Get Financial Help	
Company	*Program Name*	*Phone Number*
Bayer Corporation (acarbose)	Indigent Patient	800-998-9180
Bristol-Myers Squibb (metformin)	Patient Assistance	800-437-0994
Eli Lilly and Company (all insulin preparations)	Lilly Cares	800-545-6962
Aventis (glyburide, glimepiride, Lantus)	Patient Assistance	800-221-4025
Novo-Nordisk (insulin preparations)	Indigent Program	800-727-6500
Pfizer (glipizide, glipizide extended release, chlorpropamide)	Pfizer Prescription Assistance	800-646-4455

 What all these programs have in common is that they require you to get a prescription from your doctor. The doctor usually fills out forms that state that the patient meets the financial requirements and needs the drug. Not all companies give away free drugs for life. If you cannot afford to buy a drug that you're taking, do not hesitate to call the company and ask whether it has a patient-assistance program.

Chapter 11

Diabetes Is Your Show

· ·

In This Chapter

▶ Presenting you, the author, the producer, the director, and the star

▶ Using your primary physician — your assistant director

▶ Taking advantage of the diabetologist or endocrinologist — your technical consultant

▶ Seeing your eye doctor — your lighting designer

▶ Employing your foot doctor — your dance instructor

▶ Engaging your dietitian — your food services provider

▶ Getting information from your diabetes educator — your researcher

▶ Listening to the pharmacist — your usher

▶ Using your mental health worker — your supporting actor

▶ Inviting your family and friends — your captivated and caring audience

· ·

Shakespeare said it: "All the world's a stage." Certainly your diabetes fits that description beautifully. You have many roles in life, and one of them is the role of a person with diabetes. As with any role, you're not expected to play it alone. You have a large cast and crew, all of whom are eager to help you, but you must be willing to ask for their help and know how to use them so that they can give you their best. Believe me, as a member of that crew, everyone wants to give you their best.

The question is, do you want your play to be a comedy or a tragedy? Because you hold all the major positions, it's entirely up to you. And remember, like all plays, there is a life off of the stage. Your role as a person with diabetes is one of many, including brother or sister, mother or father, boss or employee, and so on. Fortunately, the life skills that you discover as someone with diabetes are applicable to all your other roles.

You Are the Author, the Producer, the Director, and the Star

Being the author, the producer, the director, and the star may seem like a lot of responsibility — and it is. Unlike many short-term illnesses where the doctor knows what has to be done, instructs you to do it, writes a prescription, and you're cured, diabetes is your daily companion for life. No one, not even your mother or spouse, can be with you all of the time. Therefore, you're the one who writes the script and the action. You decide whether you'll take your medication or exercise regularly. You determine whether you'll follow a diet that will control your weight and your blood glucose.

You're the one who needs to gather the resources needed to play the role properly. In this sense, you're the producer. You need your props and your theater, the equipment, the medications, and the environment in which to manage your diabetes. Your environment may be a comfortable home where you can eat the proper diet and a good exercise facility where you can burn up calories while you strengthen your heart. Or it may be the sidewalk where you can safely walk or jog.

Once you have the resources, you need to direct your cast and crew to make your play come out the way you envision it. You're the one who sees to it that the primary physician obtains a hemoglobin A1c every three or four months and that he or she sends you to the eye doctor at least once a year. The physician is dealing with many patients each day and can easily forget your specific needs. You must let the doctor know what your needs are and not expect the doctor to read your mind. You may be dealing with other doctors who treat your heart, your lungs, and other parts of you. Each doctor needs to know all the medications you take.

Finally, you're the star of the show. That role is both an honor and a responsibility. Although you may wish that you had never been chosen for this particular role, there it is. You can make of it what you will. You can learn all your lines (understand your disease) and speak them fluently (take your medications, follow your diet, and so on) or not. Obviously, not studying your lines is a lot easier, but in that case, the result can be a tragedy. Take proper care of yourself, and the smile on your face and that of all your fellow cast members and crew will clearly indicate that you have written, produced, directed, and starred in a comedy.

The Primary Physician — Your Assistant Director

Your primary physician takes on a new role in diabetes, where he or she becomes a facilitator. In the United States, where you can find numerous specialists, a specialist follows only 8 percent of people with diabetes regularly. The other 92 percent are in the hands of more general doctors who have to deal with many other illnesses besides diabetes. This is a consequence of the large size of the diabetic population and the requirements of a healthcare system with limited resources.

While using a primary physician instead of a specialist may seem not conducive to the best care, I can say many good things about it. Remember, you're a person who has diabetes. Other things can go wrong, and the primary physician can handle them as well. Your mild heart disease may not require a cardiologist, and your primary physician can also manage your bronchitis very well.

You should expect your primary physician to have a decent working knowledge of diabetes. Chapter 7 describes the proper way to follow a person with diabetes. The various tests are essential to your health, and the primary physician must know which ones to order and when to send you to a specialist because your needs are beyond his or her expertise.

The Diabetologist or Endocrinologist — Your Technical Consultant

Your diabetologist or endocrinologist should have the most in depth knowledge of the management of diabetes. He or she has had advanced training for several years after the years of training in general internal medicine and has devoted years to taking care of people with diabetes plus a few other kinds of patients. The *diabetologist* is an endocrinologist who only takes care of diabetic patients and not thyroid cases or adrenal cases or the other diseases of other glands of the body.

The person with type 1 diabetes will certainly see an endocrinologist sooner or later. If the person with type 2 diabetes gets into trouble with complications or control, the endocrinologist will be called in for consultation. You have the right to expect that this physician will be able to answer most questions that arise during the care of diabetes.

This doctor will be up on the newest treatments for diabetes, so if you have questions about the future of diabetes care, ask them here. This doctor should also have the best understanding of all the drugs currently used for diabetes, how they interact with each other, their side effects, and other drugs that interact with them.

If you're not satisfied with the answers you're getting from your primary physician, then you need to ask for a referral to a specialist. Many health plans today try to steer you away from the specialist because this doctor orders more expensive tests and costs more to see by virtue of the extra years of specialty training. Do not take no for an answer. If your primary doctor will not refer you, find one who will.

You should also be sure that any changes made with the diabetologist are reported to the primary physician. One of the big problems in medicine is the lack of communication between medical care providers of all types, not just doctors.

For your own sake, make sure that all your medical care providers know what the others are doing for you.

The Eye Doctor — Your Lighting Designer

The eye doctor *(ophthalmologist or optometrist)* is the one who ensures that your diabetes will not damage your vision. This doctor has had advanced training in diseases of the eye. Your primary care physician must see (no pun intended) to it that you have an examination by this specialist at least once a year and more often if necessary.

An ophthalmologist or optometrist must dilate the pupils of the eyes in order to do a proper examination.

The eye doctor examines you for the conditions I outline in Chapter 5. He or she must send a report to your primary care physician. He or she should also take the opportunity to educate you about diabetic eye disease.

Sometimes the good deed of restoring vision leads to unexpected, negative consequences. One ophthalmologist I talked to told me that he restored the vision of a diabetic patient, only to have the patient buy a gun and nearly shoot someone with whom he had a grievance.

The Foot Doctor — Your Dance Instructor

The foot doctor or podiatrist is your best source of help with the minor and some of the major foot problems that all people suffer. You should go to him or her with such problems as toenails that are hard to cut, corns and calluses, and certainly any ulcer or infection of your foot. This is especially true if you have any neuropathy (see Chapter 5). In that case, you're better off not trying to cut your toenails by yourself.

Foot doctors I spoke with emphasized that the earlier you see this doctor, the less likely that a minor problem will be converted into a major disaster.

The doctor can tell you which preparations you should not use on your skin. He or she can show you how important it is that you give lesions time to heal and not to rush to put weight on your injured feet. Many podiatrists also give you a list of dos and don'ts for the proper care of your feet, such as conducting daily inspections, avoiding extreme heat, and so on. Chapter 5 details all the things you need to do to preserve good foot health.

The Dietitian — Your Food Services Provider

This person serves one of the most important roles in your care. Because most diabetes is type 2 and type 2 is greatly worsened by obesity, a good dietitian can really help you to control your blood glucose both by eating the right foods and amounts and helping you to lose weight. The dietitian can also show you which foods belong to which energy source — carbohydrate, protein, and fat. (See Chapter 8 for more on your diet.)

The person with type 1 diabetes needs to know how food interacts with the insulin injections that are mandatory. The dietitian can teach you to count carbohydrates so that you know how much insulin to take for your meals. (See Chapter 10 for more on carbohydrate counting.)

A good dietitian usually holds up a mirror to you, showing you not only what you eat but how you eat as well. When do you consume most of your calories, and where do they come from? All ethnic foods can be adjusted so that you enjoy the foods you have always eaten while you stay within the bounds of a diabetic diet. A good dietitian is the best source for this kind of information.

The dietitian can also show you what a portion of food really means. This demonstration is an eye-opener in most cases. You usually find that you have been eating portions much larger than necessary. Unfortunately, when it comes to a diabetic diet, you can't have your cake and eat it, too. But you can see in the section on gourmet eating for people with diabetes (see Appendix A) that every culture makes delicious food that is actually good for the person with diabetes.

One thing you want to be sure of is that the dietitian is flexible in his or her approach to food. There are a few rules about where your calories should come from, but you have plenty of room for variation within those rules. The diet you are ultimately given should take into account your preferences as well as the fact that the amount of carbohydrate, protein, and fat is different for different individuals. Any dietitian who simply hands you a printed diet and says, "Go follow it" is doing you no favor.

The Diabetes Educator — Your Researcher

Every person in your play is actually an educator in addition to his or her other role, but this person is especially trained to teach you what you need to know about every aspect of diabetes so that you properly take care of yourself. He or she should have CDE (Certified Diabetes Educator) after his or her name. A CDE has taken extensive courses in diabetes and has passed an examination.

A diabetes educator teaches you how to take your insulin or pills, how to test your blood glucose, and how to acquire any of the other skills you need. You can find many diabetes educators in a Diabetes Education Program. Once you have gotten over the shock of having diabetes, asking your primary physician to refer you to such a program is a good idea. After you have gone through the program, go back and update yourself. New drugs and new procedures are constantly being discovered. The diabetes educator can be a wonderful source of information about these, while making sure that you continue in your good diabetic habits.

The Pharmacist — Your Usher

The role of the usher may not sound important, but how will you enjoy the play if you cannot find your seat? The pharmacist is your guide to all the medications and tools required to control your blood glucose and manage any complications that you develop. He or she ushers you into the use of all these strange and new products. You may see your pharmacist more often than you see any other of your cast and crew who are actually in the medical field.

Each time you start a new medication, a good pharmacist checks to make sure that it does not conflict with other medicines you are taking. The pharmacist tells you about side effects and makes sure that your doctor is checking you for adverse drug reactions or interactions. The pharmacist may give you a printout that you can take home and refer to, telling you all you need to know about your new medication.

Many pharmacists also prepare a list of medications that you take, telling you each drug's strengths and dosage frequency. You can carry this around in case any doctor ever needs to know what you take.

Modern pharmacists are also doing a lot of education. Posters in the pharmacy explain diseases and drugs. Pharmacists can tell you about helpful over-the-counter drugs that your doctor doesn't prescribe. They are also often aware of new drugs and treatments before they become well known. Some pharmacies have blood pressure devices that you can use for free or glucose meters.

The Mental Health Worker — Your Supporting Actor

Your mental health worker may be a psychiatrist, a psychologist, or a social worker, or your primary physician may play this role. This person comes in handy whenever you have days when you feel you just can't cope. (See Chapter 1 for more about dealing with the emotional aspects of diabetes.) The mental health worker is there at those times to support you and get you going again. Diabetes certainly proves the fact that all disease is both physical and emotional.

Your Family and Friends — Your Captivated and Caring Audience

Your audience is the people you live with, eat with, and play with. Your family and friends can be a tremendous source of help, but you must clue them to the fact that you have diabetes. If you have type 1 diabetes, you can teach them how to recognize when your glucose is too low, in case you're ever too ill to take care of yourself. If you're type 2, ask them to moderate their diet so that you can follow yours. A diabetic diet is good for anyone. Complying with your diet is difficult enough, and you don't need your family exposing you to high-calorie foods.

Your family or friends can also become your exercise partner. Sticking to a program is a lot easier when a partner is counting on you to show up to work out. Your family and friends can also accompany you when you visit the doctor and remind you to ask the doctor a question or to follow the instructions you received.

Let these people know about your diabetes and buy them a copy of this book so that they understand something about what you are going through and how they can best help you.

Chapter 12

Putting Your Knowledge to Work for You

*I*f you read this entire part, you now know as much as the experts. But knowing is often quite a distance from doing. If this fact were not the case, the world would be a much better place to live in because everyone knows what needs to be done. They just don't do it.

The key thing is to get going on it now. Don't wait another day to begin to do the things that can prolong your life and increase its quality at the same time. You don't want to regret your life the way poor George Burns did. When a beautiful girl walked into his hotel room and said, "I'm sorry, I must be in the wrong room," he told her, "No, you're not in the wrong room. You are just 40 years too late."

Developing Positive Thinking

Studies have shown fairly conclusively that if you start with a positive frame of mind, your body can work with you and not against you. Even when things go wrong, if you're optimistic, you can pick yourself up and move forward. If you're pessimistic, you can become depressed and believe that nothing will help you. That kind of attitude is not conducive to good control of your blood glucose and avoidance of complications.

I have a patient who came to me to improve his glucose control just after having a toe amputated. This is a patient who sees a lot of manure and knows there is a beautiful horse in the area. He refuses to believe that a temporary setback is a permanent defeat. I got him on a program of tight diabetic control with the newer oral medications. His eyes have gotten better and his neuropathy (see Chapter 5) has improved. He believes in his ability to control his blood glucose, and all his actions are directed toward doing just that. The result has been an amazing turnaround in his hemoglobin A1c. With his attitude, he is willing to make the changes necessary because he knows they will pay big dividends for his health.

Achieving a positive attitude has a lot to do with how you interpret problems. If you see them as permanent and unchangeable because of a flaw in your own character, then you will have trouble being positive. If you see them as temporary and the result of something you can change given enough time, you will be much more optimistic and able to solve most problems.

Monitoring and Testing

Many of my patients ask me about a cure for diabetes. One doesn't exist yet, but the future looks very promising. So far, doctors don't have a portable machine that can measure the blood glucose and respond with the right amount of insulin. Such a gadget would not be of much use for the people who take pills anyway. Therefore, you have to use your brain to make the calculation that your pancreas would do automatically if it could. The calculation is, of course, how much medicine to take for a given glucose. To make the calculation, you need to know the glucose. This is where monitoring comes in.

Without fail, you should have one of the monitors that I describe in Chapter 7. If you have type 1 diabetes, you need to monitor before meals and at bedtime at least. If you have type 2 diabetes, you can get away with a couple of tests daily and sometimes even less if you're stable.

Chapter 10 is where you can find what you should do in response to your test results. If you or your doctor are computer literate, you will do much better with a meter that can be downloaded into a computer. What you look for are trends, and the computer makes it simple to see trends. It can look at dozens of tests at once on a screen, compared to turning pages of a booklet containing your blood glucose readings.

Remember, however, that blood glucose tests are only a moment in time. What you need to know is whether you are in control 24 hours a day. That is where the hemoglobin A1c comes in. Your doctor should order this test at least every four months if you're stable and every three months if not. If you have close to normal results in this test, you do not have to worry about long-term complications (see Chapter 5) and will probably not be suffering from short-term complications (see Chapter 4) either.

Even with near-normal hemoglobin A1c results, you still want to be checked for any sign of complications. That means regular eye examinations, regular blood and urine tests for kidney damage, and regular tests for sensation in your feet. Your doctor should do this on schedule, and, if not, you have to remind the doctor.

Great treatment exists for every diabetic complication, and the earlier the treatment is started, the less likely the complication will lead to serious damage. Routine monitoring and testing allow you to discover the problem as early as possible.

Using Medications

Medications can be tricky. Some of them are very potent, but none of them work if you don't take them. Doctors use the word "noncompliance" when they talk about the tendency of patients not to take their medications. When it comes to postmenopausal women, for example, only about 30 percent take their estrogens. Not a good idea. Some of the things you need to know when you take your medications include

✔ Are you taking the right dose at the right time?

✔ Are you taking it with or without food depending upon the medication?

✔ Does it mix with your other medications?

✔ Are you aware of side effects, and are they being monitored?

✔ Can the desired effect sometimes be too strong?

✔ Do you have an antidote to its effect available if necessary?

✔ Do you need to adjust the dose when you're not feeling well?

Your doctor, your pharmacist, and your diabetes educator can all help you with your medications, but you're on your own when it comes to taking them. If you have trouble remembering, get yourself a plastic case containing seven sections with a day of the week above each section and fill them with each day's pills. You can easily see whether you took them or not.

For more on medications, see Chapter 10.

Following a Diet

If you look at Appendix A and its gourmet recipes, it should be clear to you that you're not sacrificing very much by following an appropriate diabetic diet, unless you consider avoiding overweight to be a sacrifice. You can enjoy delicious food that provides plenty of energy for your needs.

Although the emphasis in the last few years has been on reducing fat in your diets, especially cholesterol and saturated fat (see Chapter 8), when it comes to diabetes, you have to be aware of your carbohydrate intake as well. And it doesn't hurt to know something about the quality of the carbohydrate as well as the quantity. Try to choose low glycemic index carbohydrate, like basmati rice instead of white rice. Any carbohydrate with lots of fiber will be a low glycemic source. You will have a lower blood glucose as a result and require less insulin to control it. Not only does that mean better diabetic control, but your fats, particularly triglyceride, are also lower, and this will decrease the severity of the insulin resistance syndrome if you have type 2 diabetes.

Most people can make changes in their diet over the short term, but maintaining these changes over the long term is difficult. The best way to accomplish a long-term change is to have a plan and try to carry it out. It is probably the times that you are in an unplanned situation that are the most damaging to your diabetic control. For example, when you enter a restaurant, you're presented with a menu. The job of the author of that menu is to entice you by the description of the food to order that dish, just as the pictures on the food boxes in stores entice you to buy that food. If you have in mind what is good for your diabetic diet, you tend to order what helps you, not what messes up your control.

One of the things I am trying to do with the gourmet recipes is to have a section of a menu devoted to delicious diabetic meals so that you can head over there when you open the menu and avoid the temptations to be found everywhere else. Restaurants are just starting to do this, and it will take a long time to get a lot of them to offer it, not to mention the restaurants that will never do it (especially in Paris). Until then, you must go out to eat prepared to order appropriately.

The same thing holds when you eat at someone else's home. If they know you have diabetes, hopefully they will prepare something you can eat. If they do not, you must select with great care. Do not be afraid to say no. Your friendly dietitian can give you a lot of help on what to select and what to reject.

One thing that helps a lot in diabetes is if you have a fair amount of order in your life. If your life is one of disorganization, then controlling your diabetes will be much more difficult. You must take your medications at about the same time and eat at about the same time. You must test at about the same time and exercise at about the same time. But you don't have to eat the same thing all the time. An endless variety of delicious foods is available to you.

For more on your diet, see Chapter 8.

Exercising

The more you exercise regularly, the better you can control your blood glucose. This holds true for your weight as well. If you have type 2 diabetes, you need less or no medication. If you have type 1 diabetes, you need less insulin. Your exercise choices are unlimited (see Chapter 9). Yes, even a game of golf is exercise, though most people (who are not professional golfers) do not play the sport more than once or twice a week.

If you're having trouble exercising, follow these tips:

✔ **You need to do something daily, if possible, but no less than three or four times a week.** If you can't do it regularly on your own, get an exercise partner. You do not need a sports club to find step aerobics. Just walk up a few flights of stairs where you work. Go for a walk outside if the weather permits for at least 20 minutes.

✔ **Set up a program with goals so that you do not stay stuck in a low level of exercise.** If you do not know how to do this yourself, check with an exercise physiologist. If you're older than 40 and have not exercised and are overweight, check with your doctor before beginning a strenuous program.

✔ **Don't limit yourself to aerobics.** A little weightlifting a few days a week can make an amazing difference in your strength, your stamina, and your physique. If your sport is tennis, you may find that you can play that third set with much greater ease once you start on a weight program. All other sports benefit from weightlifting in a similar fashion.

Exercise is definitely a way to get high without drugs. It is good for depression or any unhappy state of mind. Don't take my word for it. Get out and find out for yourself. See Chapter 9 for more on exercise.

Using Other Expertise

People are usually eager to help you with your diabetic condition. (See Chapter 11 to find out more about your supporting cast.) So much knowledge is out there, just waiting to be tapped. The insurance companies recognize the value of these resources like the dietitian and the diabetes educator and are willing to pay for them.

You can get lots of free sources of information from your friendly pharmacist, the Internet, and other people with diabetes. You may want to be careful of these last two groups, however. A lot of misinformation is shared on the Internet and among diabetic patients. Before you make a major alteration in your treatment on the basis of uncertain information, check with your physician. (You can find out about some of fhe most common bits of misinformation in Chapters 17 and 19.)

Every time you have a question about your diabetes, write it down and save it for your next office visit with your doctor, unless it is urgent. If you don't know whether something is urgent, call your doctor and let the doctor determine the urgency of your problem.

Don't neglect your family and friends as a helpful source. These are the people who love you and know that you would help them if the tables were turned. The problem is that they cannot help you if they do not know what you're dealing with. Tell them that you have diabetes and the risks, such as hypoglycemia, that you face. Tell them how to help you if the need arises. You will find that the result will be a much closer relationship.

Part IV
Special Considerations for Living with Diabetes

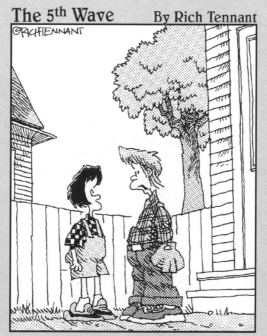

The 5th Wave   By Rich Tennant

"The way I understand it, the reason I was getting cold and tired was because my body wasn't making enough insulation."

In this part . . .

Diabetes in growing children and the elderly often produces problems that the average adult does not have to deal with. Children have to grow normally and develop sexually, while the elderly often have other illnesses and, in any case, are more frail. Both groups have emotional problems that are unique. The child is learning to fit in with peers while separating from parents. The elderly are losing friends and relatives at the same time that their mental processes are declining. This part explains their special problems and how to tackle them.

Even the middle-aged adult has unusual problems, in this case relating to insurance, both life and health, and employment. Fortunately, the barriers are rapidly coming down, but you still need to know about certain areas. Discrimination cannot be tolerated, and you can find out what to do about it here.

Finally, I tell you about the huge number of new developments, putting them into perspective as to usefulness and appropriateness. After that, I expose the false promises. So many things have been proposed for diabetes care without benefit of careful evaluation. The scientific evidence for and against is presented so that you can make up your own mind.

Chapter 13

Your Child Has Diabetes

Children with diabetes present special problems that adults with diabetes do not have. Not only are they growing and developing from babies to adults, but they have problems of psychological and social adjustment. Diabetes can add complications to a period of time that is not exactly smooth, even without it.

Many doctors believe that if a child has diabetes, the whole family really has the disease because everyone must adjust to it. Because diabetes is the second most common chronic disease in children after asthma, it is no small problem.

In this chapter, you find out how to manage diabetes in your child at each stage of growth and development. You need to remember that your child is first a child and then a child with diabetes. And you also need to remember that you are not to blame for your child's diabetes. Diabetes is not a form of retribution for your sins. It's also important to remember that your child is not to blame either.

Your Baby or Preschooler Has Diabetes

Although type 1 diabetes does not usually show up in babies, it can, and you should know what to expect when it does. Obviously, your baby is not verbal and cannot tell you what is bothering him or her. For this reason, you may miss the fact that the baby is urinating excessively in his or her diaper. The baby will lose weight and have vomiting and diarrhea, but this may be ascribed to a stomach disorder rather than diabetes. When the diagnosis is finally made, the baby may be very sick and require a stay in a pediatric intensive care unit. Do not blame yourself for not realizing that your baby was sick.

Once the diagnosis is made, the hard work begins. You must learn to give insulin injections and to test the blood glucose in a child who will be reluctant to have either one done. You have to learn when and what to feed the baby, both to encourage growth and development and to prevent low blood glucose.

At this stage, you are not as worried about tight control as you will be later on. There are several reasons for this. First, the baby's neurological system is still developing. Frequent, severe low blood glucose will damage this development, so the glucose is permitted to be higher now than later on. Second, studies show that changes associated with high blood glucose leading to diabetic complications do not begin to add up until the prepubertal years, so you have a grace period during which you can allow less tight control.

On the other hand, a small baby is very fragile. There is less of everything, so small losses of water, sodium, potassium, and other substances will more rapidly lead to a very sick baby. If you keep the baby's blood glucose around 150 to 200 mg/dl (8.3 to 11.1 mmol/L), you are doing very well.

For a time of variable duration, your child will have seemingly regained the ability to control the blood glucose with little or no insulin, the so-called "honeymoon period." This period always ends, and it isn't your fault that it does end. At this time, you have to work with the doctor, the dietitian, and the diabetes educator to find out how to control diabetes with insulin. You need to know how to do the following skills:

- Identify the signs and symptoms of hyperglycemia, hypoglycemia, and diabetic ketoacidosis (see Chapters 4 and 5)
- Administer insulin (see Chapter 10)
- Measure the blood glucose and urine ketones (see Chapter 7)
- Treat hypoglycemia with food or glucagon (see Chapter 4)
- Feed your diabetic child (see Chapter 8)
- Know what to do when your child is sick with another childhood illness

Your responsibilities as the parent of a diabetic baby or preschooler are extensive and time-consuming. Training your usual helpers to take over, even for a short time, is especially difficult. Unless you hire a professional to take over for a while, you may not get very much time away from your diabetic infant.

The honeymoon period

Given that name because it represents a period of improvement in type 1 diabetes that does not last, the honeymoon period occurs in most patients. Once the disease has been diagnosed and treated so that the blood glucose levels are close to normal, the child may require little or no insulin for a time. This is a period of remission in the disease and means there is still some function in the beta cell of the pancreas (see Chapter 2). Longer remissions are seen when:

✔ The age at onset of diabetes is older

✔ The initial presentation of the disease is milder

✔ The amount of islet cell antibody (see Chapter 2) is lower

This is a temporary remission and ends with a sudden or slowly increasing requirement for insulin. By three years after the diagnosis, there is complete loss of insulin production in young children. Older children may have some preservation of function.

Your other children may resent the attention that you pay to this one child. If your other children start to misbehave, this may be the reason.

Diagnosing diabetes if it occurs in your preschooler may be just as difficult as it is in the baby. The child may still be preverbal and is still running around in diapers. If a honeymoon period occurs after the diagnosis, this period is usually briefer than if a diagnosis is made in a teenager.

A preschooler is beginning the process of separating from its parent and starting to learn to control the environment (by becoming toilet-trained, for example). This separation process makes it more difficult for you, the parent, to give the injections and test the glucose. You must be firm in insisting that these things be done. You'll need to do them yourself because a small child neither knows how to do them nor understands what to do with the information generated by the glucose meter.

Because a child's eating habits may not be very regular, the use of very short-acting insulin like lispro is especially helpful (see Chapter 10). Very soon, people with diabetes should have a way of measuring the blood glucose in a painless fashion, which will be of great assistance in monitoring these children.

Your Primary School Child Has Diabetes

In some ways, diabetes care gets a little easier with a primary school child, but in other ways, it gets more difficult. Your child can finally tell you when he or she has symptoms of hypoglycemia, so this is easier to recognize and treat. But you must begin to control the blood glucose more carefully because your child is reaching the stage where control really counts.

You still have a child who is growing and developing, so nutrition remains very important. Enough of the right kinds of calories must be provided for this process.

As the child goes to school, he or she is interacting with other children and wants their approval and wants to fit in. Diabetes may be considered a stigma by the child. He or she may be very reluctant to share it with other children. A plan of treatment that interferes with school and friendships may be very unwelcome.

Your child is going to do more to separate from you. He or she may insist on giving insulin shots and doing blood tests. Studies again indicate that this is not a good time for you to give up these tasks, certainly not completely. Your child may not be physically capable of performing them and, in an attempt to hide the disease from peers, may not perform them at all during school. Diet may also suffer at school as the child tries to fit in and not stand out by eating the things that diabetes requires.

Because you are beginning to tighten the level of control, hypoglycemia is more of a risk, especially at night. You can avoid hypoglycemia by any or all of the following steps at this stage and from now on:

- Give a bedtime snack regularly.

- Give cornstarch at bedtime. Cornstarch is slowly broken down so that it provides glucose over a longer period of time. There is even a commercial product, called NightBite, that contains cornstarch and can be given before bedtime.

- Measure and treat a low blood glucose before bedtime.

- Occasionally check the blood glucose at 3 a.m.

- Ask about symptoms of nighttime low blood glucose, such as nightmares and headaches.

- Be sure your child does not skip meals.

- Have your child eat carbohydrate before exercising.

Some member of the family must be able to administer glucagon by injection to treat hypoglycemia should you be unable to get the child to eat or drink.

Once your child is off to school or a daycare setting, you need to address new problems. Federal laws, especially the Diabetes Education Act of 1991, specify that diabetes is a disability and that it's unlawful to discriminate against children with diabetes. If a school receives federal funding or is open to the public, it has to reasonably accommodate the special needs of the diabetic child.

The law requires that a diabetic child participate fully in all school and after-school activities. This means there must be provision for blood glucose testing, for treatment with insulin, and for taking snacks or going to the bathroom as needed.

To accomplish this, a written treatment plan is developed by your doctor, you, and the school nurse, and relevant people in the school have assigned roles. The plan must include

- Blood glucose monitoring
- Insulin administration
- Meals and snacks
- Recognition and treatment of hypoglycemia
- Recognition and treatment of hyperglycemia
- Testing of urine ketones as indicated

As the parent, you are responsible to provide for all supplies for testing and treatment. It is the responsibility of a school provider to understand and treat hypoglycemia, to test the blood glucose and treat when the level is outside certain parameters, to coordinate meals and snacks, and to permit excused appointments to the doctor as well as restroom use. There is no reason that your child should not participate fully in school.

Your Adolescent Has Diabetes

Your adolescent or teenager with diabetes will provide some of your biggest challenges. This is the time that most childhood diabetes begins. The Diabetes Control and Complications Trial showed that tight control can be accomplished beginning at age 13, and that this control can prevent complications. The higher frequency of severe hypoglycemia that accompanies tighter control was not found to be damaging to the brain of the child at this age. However, children at this age do not think in terms of long-term blood glucose control and prevention of complications. So they're not willing to do many of the tasks required to control their diabetes on a regular basis.

The goal of treatment at this stage is a hemoglobin A1c between 7 and 9 percent. A value above 11 percent is poor control. This is not true for smaller children, who are allowed to have a higher hemoglobin A1c.

This stage is when your child is most eager to become independent. You don't want to give up all control at this time for several reasons:

- ✔ Your child actually does better if he or she has limits that are clearly stated and enforced.

- ✔ The "shame" of diabetes may cause the child to skip shots and food, especially around friends.

- ✔ The problem of eating disorders (see Chapter 8) may pop up at this time, especially among the girls trying to maintain a slim body image. Diabetic girls know that if they skip their injections, they will lose weight. They ignore the high blood glucose that results.

- ✔ Teenagers with diabetes may still be unable to translate levels of blood glucose into appropriate action.

The hormonal changes that occur in puberty are often associated with insulin resistance. This may be the source of loss of control rather than any failure of your child to follow the diabetic treatment plan. Upward adjustment of the insulin may overcome this problem.

Your Young Adult Child Has Diabetes

When your child becomes a young adult, you definitely want to give up the control that has helped your child to thrive up to this point. Your child should be doing his or her own testing. He or she is ready to leave the pediatric level and begin to work with doctors who care for adults. This means that you are probably out of the loop. Your child should now have the skill to choose appropriate insulin treatment based upon blood glucose levels and calories of carbohydrate consumed (see Chapter 10).

Your child now has new challenges, including finding work, going to college, finding a future mate, and finding a place to live independently. At the same time, the reluctance to admit to diabetes and the desire for a thin body continue to complicate care.

Diabetes care must be intensive at this point (see Chapter 10). Multiple shots of intermediate and short-acting insulin are taken. Your child must follow a diabetic diet (see Chapter 8). An exercise program is essential (see Chapter 9). The rest of this book really has to do with the tasks that your young adult child with diabetes faces.

Obesity and Type 2 Diabetes in Children

The epidemic of obesity, which has spread to children in the United States in the past few decades, has led to a much higher prevalence of type 2 diabetes in children than was ever seen before. Even without diabetes, obesity is a burden for children. The obese child has severe psychological and social consequences:

- Lower respect from peers than other disabled children get
- Less comfortable family interactions
- Poor body image
- Low self-esteem

Adding type 2 diabetes into this mix can be devastating. The consequences of the preceding problems may lead to failure to manage the diabetes because the child wants to avoid any activity that will make him or her even more different from his or her peers.

Overweight or obesity is present in as many as 25 percent of all children. Only a fraction of these children go on to develop diabetes, but it is important to separate type 1 diabetes from type 2 because the disease is milder in type 2. The key differences that suggest type 2 in children are

- A family history of type 2 diabetes
- Belonging to certain ethnic groups such as American Indian and Mexican American
- Obesity
- No evidence of autoimmunity (see Chapter 2)
- Extremely rare ketoacidosis (see Chapter 4)
- A velvety darkening of the skin, especially under the arms, called *acanthosis nigricans*
- A reserve of insulin in the body, as shown by a C-peptide level in the blood that is normal or elevated (C-peptide is made every time insulin is produced, so its presence indicates that the body is making insulin)

The child with type 2 diabetes has milder diabetes and can be treated with pills or diet and exercise alone. However, because children do not appreciate long-term consequences of their actions, you often have the problem of compliance.

You must help your obese child to lose weight because most obese children will become obese adults. With the assistance of a dietitian, you can figure out the food that your child can eat to maintain growth and development without further weight gain. One of the most helpful techniques is to take the child into the supermarket and point out the difference between empty calories and nourishing calories. Another is never to make high-calorie food like cake and candy a reward. Finally, if you keep problem foods out of the house, there is much less likelihood that your child will eat them.

Sick Day Solutions

Your child is susceptible to all the usual childhood illnesses, but diabetes complicates your care. An illness can affect diabetes in opposite ways. An infection may increase the level of insulin resistance so that the usual dose of insulin is not adequate. Or it may cause nausea and vomiting so that no food or drink can stay down, and the insulin may cause hypoglycemia. For this reason, you need to measure the blood glucose in your sick child every two to four hours. If the glucose is over 250 mg/dl (13.9 mmol/l), you need to give extra short-acting insulin. If it's under 250, you give more carbohydrate-containing nutrients.

Ketones in the urine (see Chapter 7) are also tested when your child urinates. If these become elevated, you need to discuss the situation with your doctor.

You should probably feed the child with clear liquids like tea and soda during the sick days. Milk is excluded because it upsets the stomach. As long as your child can hold down clear liquids, you can continue to take care of him or her. If clear liquids cannot be held down, you must contact your doctor and bring your child to the hospital.

While the blood glucose remains over 250 mg/dl use tea, water, and diet soda so as not to add calories of carbohydrate. When the blood glucose is less than 250 mg/dl, you can use regular soda or glucose drinks.

The Extra Value of Team Care

Especially when your child is first diagnosed with diabetes, the stress can be overwhelming. The guilt that comes with this diagnosis may leave you unable to help your child much at first and certainly unable to learn all that you need to know to master all of the areas of importance to the health of your child. Here is where you must depend upon the help of the diabetes care team, more at the beginning, but throughout the duration of his or her childhood.

The pediatrician can show you how to administer insulin and test the blood glucose. This doctor can also explain how to use the information to determine an insulin dose. The dietitian can show you how many calories of which foods are needed for growth and development. The diabetes educator can explain the short- and long-term complications of diabetes and how your child can avoid them. The mental health worker can help you deal with the psychological issues at each stage of your child's development. One of these people can help you with an exercise program for your child.

One resource that can be tremendously valuable for you and your child is the diabetes summer camp. These camps are located all over the country and provide a safe, well-managed place where your child can go and be in the majority. He or she can learn a great deal about diabetes while enjoying all the pleasures of a summer camp environment. (Certainly not a minor benefit is the opportunity for you to have time off for perhaps the first time in years.)

You can find an extensive list of camps for diabetic children throughout the United States by going to the Web site www.childrenwithdiabetes.com/index_cwd.htm.

This is one of the many services of the Web site Children With Diabetes.

In Chapter 11, I compare diabetes to a stage play. There, the person with diabetes was the author, the producer, the director, and the star. When you have a child with diabetes, he or she is the star, but you take on the roles of author, producer, and director. You obviously have a great responsibility but one that I feel certain you can handle. Just don't try to do it alone. Use your medical experts as well as your family and friends to make it manageable.

Chapter 14

Diabetes and the Elderly

. . . .

In This Chapter

▶ Diagnosing diabetes in the elderly

▶ Coping with intellectual functioning in the elderly

▶ Dealing with dietary considerations

▶ Focusing on unique eye problems of the elderly

▶ Solving urinary and sexual problems

▶ Individualizing treatment considerations

▶ Understanding the new Medicare law

. . . .

Everyone wants to live a long time, but no one wants to get old. Nevertheless, getting old is better than the alternative. Woody Allen says the one advantage of dying is that you don't have to do jury duty. I think I would rather do jury duty.

Defining "elderly" is the first problem. Every year my definition seems to change, but I think it's fair to talk about the age of 70 as the beginning of elderly. By that definition, by the year 2020, more than 20 percent of the population in the United States will be elderly. As many as one-fifth of that population will be elderly people with diabetes.

Elderly people with diabetes have special problems. They're hospitalized at a rate that is 70 percent higher than the general elderly population. Even without hospitalization, elderly people with diabetes have special problems. In this chapter, you find out about those problems and the way to handle them.

Diagnosing Diabetes in the Elderly

The incidence of diabetes in the elderly is higher for many reasons, but the main culprit seems to be increasing insulin resistance with aging, even if the elderly person with diabetes is not particularly obese or sedentary. Doctors do not yet understand why insulin resistance increases. When they look at the pancreas, it seems to be able to make insulin at the usual rate. The fasting blood glucose actually rises very slowly as you get older. It's the glucose after meals that rises much quicker and leads to the diagnosis. Because the fasting blood glucose is usually normal, some doctors recommend using the hemoglobin A1c to help to make the diagnosis in the elderly population. A hemoglobin A1c that is 1½ percent higher than the upper limit of normal for that lab is considered diagnostic of diabetes. Because most labs have a normal of up to 5.4 percent, a value of 7 percent or greater is probably diabetes. Between normal and that value is a gray zone that is probably impaired glucose tolerance (see Chapter 2).

Elderly people with diabetes often do not complain of any symptoms. When they do, the symptoms may not be the ones usually associated with type 2 diabetes or they may be confusing. Elderly people with diabetes may complain of loss of appetite or weakness, and they may have lost weight rather than become obese. They may have incontinence of urine, which is usually thought of as a prostate problem in elderly men or a urinary tract infection in older women. Elderly people with diabetes may not complain of thirst because their ability to feel thirst is altered.

Evaluating Intellectual Functioning

You need to evaluate the intellectual function of an elderly person with diabetes because management of the disease requires a fairly high level of mental functioning. The patient has to follow a diabetic diet, administer medications properly, and test the blood glucose. Studies have shown that elderly people with diabetes have a higher incidence of *dementia* (loss of mental functioning) and Alzheimer's disease than nondiabetics, making it much harder for them to perform those tasks.

The patient can take *cognitive screening tests* to determine his or her level of function. Testing makes it easier to tell whether the patient can be self-sufficient or will need help. Many older people now living alone with no assistance really require an assisted-living situation or even a nursing home.

Preparing a Proper Diet

In addition to the intellectual function required to understand and prepare a proper diabetic diet (see the preceding section), the elderly have other problems when it comes to proper nutrition:

- They may have poor vision and be unable to see to read or cook.
- They may have low income and be unable to purchase the foods that they require.

> ✔ Their taste and smell may be decreased, so they lose interest in food.
>
> ✔ They often have a loss of appetite.
>
> ✔ They may have arthritis or a tremor that prevents cooking.
>
> ✔ They may have poor teeth or a dry mouth.

Any one of these problems may be enough to prevent proper eating by the elderly person with the result that the diabetes is poorly controlled.

Dealing with Eye Problems

Elderly people with diabetes have the eye problems that are brought on by diabetes earlier, and they can affect all aspects of proper diabetes care. They get cataracts, macular degeneration, and open angle glaucoma in addition to diabetic retinopathy. (See Chapter 5 for more information on these eye problems.)

One of biggest failures in diabetes care is that as many as one-third of the elderly never have an eye examination at all. How can disease be found when it is early enough to treat if no examination is done?

Once these problems are detected, they can be treated and save vision.

Coping with Urinary and Sexual Problems

Urinary and sexual problems are very common in elderly people with diabetes and greatly affect quality of life. It is not uncommon for an older person with diabetes to have paralysis of the bladder muscle with retention of urine followed by overflow incontinence when the bladder fills up. An older person may be unable to get to the bathroom fast enough. Sometimes spasms in the bladder muscle lead to incontinence. The result may be frequent urinary tract infections.

Almost 60 percent of men over the age of 70 are impotent, and 50 percent have no *libido,* a desire to have sex. These problems can have many causes (see Chapter 6), but older men are especially likely to have blockage of blood vessels with poor flow into the penis. The elderly take an average of seven medications daily, many of which affect sexual function.

To have sex at any age, you need sexual desire and the physical ability to perform, you need a willing partner, and you need a safe, private place. Any or all of these may be missing for the elderly.

It is not always necessary to treat sexual dysfunction if the male and his partner are okay with the situation as it is. If not, Chapter 6 points out a number of treatments for potency problems.

Considering Treatment

When deciding upon treatment, you first have to consider your goals. Do you have a very elderly person with diabetes with a low life expectancy, or do you have a person with diabetes who is elderly but physiologically young and could live for 15 or 20 more years? A person who has lived to age 65 has a life expectancy of at least 18 more years, plenty of time to develop complications of diabetes, especially macrovascular disease, eye disease, kidney disease, and nervous system disease (see Chapter 5). Most people who are discharged from a nursing home die within one year after discharge, so treatment decisions are different for them.

The level of care may be basic or intensive.

- **Basic care** is meant to prevent the acute problems of diabetes like excessive urination and thirst. You can accomplish this goal by keeping the blood glucose under 200 mg/dl (11.1 mmol/l). Basic care is used for an elderly person with diabetes not expected to live very long because of the diabetes or other illnesses.

- **Intensive care** is meant to prevent diabetic complications in an elderly person expected to live long enough to have them. The goal here is to keep the blood glucose under 140 mg/dl (7.7 mmol/l) and the hemoglobin A1c as close to normal as possible while avoiding frequent hypoglycemia.

Treatment always starts with diet and exercise, but exercise may be limited in the elderly person with diabetes. You need to remember that exercise is helpful, even in the very old, as recent studies have shown. Exercise reduces the blood glucose and the hemoglobin A1c. Because elderly patients have more coronary artery disease, arthritis, eye disease, neuropathy, and peripheral vascular disease, exercise just may not be possible. (See Chapter 9 for more on exercise.)

The diet for the elderly person with diabetes is basically the same as the younger person with diabetes. (See the section "Preparing a Proper Diet," earlier in this chapter, and Chapter 8.)

Education for the patient who can benefit can be of great value, especially if the spouse is also involved.

Once diet and exercise have been found to be inadequate, medications must be added. This is complicated by a number of considerations special to the elderly:

- ✔ The patient may not be able to see the correct dosage.
- ✔ He or she may be mentally unable to take the medicine properly.
- ✔ Physical limitations may prevent medication taking, especially insulin.
- ✔ Multiple other drugs may interact with the diabetes medicine.
- ✔ Elderly patients have decreased kidney and liver function, making some diabetic drugs last longer.
- ✔ Poor nutrition may make them more prone to hypoglycemia.

I explain medication usage in Chapter 10, but, again, drugs in the elderly must be handled more carefully. Of the sulfonylurea drugs, chlorpropamide is the longest acting and can cause very prolonged hypoglycemia, so it's not used often after the age of 65. Most doctors use the newer sulfonylureas like glipizide and glyburide, but they don't seem to have any great advantage over the older drugs besides their newness.

Metformin can lower the blood glucose without the fear of hypoglycemia and can be very useful in an older population for this reason. It often causes weight loss, which may be helpful for many patients, but I have seen it cause very excessive weight loss in certain elderly patients. Because the elderly have diminished kidney function, metformin must be used with care in them and not used at all when alcoholism, liver disease, or acute infection exists.

Rosiglitazone is the first of a group of drugs that actually reverses the lesion that makes diabetes so prevalent in older people — the insulin resistance. Rosiglitazone or pioglitazone, the other drug in this class, may play a huge role in the future in preventing diabetic complications as well as the transformation from impaired glucose tolerance to diabetes in the elderly.

Insulin is added when the oral drugs have failed. For basic treatment, a nighttime shot of insulin glargine, along with a daytime pill, may be all that is needed. For intensive treatment, multiple shots of short-acting insulin, plus a nighttime shot of insulin glargine, will be needed, along with frequent monitoring of the blood glucose. This may be hard to accomplish in a very elderly patient outside of an institution.

A patient who is transferred from self-care to institutional care may require a significant reduction in medication because he or she may not have been taking the medication properly.

Understanding the New Medicare Law

As of July 1, 1998, the federal government began to offer new benefits for the 4.2 million Medicare (over age 65) people with diabetes. Under the policy, all people with diabetes enrolled in Medicare Part B or Medicare managed care are eligible to receive coverage of glucose monitors, test strips, and lancets. It does not matter which method they use to control their disease.

If you're enrolled in Medicare, you can get these benefits by having your physician prescribe the supplies and document how often you use them.

The Health Care Financing Administration, which administers Medicare, has also passed regulations that permit people with diabetes to get reimbursed for education programs. In addition, if you have Medicare insurance and have type 1 diabetes, you are eligible for Medicare to pay for your insulin pump.

Chapter 15

Occupational and Insurance Problems

*A*fter we got his diabetes under control, one of my patients wrote to his mother, "Dear Mom, I'm not working, but my pancreas is." Most people need to work, and some people even want to work. People need to work for the same reason that a certain man did not turn in his brother-in-law who thought he was a chicken. We need the eggs (though not too many).

As a person with diabetes, when you try to get a job, you may run into various forms of discrimination. Part of it has to do with the fear that the company will have to pay higher insurance premiums if they hire a person with a chronic illness. Part of it has to do with a lack of understanding of the great strides that have been made in diabetes care so that a person with diabetes often has a better record of coming to work than a nondiabetic.

In this chapter, you find out what you need to know when you apply for work, health insurance, and life insurance. You discover how to work the health care "system" so that you derive the greatest benefits possible at the lowest cost.

(You will save so much money that I am sure you will want to send a donation to the American Diabetes Association for the great work they have done and are doing on your behalf.)

Where They Won't Hire You

You may have grown up watching Eliot Ness on television and had your heart set on being a member of the Federal Bureau of Investigation. Forget it if you require insulin. This policy of the FBI is called a *blanket ban* on hiring a certain group of people, in this case people with diabetes who take insulin. A blanket ban does not take into account the condition of the individual, the past employment history, the way the person manages his or her diabetes, or the responsibilities of the position. It simply says, you've got the disease, you can't work here. It's a throwback to the days before 1980, when a person with diabetes could never be sure what his blood glucose was doing.

Another important area that has a blanket ban in place is the United States military. If you have any kind of diabetes, you are not eligible to serve. If you develop diabetes after you've been in the military, you will probably be given a discharge. This does not make a lot of sense because many countries have people with diabetes in their military forces and have no difficulty with them. And so it goes.

But fortunately, blanket bans are falling faster than Barry Bonds home runs. Even the Department of the Treasury lifted a blanket ban on becoming a member of the Bureau of Alcohol, Tobacco, and Firearms if you had insulin-requiring diabetes. Recently, several states lifted a ban on hiring people with diabetes to be school bus drivers. This was the result of lawsuits against several school districts when they fired their drivers with spotless driving records just because they had diabetes. This does not mean that there are no safeguards against risky drivers. Drivers are evaluated on a case-by-case basis before they are accepted to drive children. This is fair.

The situation for drivers is not all rosy, however. People with diabetes who take insulin cannot receive a license for commercial interstate driving (truck drivers). It does not make a lot of sense that a driver can get to the state line but can't cross it, but there it is.

Another blanket ban that is falling is the ban on piloting airplanes. For 37 years, a person who took insulin could not fly a plane. In 1996, the Federal Aviation Administration reconsidered based upon the great advances in controlling diabetes. They decided to permit people to fly privately but not for commercial airlines, again on a case-by-case basis.

Is there ever a justification for a blanket ban? The answer is no, and it has been proved in a number of studies. In one study of accidents of all kinds, people with diabetes actually had fewer accidents, including automobile accidents, than groups of people without diabetes. In another study of people over age 65 with diabetes, the rate of automobile accidents was no greater than that of the nondiabetic groups.

Flying a plane: It's not easy, but it's worth it

Getting a pilot's license is not easy but is well worth it for the person who loves to fly. You must have no other disqualifying conditions like arteriosclerotic disease of the heart or brain, diabetic eye disease, or severe kidney disease (see Chapter 5). You must have had no more than one hypoglycemic reaction with loss of consciousness in the last five years and at least a year of stability after that. You must be evaluated by a specialist every three months after you get the license and measure your blood glucose multiple times a day. You must carry a glucose meter and meter supplies in flight along with supplies for rapid treatment of hypoglycemia. Your blood glucose must be between 100 and 300 mg/dl (5.5 to 16.6 mmol/l) a half hour before take off, every hour of the flight, and a half hour before landing. However, you're not expected to measure your blood glucose in flight if it interferes with properly flying the plane. Phew! Lindbergh would never have made it to Paris.

The Law Is On Your Side

A number of laws protect you in the workplace, but the most important is probably the Americans with Disabilities Act of 1990. This act states,

> *The determination that an individual poses a 'direct threat' shall be based on an individualized assessment of the individual's present ability to safely perform the essential functions of the job.*

In 1998, the U.S. Court of Appeals ruled that the ADA applied to Americans with diabetes. As a result, you are qualified for a particular job if you can perform the essential functions of the job as determined by the employer, with or without reasonable accommodation. That means you can't be discriminated against in hiring, firing, promotion, training, pay, or any other aspect of employment because you have diabetes. Your boss cannot ask whether you have diabetes but can expect you to pass a physical examination to verify that you are well enough to do the job.

The Federal Rehabilitation Act of 1973 is an important law that protects you when you apply for a federal job or a job in a company that receives federal assistance. A person with diabetes is specifically protected under this law. The most important provision states,

> *No otherwise qualified handicapped individual in the United States shall, solely by reason of his handicap, be excluded from the participation in, be denied the benefits of, or be subjected to discrimination under any program or activity conducted by the Executive agency. . . .*

Federal agencies have to prove that you will not be able to perform safely if given the job. That is hard to do and puts the burden on them, not you. They must decide on a case-by-case basis.

What can you do if you run into discrimination on the job due to your diabetes? You can contact the U.S. Department of Justice by calling 800-514-0301 to find out more about the Americans with Disabilities Act. If you have a complaint to file, send it to the U.S. Department of Justice/Disability Rights Section, P.O. Box 66738, Washington, DC 20035-6738.

You and the Medical Insurance System

If you or your child has diabetes, you can count on several things being true when you interact with the medical insurance system in the United States. It will cost you more out-of-pocket than families without diabetes even when you have coverage. You may be denied coverage more often.

If you are an older adult with diabetes, you can expect to spend one and a half times as much for medical care as a person without diabetes, although Medicare pays for much of it. You want to be sure that you are not medically shortchanged in an effort to save money.

The good news is that you can get health insurance just as often as the person who does not have diabetes, although you may be turned down more often. And the type of insurance you will have is the same as the nondiabetic population: Blue Cross/Blue Shield, Health Maintenance Organizations (HMOs), CHAMPUS, and so on.

In order to get the most for your money, you need to understand how this so-called health insurance system works and how to interact with it. I say "so-called" because there are so many variations that there is really no one system at all.

Currently, there are two major forms of payment for medical care — fee-for-service and capitated payment — with a lot of hybrids in between. The old *fee-for-service* method pays the medical provider, whether a physician, a lab, or a hospital, based on the number of services provided. More services and procedures mean more profit for the provider. So the incentive is to do more in order to make more money. (Not that providers would ever do more than is necessary for the money.)

The other main method of reimbursement is *capitation*. Here the provider gets a fixed amount of money for each patient. The risk is divided among many patients so that if one costs more, hopefully another will cost less. This is the basis of the Health Maintenance Organization (HMO), which hires physicians to provide the care. HMOs look to enroll people who cost as little as possible for their medical care. The incentive is to do less in order to save money, which is then kept by the provider. (Not that providers would ever do less than is necessary for the money.)

Because they seem to end up costing less money overall, capitation plans are growing while fee-for-service is declining. The government is even encouraging HMOs to enroll Medicare recipients in order to reduce costs. At the same time, it is requiring them to enroll people who cost more, like most people with diabetes.

As a consumer of medical care, you want to look for a large group because such a group can spread out your extra expenses among many people who don't consume as much medical care. You need to ask several questions before you sign up:

- ✔ What is your total annual cost, and how often is a payment required?

- ✔ Is there a deductible where you have to pay the first so many dollars before the insurance starts paying?

- ✔ Is there a *co-payment* (which means every time you use a provider, you have to pay some dollars)?

- ✔ Does your plan pay for durable medical equipment like an insulin pump (see Chapter 10), which can be very expensive, although when you sign up you may not foresee a need for it?

- ✔ Will your plan pay for your diabetes medication and diabetes supplies and to what extent?

- ✔ Can your physician order any medications you need, or is he or she restricted to certain medications?

- ✔ How often will you need to travel to the pharmacy to pick up medications? (Some plans make you go back every 30 days.)

- ✔ Are you covered for specialists, particularly eye doctors and foot doctors?

- ✔ Are you limited to certain hospitals, certain physicians, and certain laboratories (which may make it much more inconvenient for you, not to mention requiring you to change from a physician with whom you are very comfortable)?

- ✔ Is home health care included in the plan and to what extent?

Once you have signed up for a plan, you need to be vigilant to be sure you are getting what you paid for. Very often it will take a number of calls by you and your physician to get what you need, but if you persist you can often come away with a "Yes." Even goods and services that are excluded in your original contract may be provided by the insurance company if you are persistent.

Changing or Losing a Job

One of the major reasons people with diabetes used to stay in jobs they did not care for was their fear of losing their health insurance. This does not have to stop you in today's job market. Several laws protect you from the loss of health insurance if you change or lose your job.

The *Consolidated Omnibus Budget Reconciliation Act* (COBRA) stipulates that your employer must keep you on your current health insurance for as long as 18 months after your job ends and longer if you are disabled. If your child is at the age when he or she is no longer covered under your policy, the child's coverage can continue for up to three years. You, rather than your employer, will have to pay the premiums for this continued insurance.

If you are leaving work because of retirement at age 65, sign up for Medicare without fail. It is a generous program (which you supported while you were working) that recognizes the specific needs of people with diabetes. Since July 1, 1998, it has expanded its coverage to blood glucose monitors and test strips once your physician certifies the need. It also offers payment for out-patient diabetes education programs as long as they are considered necessary by your physician within very specific limitations. The program is not entirely enlightened, however, because it still does not cover insulin and syringes, annual eye examinations, and nutrition counseling. To find out more about Medicare, call the Medicare Hotline at 800-638-6833.

Some employers have conversion policies that allow you to stay with your insurance company if you leave work, but with individual rather than group coverage. These policies can be pretty expensive.

Some states offer "Pooled Risk" health insurance for people who have lived in the state a certain number of months but can't get group or individual coverage. Check with your state insurance office.

Life Insurance

As you might expect, the situation with life insurance and the person with diabetes is in a state of flux. Insurance companies like to calculate your chance of dying and charge you or turn you down based upon those calculations. Many companies are using calculations based on the life span of people with diabetes in 1980 or before. Using those statistics, diabetics clearly died earlier than their nondiabetic friends. Thus, the cost of life insurance is greater for people with diabetes than nondiabetics.

As new studies are done, they should indicate that the life spans of people with diabetes and nondiabetics are approaching equality. In some cases, people with diabetes, who take better care of themselves than people without a chronic illness, are living even longer. So the situation is improving and insurance companies will catch up sooner or later. Can you imagine the surprise if insurance companies were ever to charge people with diabetes less than others because of their good habits?

Chapter 16

What's New in Diabetes Care

*W*hen I think of heaven, I think of a wonderful place of great beauty and brightness and pleasure. I hope that everyone will all go there some day. More and more, you will discover there is a state of mind here on Earth that I call "Diabetes Heaven." The products, tests, and treatments I describe in this chapter can speed you on your way to that state.

Between 1921, when insulin was isolated and used for the first time, and 1980, when blood glucose meters began to be available, relatively little was discovered to improve diabetes care. Since 1980, and until about 1995, the same thing could be said. But since 1995, the pace of discovery of new tests, new treatments, and other products for diabetes is astonishing.

Discoveries like metformin and pioglitazone have become established in diabetes care. Doctors and other scientists are aware of the huge need for new therapies to address the growing problem of diabetes. Their response is truly remarkable.

Diabetes used to be thought of as a progressive disease. Right now, you and your doctors have all the tools necessary to turn diabetes into a nonprogressive disease. The tools I describe in this chapter make it more and more simple for you to accomplish that task.

Choosing from the New Monitoring Devices

Available devices for monitoring blood glucose are a great advance, but they have their problems. Testing may be painful. Monitoring may be inconvenient. Certain people may have a hard time monitoring because of physical handicaps. The followings devices are designed to overcome these limitations.

- **New types of lancet devices:** Many patients complain about the difficulty of sticking the fingertips again and again. The Auto-Lancet Mini, sold by Palco Laboratories (800-346-4484), provides five different depths of penetration of your finger, depending upon your needs. The Gentle Lance Lancing Device, sold by Futura Medical Corporation (800-631-0076), also offers five adjustable settings. It can be used with most lancets.

- **New types of meters still using blood:** The InDuo System is a joint collaboration between Novo Nordisk and Lifescan. This new meter is an attempt to integrate testing blood glucose with giving insulin in one product. The meter requires a tiny amount of blood for testing and gives a result in five seconds. The meter also remembers the amount of insulin given and the time of the last insulin injection. The insulin to be given is dialed up like other pen devices.

- **Non-invasive meters:** The dream of glucose-testing without sticking the skin is just around the corner. A number of companies are developing devices that are available or may come to market soon.

  Cygnus, Inc., has a GlucoWatch Biographer, which looks like a wristwatch. A low level of electric current painlessly draws glucose into a patch that is on the skin. A reaction takes place depending on the amount of glucose that generates electrons. The GlucoWatch displays the results of measurements every 20 to 30 minutes. The company is working on calibrating the patch at the present time.

  Another company, Technical Chemicals and Products, Inc., has a product called the TD Glucose Meter, which painlessly draws body fluid to measure the glucose in it. The meter doesn't use blood, and the company is trying to correlate the level of glucose in the fluid with the level of glucose in the blood at the present time.

  CME Telemetrix, Inc., is developing a different technology for non-invasive monitoring, which uses a beam of infrared light passed through a finger. Different compounds like glucose absorb infrared at different levels, and the device measures the amount absorbed at the level of glucose. The presence of so many other substances makes this a little tricky.

New Oral Agents

Pharmaceutical companies are looking for newer versions of older agents (which may be more effective and have fewer side effects) as well as entirely new agents with different mechanisms of actions. This area is literally exploding, and you are the beneficiary.

Drugs to slow glucose absorption

Acarbose is known for its ability to slow the absorption of glucose, thus lowering after-meal glucose levels (see Chapter 10). Now Pharmacia & Upjohn has come out with miglitol, which it calls Glyset. Because Glyset works just like acarbose by blocking an enzyme that breaks down complex carbohydrate in the intestine, the result is a lot of carbohydrate lower down in the intestine and lots of gas, diarrhea, and abdominal pain.

My patients generally did not like the side effects of acarbose and the glucose-lowering effect is modest at best. Therefore, I do not use acarbose in my practice, and I see no reason why miglitol should receive a better fate.

Drugs to encourage weight loss

Because most people with type 2 diabetes are obese and their glucose control improves with weight loss, the search for weight-lowering drugs has been enthusiastic, to say the least. Such drugs can have an enormous impact, not only on people who have diabetes but on the huge, nondiabetic obese population.

Roche Pharmaceuticals, Inc., has developed orlistat, which it calls Xenical. *Orlistat* is a gastrointestinal lipase inhibitor, which means that it reduces dietary fat absorption. Because the fat remains in the intestine, it reaches the stool, and some patients complain of gas, oily bowel movements, and even bowel incontinence. Usually these side effects disappear after a few weeks, but a few people stopped taking the drug because of this effect.

In a two-year study funded by the drug company, the people on orlistat lost considerably more weight than those who did not take the drug. Both groups were given a diet. Once they had lost weight, the patients showed a drop in blood pressure, bad cholesterol, and the need for insulin to control the blood glucose.

In another study also funded by the company, this time specifically of people with diabetes, the orlistat group lost much more weight than the non-orlistat group. The orlistat users were able to reduce their blood glucose, their hemoglobin A1c, their need for oral sulfonylurea medication, as well as their bad cholesterol levels. Very few of the orlistat-takers stopped the drug and left the study because of intestinal or bowel problems. Orlistat could be a major new weapon against the obesity that worsens diabetes and coronary artery disease.

Another drug that has shown some promise of weight loss in studies is leptin, which is made by Amgen, Inc. Leptin was discovered to be present in fat cells. As fat cells increase, more leptin is made, and it tells the brain to reduce food intake. In a small study of about 120 people, leptin, which must be given by injection, was given to one group and no leptin to the other. Both were put on a weight-loss diet. Those on leptin lost much more weight (four pounds compared to less than one pound on average) than those who did not take the drug. None of the people in this study had diabetes. Much more work needs to be done on this drug, and the problem of the need for injections is considerable.

A unique new drug that reduces glucose

About ten years ago, it was discovered that when insulin is secreted by the pancreas, another compound, now called *amylin,* is secreted at the same time. Amylin acts within the brain to slow the intestine, thus slowing the uptake of glucose after a meal. It also signals the liver to reduce liver output of glucose after eating, probably by suppressing production of glucagon, another hormone from the pancreas that helps to raise glucose when needed. Amylin is not working correctly in both type 1 and type 2 diabetes. In type 1, it is not present at all, and in type 2 it does not rise when food is eaten.

A company called Amylin Pharmaceuticals has developed an injectable form or amylin called *pramlintide.* A study has been done where pramlintide is injected along with insulin before meals in type 1 diabetes. Those who took the drug showed improvement in glucose compared to those who did not. Their diabetes became much easier to manage. In another study in type 2 diabetes, pramlintide has lowered blood glucose and hemoglobin A1c.

There have been problems in that the highest dose did not always lower glucose the most, but there have been few side effects other than nausea, which does not last. One potential benefit of pramlintide is its tendency to cause weight loss. The drug does not worsen hypoglycemia, but it must be given by injection, although it can be mixed with the insulin injection.

New drugs for neuropathy

Two drugs may improve the symptoms of neuropathy (see Chapter 5 for more on this condition). Both have been on the market for some time for the treatment of other conditions, but a new use may exist for them.

- ✔ **Gabapentin:** Manufactured by Parke-Davis for the treatment of seizures, gabapentin has been shown to significantly reduce the pain of diabetic neuropathy. Called Neurontin by the company, this drug not only improves diabetic neuropathy but the pain of other forms of neuropathy as well. Patients were able to sleep better because diabetic neuropathy is often worse at night. The drug may work as soon as two weeks after starting treatment.

  Gabapentin does have some side effects, namely sleepiness, dizziness, loss of balance, and fatigue.

- ✔ **Memantine:** Doctors have used this other promising drug in AIDS treatment. Memantine seems to reduce the pain of neuropathy, especially neuropathy at night. It does not appear to have any serious side effects, but more study is needed for this drug.

Improving Insulin Delivery

The biggest barrier that arises when I tell a patient that he or she needs to be on insulin is the fear of taking multiple shots. Drug companies are working on ways to deliver insulin without needles. This section provides the latest information about new ways to deliver insulin, many of which are on the verge of coming to market.

- ✔ **Oral insulin:** The difficulty with taking insulin by mouth is that it is a large protein and proteins are broken down by digestive enzymes into individual amino acids. In order to take insulin by mouth, you need a device to protect the insulin from those digestive enzymes. One way that this can be done is by packaging the insulin in "biologically erodable microspheres." These tiny round packages can carry insulin through the intestinal lining, where it's released in an active form into the circulation. The packages break up and leave the body. This work is fairly new and far from the market, but you should know about it because you may be taking insulin this way in the future.

- ✔ **Inhaled insulin:** Inhaled insulin is much closer to your medicine cabinet than oral insulin. Inhaled insulin will probably hit the market in the next couple of years. It will be a major improvement in diabetes care when it does. Studies have shown that it's just as effective as injected insulin in controlling the blood glucose in both type 1 and type 2 diabetes. A group receiving inhaled insulin had a lowering of hemoglobin A1c that was equal to a group using injections. Inhaled Therapeutics Systems, Inc., developed the device that delivers the insulin, and Pfizer, Inc., will probably market it.

The device is taken into the mouth, and the insulin is delivered in a dry powder into the lungs where it gets into the bloodstream. It has not resulted in problems in the nasal passages or lungs. The lowering of glucose by different doses of inhaled insulin is fairly consistent. People have used it for more than a year, and most of them chose to stay on it when the study was over.

The study used a form of rapid-acting insulin as the inhaled insulin. The patients still took a shot of long-acting insulin at night, so not all shots have been eliminated yet.

✔ **An implantable insulin pump:** This device is implanted under the skin and delivers insulin either to the abdominal cavity or into a vein. Studies of about 70 patients have shown that the pump can deliver insulin successfully for up to four years or longer. The patients had good metabolic control without a lot of weight gain. The major problem has been obstruction of the tube carrying the insulin, but this has been managed without surgery in most cases. More work needs to be done before this device is ready for patients.

Developing a New Form of Insulin

When it comes to rapid-acting insulin, which is needed for the glucose in a meal, lispro insulin (brand name Humalog) is an excellent form (see Chapter 10). Lispro insulin is made by Eli Lilly and Company. A new short-acting insulin, insulin aspart, is coming to market from Novo Nordisk under the brand name NovoLog. Insulin aspart is active almost instantly after the injection is taken, same as lispro insulin. It acts rapidly and is gone about the time the absorption of food from the meal is ending. There is less hypoglycemia with insulin aspart than regular insulin. Exactly how insulin aspart differs from lispro insulin is not clear yet.

Testing in New Ways

Becton Dickinson has come out with a home test for hemoglobin A1c, called the A1c At Home Test kit, which you can purchase at a pharmacy. At home, you obtain two drops of blood and put them on a treated test strip, which is then sealed in an envelope and mailed to a specific lab. Within seven to ten days, you receive your result.

You can sign up to have the kit sent to you automatically every three or six months. This is a valuable way to follow the progress of your diabetes care. Your doctor receives a copy of the test results when you do.

Transplanting of the Pancreas or Insulin-Producing Cells

If you have type 1 diabetes, all you need is a new pancreas, and you're cured. If it were only that simple. The problem is that your body does not like to have someone else's pancreas inside it. It tends to reject the foreign tissue and destroy it. The only way to protect the new organ is to block the body's response, called the immune response. Several drugs can do that, but they create their own problems. For example, steroids block immunity but raise the blood glucose.

One treatment for kidney failure is transplantation of a new kidney (see Chapter 5). If a person with diabetes needs to have a kidney transplant, that may be the best time to do a pancreas transplant as well because the kidney is going to require immunosuppression anyway. Pancreas transplantations have many benefits:

✔ The new kidney is exposed to normal blood glucose levels.

✔ Progression of complications already present may be slowed or stopped.

✔ Patients suffering from hypoglycemia, hyperglycemia, or autonomic problems (see Chapter 5) have an improved quality of life.

The choice of the recipient of the transplant is important because certain factors lead to greater success:

✔ Older age (greater than 45) confers a worse prognosis.

✔ Hardening of the arteries already present is a negative factor.

✔ Congestive heart failure results in a poor prognosis.

✔ Obesity increases the risk of transplant loss.

✔ Hepatitis C infection also increases the risk of transplant loss.

Simultaneous kidney and pancreas transplantation is, therefore, a definite choice for a younger person without the preceding risk factors or a person with life-threatening lack of awareness of hypoglycemia or poor quality of life due to uncontrolled diabetes.

Another approach is the use of *microencapsulated pancreatic islets,* which are injected into the person who requires insulin. The idea is to surround the insulin-producing cells with a protective capsule so that the cells in the body that want to destroy these injected foreign cells cannot get to them. So far, this approach has not been very successful. Although the cells continue to work and make insulin, they become covered with a layer of other cells. The process is called *fibrosis.* The result is that the blood glucose cannot get in to trigger insulin production and release, and the insulin cannot get out.

Some studies of microencapsulation have been successful in animals. No immunosuppression is needed, and the blood glucose remains normal. The microencapsulated cells rarely function for more than a year, however.

The most promising results have come from the University of Alberta in Edmonton, Canada. They are using new drugs to block the autoimmune destruction of islet cells taken from the pancreas of people who have recently died. Starting in 1999, they were able to transplant these cells into the liver of ten people with type 1 diabetes and these people were able to stop insulin injections entirely. As they have used the technique on more patients, the results have not been quite as good, with some patients requiring insulin, but not as much as before the transplantation. These results are so promising that the National Institutes of Health in the United States is funding a multi-center study to see if their results can be duplicated in other diabetes programs.

A New Hormone Linking Obesity to Diabetes

A study in *Nature* in January 2001 reports the discovery of a hormone called *resistin*. This hormone is made by fat cells and causes insulin resistance, which explains why insulin resistance increases with obesity. Resistin is suppressed by the drug that improves insulin resistance, rosiglitazone. Scientists have also begun to manufacture resistin. When resistin is injected into mice, it causes increased insulin resistance. When antibodies that oppose resistin are given to the mice, insulin resistance improves. This shows that other agents, besides the glitazone class of drugs, may help to improve type 2 diabetes by blocking resistin.

Getting Intestinal Cells to Make Insulin

A new technique to get intestinal cells to produce insulin has been described by Dr. Ira Goldfine and his colleagues at the University of California in San Francisco. They took the gene that is responsible for producing insulin in mice, broke it into small fragments, and fed it to the mice. The cells of the intestine of the mice were able to incorporate the fragments into their DNA and begin to synthesize insulin. The result is not a cure for diabetes because the intestinal cells live only a few days, so a pill would have to be taken regularly. Testing of this new treatment will take at least three to five years, but the immediate results are very promising.

Chapter 17

What Doesn't Work When You're Treating Diabetes

. . . .

In This Chapter

▶ Recognizing the signs that a treatment won't work

▶ Identifying drugs, diets, and other treatments that don't work

. . . .

*E*veryone wants a quick and easy solution to their problems. For every problem, five people offer a quick and easy answer. Just send in the money. These cheats have got what it takes to take what you've got.

Being fooled by these claims may be a lot more serious for you than the person who walked up to the man dressed as a polar bear who was promoting soft drinks in a shopping center. The first man said: "Don't you feel foolish, dressed like a bear?" The "bear" replied: "Me, foolish? You're the one talking to a bear."

The purpose of this chapter is to tell you as much as I know about the tests and treatments that don't work. Don't expect to find everything you have heard or read about that is "the new wonder cure" for diabetes. As soon as this book is published, new, more seductive claims will be made. I hope that you will remain skeptical, use the information, especially in the first section to test them out, and check with your doctor before you stop what works and try something that may do more harm than good.

How to Tell What Will Work for You

Many clues can alert you that a treatment may not work. Here are some of them:

✔ **If a treatment is endorsed by a Hollywood star or a basketball player or other sports figure, be highly skeptical.** Always consider the source and make sure that it's reputable. In this case, it's the fame of the star that is being used to convince you, not any special knowledge that he or she possesses.

Your health and the Internet

The Health on the Net Foundation has established a set of principles that any site on the Internet can adhere to. A site that follows the HONcode principles has agreed to the following principles:

Principle 1: Medical advice will be given by qualified professionals, or it will be stated that this is not the case.

Principle 2: The information supports but does not replace the patient-physician relationship.

Principle 3: Confidentiality of visitors to the site is respected.

Principle 4: Information is supported by references.

Principle 5: Claims about the benefit of specific treatments are supported by references.

Principle 6: Information is provided in the clearest possible manner with contacts provided for more information, including the Webmaster's e-mail address.

Principle 7: Support for the site is clearly identified, especially commercial support.

Principle 8: If supported by advertising, it is clearly stated, along with the advertising policy. Advertising is clearly differentiated from non-advertising material.

If a site agrees with these principles, you can bet the information on it is very reliable. I describe many of the HONcode sites in Appendix C.

- **If the treatment has been around for a long time but is not generally used, don't trust it.** Treatments that really work that have been around will have been tried in an experimental study where some people take it and some don't. Doctors and medical texts recommend drugs that pass that test.

- **If it sounds too good to be true, it usually is.** An example would be the claims about chromium improving blood glucose levels. The study that "proved" it was done on chromium-deficient people, a situation that does not exist in the United States.

- **Anecdotes are not proof of the value of a treatment or test.** The favorable experiences of one or a few people is not a substitute for a scientific study. If they did seem to respond to the drug, it may be for entirely different reasons.

A lot of the information comes from the Internet, specifically, the World Wide Web. In Appendix C, I provide the best resources currently available for diabetes from this amazing source. The same rules apply when you consider the validity of claims made on the Web with a few new rules thrown in:

- ✔ **Don't rely on search engines.** Search engines do not check claims for validity.

- ✔ **Go to the site of the claim and check to see whether most of the information there makes sense.** A lot of silly information should alert you. If you still feel the treatment might work, ask the Webmaster for references. If none are forthcoming, forget about the idea.

- ✔ **Go to sites that you know are reliable to see whether you can find the same recommendations.** The treatments on sites like the American Diabetes Association and the Diabetes Monitor can be relied upon. When there is uncertainty, these sites can usually tell you.

- ✔ **Go to conferences put on by reputable experts.** One reliable source is a book by Warner V. Slack, *Cybermedicine, the Computer as a Cure for Modern Medicine.*

Drugs That Don't Work

In the last decade so many drugs have been touted as the cure for diabetes, you would think everyone would all be cured by now. The fact is, as I have said again and again, you do have the tools right now to control diabetes, but it is not so simple as taking a pill. If it were, this book would not be necessary. In this section, I tell you about some drugs that have usually become well known because they "worked" in a few people.

A system is in place to protect you in clinical research studies. Make sure that your study has been approved by a review board in an institution that has been approved to do the research. (See the sidebar "How the ADA evaluates new drugs" for more on how the ADA evaluates new treatments.)

Chromium

You can find articles singing the praises of chromium for controlling the symptoms of diabetes in all kinds of magazines, newspapers, and on the Internet. Should you take supplements of chromium?

The strongest case for chromium comes from a study of people with type 2 diabetes in China. They were given high doses of chromium and were found to improve their hemoglobin A1c, blood glucose, and cholesterol while reducing the amount of insulin they had to make. However, these people were found to be chromium deficient in the first place. People in the United States and other countries where the diet is sufficient in chromium do not show chromium deficiency and do not show improvement in glucose tolerance when they take chromium. In addition, chromium is present in such small amounts normally that it is hard to measure even in people without chromium deficiency.

The amount of chromium needed by a person in his or her diet is uncertain but is estimated to be 15 to 50 micrograms daily. People given much more than that tend to accumulate it in their liver, where it can be toxic. Some studies suggest that chromium can cause cancer in high doses.

For now, the answer is that the evidence does not support the use of chromium in diabetes except where the person is known to be chromium deficient.

Aspirin

People who take the sulfonylurea drugs (see Chapter 10) sometimes have a greater drop in blood glucose when they take aspirin. This is because aspirin competes with the other drug for binding sites on the proteins that carry sulfonylureas in the blood. When they're bound to protein, the sulfonylureas are not active but when they're free, they are. Aspirin knocks the sulfonylureas off so that they're free. As a result, aspirin has been recommended as a drug to lower blood glucose.

By itself, aspirin has little effect on blood glucose. Its effect with sulfonylureas is so inconsistent that it can't be reliably depended upon to lower the blood glucose.

Pancreas formula

Pancreas formula is sold on the Internet as a mixture of herbs, vitamins, and minerals that help diabetes. No clinical or experimental evidence shows that pancreas formula does anything of value in the human body. The claims that are made for this "treatment" are not supported by factual evidence. Look for references in respected journals, and you will not find them. Save your money.

Fat Burner

You will hear and read a lot of advertising for the Fat Burner product in reputable newspapers and on reputable radio stations. Advertising claims that you can "burn fat without diet or exercise," and they will even throw in, ABSOLUTELY FREE, a bottle of Spirulina to enhance your Fat Burner weight control program. If you believe this is possible, I have a bridge I would like to sell you, CHEAP. In order to burn fat, you must exercise and stop taking in large amounts of carbohydrates.

How the ADA evaluates new drugs

The American Diabetes Association evaluates new therapies and places them in one of four categories:

✔ Clearly effective

✔ Somewhat/sometimes effective or effective for certain categories of patients

✔ Unknown/unproven but possibly promising

✔ Clearly ineffective

If you're about to try a new therapy that has not been recommended by your doctor and it is not discussed in this book, you may want to contact the ADA and find out its position on the treatment. Of course, if you're involved in a clinical trial that is trying to determine the effectiveness of a therapy, no one will know whether it works or not.

Ki-Sweet

The literature for Ki-Sweet is another lesson in being skeptical. The creators of this "miracle" sweetener claim that it has a "special designation from the American Diabetes Association." The ADA denies the claim, but how many people will buy something when they see ADA approval and not bother to see whether it's true? There is no evidence that Ki-Sweet, made by squeezing the juice of kiwi, has any advantages over other sweeteners.

Gymnema silvestre

Gymnema silvestre is a plant found in India and Africa. It's promoted as a glucose-lowering agent as part of a type of alternative medical treatment called Ayurvedic medicine. (For more on alternative treatments, see *Alternative Medicine For Dummies* by James Dillard, M.D., D.C., C.Ac., and Terra Ziporyn, Ph.D. [Hungry Minds, Inc.].) Gymnema silvestre has never been tested in a controlled study in humans. One statement in its advertising is, "For most people, blood sugar lowers to normal levels." There is no evidence that this is the case.

Aspartame

You will find the statement that aspartame causes cancer in many news sources. Because aspartame is used so much in diabetes and by nondiabetics, I want to emphasize the following:

Aspartame is an acceptable artificial sweetener with no known dangers to human beings. No evidence shows that aspartame causes cancer when used in normal amounts. The Food and Drug Administration has an acceptable daily intake for food additives, including a 100-fold safety factor. It is inconceivable that anyone would use more than that.

Diets That Don't Work

For the overweight person with type 2 diabetes, any diet that causes some weight loss helps for a time. But you have to ask yourself the following questions:

- ✔ Am I prepared to stay on this diet indefinitely?
- ✔ Is it a diet that is healthy if I stay on it?
- ✔ Will it combine all the features I need, namely weight loss, reduction of blood glucose, and reduction of blood fat levels with palatability and reasonable cost?

If you can say yes to all those questions, then the diet will probably work for you. If you walk into a reasonably large bookstore, you will be overwhelmed by the number of titles of diet books. It may be a fair statement that the more books that are written about a subject, the less that is known for certain about that subject. Why would authors bother to come up with ten new books on dieting each year, if the solution rested in some older book? You can bet that word of mouth would have made that book the all time bestseller in any category.

The books are way too numerous to list here, but they can be broken down into a few categories:

- ✔ **Diets that promote a lot of protein with little carbohydrates:** The trouble with these diets is that they're not a healthy and balanced approach. Unless you use tofu as your source of protein, you will be getting a lot of fat in your diet, much of it saturated fat. That is not good for you. The diet is lacking in vitamins that a supplemental vitamin pill may or may not provide. Very few people stay on such a diet for long. How many people can eat chicken for breakfast, lunch, and supper? The diet is also lacking in potassium, an essential mineral.

    People who do follow this kind of diet for a long time also find that they have problems with hair loss, cracking nails, and dry skin. Their breath and their urine smell of acetone because of all the fat breakdown. They become very dry and need to drink large quantities of beverages.

I see a place for this diet as a starter. Some people with type 2 diabetes who have high blood glucose levels show rapid improvement when started on a diet like this. As the glucose comes under control, the diet can be changed to a more balanced one.

✔ **Diets that promote little or no fat:** The people who can follow a diet that is less than 20 percent fat deserve a new designation — fatnatics (fat fanatics). This kind of diet is extremely difficult to prepare and perhaps even more difficult to eat unless you're a squirrel. In order to make up the calories, people on this diet eat large amounts of carbohydrates. Chapter 8 makes it clear why this is not a good idea for people with diabetes.

Like the protein diet, this diet may be lacking in essential vitamins and minerals, especially the fat-soluble vitamins. It is rare that a person will stay on such a diet after he or she has left the confines of the spa or other sanctuary where the diet is promoted. It, too, may be a good way to start a dietary program for a person with type 2 diabetes, as long as the total calories are not greater than the daily needs of that individual.

✔ **Very low calorie diets:** These diets, in the form of little food or a liquid containing calories (which generally does not taste very good) are lacking in many essential nutrients. They must be supplemented by vitamins and minerals. They cannot form the basis of a permanent diet because the dieter would eventually become emaciated. Dieters who start this kind of program do not last on it and regain every ounce they have lost and then some. (There are always exceptions, of course.)

I do not like this kind of diet even as a starter diet because it is so unlike our usual eating habits that people rapidly find it to be intolerable. Eating is a basic part of human existence. Eating can be done alone, but it's more enjoyable in company. It's a source of great pleasure for human beings and other animals. A diet that takes away this fundamental activity will not be tolerated for very long.

The transition from a very low calorie diet to a balanced diet is a very difficult one and rarely succeeds.

What about hypnosis?

As respected a source as the National Institutes of Health has listed hypnosis as a treatment for "stabilization of blood sugar in diabetes." Although it has a disclaimer that says that publishing this statement does not imply endorsement of the treatment, the fact that it comes from the NIH gives it credibility. The only trouble is that there is no experimental evidence that proves the usefulness of hypnosis. So you have to be wary, even when the advice comes from the most respected of sources.

Part V
The Part of Tens

The 5th Wave   By Rich Tennant

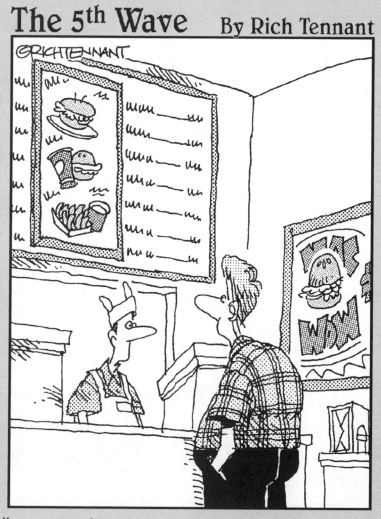

"Sorry sir—we don't currently offer
a 'Happy Hemoglobin Meal'."

In this part . . .

In this part, you find key techniques for managing diabetes. With just a little background from the other parts, you can use this section to really fine-tune your diabetes care. You find the ten commandments of excellent care, along with ten major myths about diabetes that you can discard. Finally, you find out how to utilize the skills and knowledge of the people around you, both the diabetes experts and your friends and family.

Chapter 18

Ten Ways to Prevent or Reverse the Effects of Diabetes

*I*f you read everything that came before this, congratulations. But I didn't expect that you would (and besides, this is a reference book, not a novel) and that's why I wrote this chapter. Follow the leader's (my) advice in this chapter, and you can be in great diabetic shape.

Major Monitoring

You have your glucose meter. Now what do you do with it? Most people do not like to stick themselves and are reluctant to do so at first. But you can do this in so many ways, almost without pain, that you have no excuse for not using this great advance in diabetes care. How often you test is between you and your doctor, but the more you do it, the easier it will be to control your diabetes. Monitoring gives you more insight into your particular body response to food, exercise, and medications. (See Chapter 7 for more on monitoring.)

People with type 1 diabetes need to test before meals and at bedtime because their blood glucose level determines their dose of insulin. People who have stable type 2 diabetes may test once a day at different times or twice a day. If you're sick or about to start a long drive, you might want to test more often because you don't want to become hypoglycemic — or hyperglycemic for that matter. The beauty of the meter is that you can check your blood glucose in less than 30 seconds any time you feel it's necessary.

Devout Dieting

If you are what you eat, then you have the choice of being controlled or uncontrolled depending upon what you put into your mouth. If you gain weight, you gain insulin resistance, but it does not take a lot of weight loss to reverse the situation. The main point you should understand about a "diabetic diet" is that it's a healthy diet for anyone, whether they have diabetes or not. You should not feel like a social outcast because you're eating the right foods. You don't need special supplements; the diet is balanced and contains all the vitamins and minerals you require (although you want to be sure you're getting enough calcium).

You can follow a diabetic diet wherever you are, not just at home. Every menu has something on it that's appropriate for you. If you're invited to someone's home, let them know you have diabetes and that the amount of carbohydrate and fat that you can eat is limited. If that fails, then limit the amount that you eat. And if that is somehow not possible, then accept the fact that your diet will not always be perfect and go on from there. (See Chapter 8 for more on your diet.)

Tenacious Testing

The people who make smoke detectors recommend that you change the battery without fail each time that you have a birthday. You should use the same simple device to remember your "complication detectors." Make sure that your doctor checks your urine for tiny amounts of protein and your feet for loss of sensation every year around the time of your birthday. It takes five to ten years to develop complications. Once you know the problem is present, you can do a lot to slow it down or even reverse it. Never has it been truer that "an ounce of prevention is worth a pound of cure." (For more on complications you may develop, see Chapter 4 and 5.)

I've made it very easy for you to get the tests you need at the time you need them. The Cheat Sheet at the front of this book gives you the current testing recommendations. Check out these recommendations and make a copy for your doctor if he or she does not already have such a list. Demand that you get the tests when they are due. A doctor with a busy medical practice may forget whether you have had the tests you need, but you don't have an excuse for forgetting.

Enthusiastic Exercise

When you take insulin, controlling your diabetes is a little harder than taking pills because you have to coordinate your food and the activity of the insulin. But I have patients who have had diabetes for decades and have little trouble balancing their food and insulin. They are the enthusiastic exercisers. They use exercise to burn up glucose in place of insulin. The result is a much more narrow range of blood glucose levels than is true of the insulin takers who do not exercise. They also have more leeway in their diet because the exercise makes up for slight excesses.

I am not talking about an hour of running or 50 miles on the bike. Moderate exercise like brisk walking can accomplish the same thing. The key is to exercise faithfully. (For more on exercise, see Chapter 9.)

My practice is among the hills of San Francisco. My patients really enjoy the ability to climb those hills with ease, a major benefit of a lifelong exercise program.

Lifelong Learning

When I see a patient new to me who has had diabetes for some time, I am amazed at the lack of knowledge of many fundamental areas of their disease. You would think that they would want to know anything that might help them to live more comfortably and avoid complications.

So much is going on in the field of diabetes that I have trouble keeping up with it, and it's my specialty. How can you expect to know when the doctors come up with the major advances that will cure your diabetes? The answer is lifelong learning. Once you have gotten past the shock of the diagnosis, you are ready to learn. This book contains a lot of basic stuff that you need to know. You can even take a good course in diabetes. Then you need to keep learning. Go to meetings of the local diabetes association. Become a member of the American Diabetes Association and get their terrific magazine called *Diabetes Forecast,* which usually contains the state of the art. Go to the Web sites that I discuss in Appendix C.

Remember that there is a lot of misinformation on the Web, so you must be careful to check out a recommendation before you start to follow it (see Chapter 17). Even information on reliable sites may not be right for your particular problem.

Above all, never stop learning! The next thing you learn may be the one that will cure you.

Meticulous Medicating

Compliance, which means treating your disease in accordance with your doctor's instructions, is a term that has special relevance for the patient with a chronic disease like diabetes who must take medications day in and day out. Sure, it's a pain (even if you could take insulin by mouth and not by injection). But the basic assumption in diabetes care is that you're taking your medication. Your doctor bases all his or her decisions on that assumption. Some very serious mistakes can be made if that assumption is false. Diabetes medications are pretty potent, and too much of a good thing can be bad for you. (For more on medications, see Chapter 10.)

Every time a study is done on why patients do not do better, compliance is high up or leads the list of reasons. Do you make a conscious decision to skip your pills, or do you forget? Whatever the reason, the best thing to do is to set up a system so that you're forced to remember. Keeping your pills in a dated container quickly shows you if you have taken them or not. You might even divide the pills by time of day. Make the system simple so that it will work for you.

Appropriate Attitude

Your approach to your disease can go a long way toward determining whether you will live in diabetes heaven or diabetes hell. If you have a positive attitude, treating diabetes as a challenge and an opportunity, not only is it easier for you to manage your disease, but your body actually produces chemicals that will make it happen. A negative attitude, on the other hand, results in the kind of pessimism that leads to failure to diet, failure to exercise, and failure to take your medications. Plus, your body makes chemicals that are bad for you.

Diabetes is a challenge because you have to think about doing certain things that others never have to worry about. It brings out the quality of organization, which can then be transferred to other parts of your life. When you're organized, you accomplish much more in less time.

Diabetes is an opportunity because it forces you to make healthy choices for your diet as well as your exercise. You may well end up a lot healthier than your neighbor without diabetes. As you make more and more healthy choices, you feel and test less and less like a person with diabetes. Does this mean that at some point you can give up your treatment? Probably not, although you will certainly take less medication.

Does diabetes mean that you cannot do what you want to do in your life? The person with diabetes has only a few legal restrictions, and they're disappearing fast. (See Chapter 15 for more on these restrictions.)

Preventive Planning

Life is full of surprises. Like the sign on a display of "I Love You Only" Valentine cards: Available in Multipacks. You never know when you will get more than you bargained for. That is why having a plan to deal with the unexpected is so important. Say you're invited to someone's home, and they serve something that you know will raise your blood glucose significantly. What do you do? Or you go out to eat and are given a menu of incredible choices, many of which are just not for you. How do you handle that? You run into great stress at work or at home. Do you allow it to throw off your diet, your exercise, and your drug taking?

The key to these situations is the realization that it's not possible for everything to go right all the time. You must be prepared for the times when things go wrong. In the case of the friend who cooked the wrong thing for you, you can at least eat a small portion to limit the damage. At the restaurant, you should come prepared with the food choices you know will keep you on your diet. It might be better not to look at the menu and simply discuss with your waiter what they have from your list of correct foods (unless, of course, you go to a restaurant that features "diabetes delicious" recipes). And if you allow stress to throw you off, you add the problems of poor diabetic control to your other stress, making it considerably worse.

This book is all about "what to do if." The more you understand the information available in this book, the less often you will find yourself in a situation that you cannot handle.

You might even do a "dry run." Go to a restaurant that you might like to try and read their menu. Carefully select the foods that will help you to stay in control. Practicing handling these situations before they arise makes it a lot easier to function when you are faced with the real thing.

Fastidious Foot Care

A recent headline read: "Hospital sued by seven foot doctors." I would certainly not like to treat any doctor with seven feet or even a doctor who is seven feet tall. Whether you have two feet or seven feet, you must take good care of them. The problem occurs when you can't feel with your feet because of neuropathy (see Chapter 5). You can easily know when this is present just by checking with a 10-gram filament. If your feet cannot feel the filament, they will not feel burning hot water, a stone, a nail in your shoe, or an infected ulcer of your foot.

When you lose sensation in your feet, your eyes must replace the pain fibers that would otherwise tell you there is a problem. You need to carefully examine your feet every day, keep your toenails trimmed, and wear comfortable shoes. Your doctor should inspect your feet at every visit.

Although diabetes is the primary source of foot amputations, it's entirely preventable, but you must pay attention to your feet. Test bath water by hand, shake your shoes out before you put them on, wear new shoes only a short while before checking for pressure spots, get a 10-gram filament and see whether you can feel it. The future of your feet is in your hands.

Essential Eye Care

You're reading this book, which means you are seeing this book. So far, there are no plans to put out a Braille edition, so you had better take care of your eyes or you will miss out on the wonderful gems of information that brighten every page.

Caring for your eyes starts with a careful examination by an ophthalmologist or optometrist. You need to have an exam at least once a year (or more often if necessary). If you have controlled your diabetes meticulously, the doctor will find two normal eyes. If not, signs of diabetic eye disease may show up (see Chapter 5). At that point, you need to control your diabetes, which means controlling your blood glucose. You also want to control your blood pressure because high blood pressure contributes to worsening eye disease.

Although the final word is not in on the effects of smoking and excessive alcohol on eye disease in diabetes, is it worth risking your sight for another puff of a cigarette? Even at this later stage, you can stop the progression of the eye disease or reverse some of the damage.

Chapter 19

Ten Myths about Diabetes That You Can Forget

Myths are a lot of fun. They're never completely true, but you can usually find a tiny bit of truth in a myth — which is one reason (and the need for an explanation when "science" fails to provide one) so many myths are believed.

The trouble is that some myths can hurt you if you allow them to determine your medical care. This chapter is about those kinds of myths — the ones that lead you to fail to take your medication or stay on your diet or even take things that may not be good for you. The ten myths in this chapter are only a small sample of all the myths that exist about diabetes. You probably know a few yourself, and I encourage you to send them to me. They could take up a whole book on their own. But the myths I describe in this chapter are some of the more important ones. Realizing that these myths are false can help prevent you from making some serious mistakes about good diabetes care.

Perfect Treatment Yields Perfect Glucoses

Doctors are probably as responsible as their patients are for the myth that perfect treatment results in perfect glucoses. For decades, doctors measured the urine glucose and told their patients that if they would just stay on their diet, take their medication, and get their exercise, the urine would be negative for glucose. Doctors failed to account for the many variables that could result in a positive test for glucose in the urine, plus the fact that even if the urine was negative, the patient could still be suffering diabetic damage (because the urine becomes negative at a blood glucose of 180 mg/dl (10 mmol/L) in most people, a level that still causes damage).

The same thing is true for the blood glucose. Although you can achieve normal blood glucose levels most of the time if you treat your diabetes properly, you can still have times when the glucose is not normal for any apparent reason. So many factors determine the blood glucose level at any given time that this should hardly be a surprise. These factors include

✔ Your diet

✔ Your exercise

✔ Your medication

✔ Your mental state

✔ Other illnesses

✔ The day of your menstrual cycle (if a woman)

The miracle is that the blood glucose is what you expect it to be as often as it is. Don't allow an occasional unexpected result to throw you. Keep on doing what you know to be right, and your overall control will be excellent.

Eating a Piece of Cake Can Kill You

Some people become fanatics when they develop diabetes. They think that they must be perfect in every aspect of their diabetes care. They often drive their family crazy with their demands for exactly the right food at exactly the right time. Doctors, again, can be blamed for the perpetuation of this myth. They told their patients that they must avoid sugar at all costs. Now, as Chapter 8 shows, doctors understand that a little sugar in the diet is not harmful, and that some foods, thought to be safe because they were "complex" carbohydrates, can raise the blood glucose just as rapidly as table sugar.

This myth goes back again to the fact that science does not have all the answers. Knowledge is still evolving. It may never reach the point where the statement made to Woody Allen's character in the movie *Sleeper* is true. He wakes up after sleeping for 100 years and is told that scientists now realize that milk shakes and fatty meats are good for you. But who knows?

Unorthodox Methods Can Cure Diabetes

In Chapter 17, I talk about some treatments that don't work. Those treatments were just the tip of the iceberg. Many treatments will not help you and may hurt you. Whenever a problem affects a huge number of people, others are eager to exploit this potential gold mine.

How can you know if what you read in your favorite magazine or see on the Internet is actually useful? Check it out with your physician, your diabetes educator, or other members of your team (see Chapter 11). They will know or can find out for you about any appropriate treatment. To date, diabetes has no simple cures. A book or organization that promises an easy cure is not doing you any favor.

Diabetes Ends Spontaneity

You may think that your freedom to eat when you want and come and go as you please is gone once you have diabetes. This myth is far from the truth. If you have type 1 diabetes, you need to balance your insulin intake with your food intake, but the availability of newer insulins means you can eat just about when you want and take your short-acting insulin (see Chapter 10) just before or even during or right after you eat. If you're a heavy exerciser, even the need for much insulin may not be true. One of my type 1 patients takes only a few units of insulin because he is so physically active. The result is that he requires little insulin, and his blood glucose stays in a very normal range most of the time.

Newer oral agents for type 2 diabetes allow you to eat when you want and anticipate that the blood glucose will remain normal. Exercise helps the type 2 patient as well.

Can you travel where you want with diabetes? Most certainly. You need to start a trip in good blood glucose control. You also need to make sure that you keep your medications with you so that if your luggage gets lost, your medicine does not go with it. In addition, find out about doctors who speak your language where you're going. These three things are now simple to do and ensure that diabetes will not affect your trip.

Should you dance the night away even though you have diabetes? If you can dance, I see no practical reason not to. Cut back on your insulin because you'll be doing so much exercise and check your blood glucose once or twice during the night. Otherwise, go for it!

Hypoglycemia Kills Brain Cells

Because hypoglycemia often comes on so fast and leaves you with a headache or a general feeling of weakness and sometimes confusion, it has been thought that low blood glucose (see Chapter 4), especially if it occurs repeatedly, may destroy mental functioning. Tests of people who have had repeated episodes of hypoglycemia have shown no loss of mental functioning. Children, on the other hand, may have different results because their brains are still developing, but adults will have no loss of mental functioning.

Fortunately, your body is supplied with hormones to reverse hypoglycemia. You need to check your blood glucose prior to heavy exercise and keep a supply of rapidly absorbable glucose nearby. Also let coworkers and loved ones know about your diabetes and how to recognize hypoglycemia. If you're prone to frequent low blood glucose, wear an ID bracelet. But you do not have to fear for your grey matter. It can withstand some pretty low levels of blood glucose without complaint.

Needing Insulin Means You're Doomed

Many people with type 2 diabetes believe that once they have to take insulin, they're on a rapid downhill course to death. This is not so. Once you're using insulin, it probably means that your pancreas has pooped out and cannot produce enough insulin to control your blood glucose, even when stimulated by oral drugs. But taking insulin is no more a death sentence for you than it is for the person with type 1 diabetes.

First of all, using insulin is often a temporary measure for when you're very sick with some other illness that makes your oral drugs ineffective. Once the illness is over, your insulin needs end.

Secondly, I see more and more people with diabetes who have been on insulin for some time after "failing" oral agents, who can be taken off the insulin and given one of the newer oral agents, which actually controls their glucose better than the insulin. One typical patient came to me on 60 units of insulin weighing 180 pounds with a hemoglobin A1c of 7.4. I gradually lowered his insulin as I added rosiglitazone to his treatment. He lost 22 pounds, came off of insulin entirely, and now has a hemoglobin A1c of 6.

Thirdly, elderly people with diabetes may need insulin to keep their blood glucose at a reasonable level but do not need very tight control because their probable life span is shorter than the time it takes to develop complications. Their treatment can be kept very simple. The insulin is being used to keep them "out of trouble," not to prevent complications.

Finally, people with type 2 diabetes who truly need to be on insulin intensively need to check their blood glucose more often and live more like a person with type 1 diabetes. Hopefully, you realize that with today's methods, this level of intensive treatment means a much higher quality of life than it used to.

People with Diabetes Shouldn't Exercise

If any myth is really damaging to people with diabetes, it is this one: People with diabetes shouldn't exercise. The truth is exactly the opposite. Exercise is a major component of good diabetes management, one that, unfortunately, all too often gets the least time and effort on the part of the patient as well as his or her care providers.

Sure, if you have certain complications like hemorrhaging in your eye or severe neuropathy, you need to take precautions or not exercise at all for a time. Certainly, if you're older than 40 and have not exercised, you need to have an examination and start gradually. But except for these and a few other reasons (see Chapter 9), exercise ought to be done regularly by every person with diabetes.

And I'm not just talking about aerobic exercise where your heart is beating faster. Some form of muscle strengthening needs to be a part of your lifestyle. (See Chapter 9 to find out the benefits of muscle strengthening.)

If you have a muscle that you can move, move it!

You Can't Get Life and Health Insurance

I devote Chapter 15 to show you that you *can* get life and health insurance. As the insurance industry recognizes that people with diabetes take better care of themselves than the general population does, it is more and more willing to insure them. Some unenlightened insurance companies still exist, but most are seeing the light as the vital statistics of the diabetic population improves.

The old problem of a "preexisting condition" seems to be disappearing as well. Insurance companies are not being allowed to use this excuse to block you from getting new insurance when you change jobs.

One thing that is true is that the cost of medical care is significant and is not declining. You don't want to be without medical insurance for any length of time. You may have to look a little longer than the person without diabetes, but you can eventually get insurance, and the price will be no higher than anyone else is paying.

Most Diabetes Is Inherited

Although type 2 diabetes runs in families, type 1 diabetes more often occurs as an isolated event in a family rather than being handed down from parent to child. (Chapter 3 explains why this is the case.) Even type 2 diabetes does not come out in every family member. It depends on such things as body weight, level of activity, and other factors.

A parent should not feel guilty if their small child develops diabetes. Such feelings make it harder to perform the necessary functions that the parent must do until the child can do them.

Diabetes Wrecks Your Sense of Humor

After the initial stages of accepting diabetes, your sense of humor should return. (See Chapter 1 for more on dealing with diabetes.) If your humor doesn't return, it's no laughing matter.

Dr. Joel Goodman, director of The HUMOR Project, pointed out in a lecture I attended that you "jest for the health of it." Numerous scientific studies have shown the health benefits of laughter.

The comedian, Steve Allen, pointed out in an interview performed by Dr. Goodman that there is humor in every aspect of life. You just have to look for it. If you keep your eyes and ears open, you will see and hear much to laugh at.

The saying goes "Someday we'll laugh about this." The question is "Why wait?"

My diabetic patients have been the source of many funny stories, some of which I have told in this book. I want to give you the assignment of coming up with at least one (or more) funny story from your diabetic past. Send me an e-mail at mellital@ix.netcom.com or write me a note about it. Remember that what you think is funny may not be funny to someone else. This is clearly shown by our individual preferences in comedians. Ask ten of your friends (do you have that many?) who their favorite comedian is and see if you don't come back with 12 answers.

Chapter 20

Ten Ways to Get Others to Help You

Diabetes is a social disease. No, I don't mean that you catch it like herpes. I mean that you can't continue very long with diabetes without calling on the help and expertise of others. Asking for help is not such a bad thing. People who regularly interact with others seem to live longer and have a higher quality of life.

In this chapter, you discover how to make use of the great resources that are available to people with diabetes. So many knowledgeable people are out there. It is a shame not to utilize their information. (Why, even I use my colleagues' knowledge on very rare occasions!)

Teach Hypoglycemia to Significant Others

If you take either insulin or one of the sulfonylurea medications (see Chapter 10), you may become hypoglycemic. Occasionally, hypoglycemia can be so severe that you're unaware of the problem. At that point, someone in your environment needs to know the symptoms of hypoglycemia and how to treat it. Chapter 4 contains all that information.

You may want to make a list of the signs and symptoms of hypoglycemia and pass it around to your family and friends. You should keep that list and an emergency kit to treat hypoglycemia at home and at work. You may even want to wear a medical alert bracelet so someone can identify your problem when none of these people are around.

Follow the Standards of Care

Decades of following diabetes patients along with increasing scientific knowledge have led to the establishment of "standards of care" for the person with diabetes. These recommendations usually appear in a supplement to the January issue of *Diabetes Care,* a journal of the American Diabetes Association. I outline these standards in Chapter 7 and on the Cheat Sheet at the front of this book. By following the standards of care, you have a good chance of avoiding the short- and long-term complications of diabetes. If these complications have already occurred, you have a good chance of having them diagnosed while they are still treatable.

You are the one who needs to make sure that you get an annual eye examination, get your urine tested for microalbumin and your nerves tested for sensation, not to mention all the other tests and studies that must be done regularly and routinely. (See Chapter 7 for more on these tests.) You can't do these tests alone, however. You need your physician to order the tests and send you to the eye doctor. Don't expect your physician to remember all these details. Just as you have trouble keeping to a program of care over a lifetime, your physician does much better with acute illnesses than chronic ones.

Make up a flow sheet with a list of the important tests and studies in one column. The next columns are the dates on which these things have been done or will be done on a regular basis. Blank spaces on the flow sheet should be obvious.

The standards of care include goals of treatment. If the standards are followed, the goals can be achieved. The goals of treatment give you a way of comparing your treatment with what is possible (though not necessarily certain).

Find an Exercise Partner

Few people (and I certainly count myself among this group) continue a regular exercise program completely on their own. However, when you know that someone is waiting for you, you tend to perform the exercise much more regularly. In my practice, I have many patients who are regular exercisers because I emphasize exercise so much. All of them exercise with a partner.

If you belong to a club, finding an exercise partner is easy. First, you select the sport and then hang out in the place where the sport is played. If the sport is a racket sport, you will soon find others at about your level. If the sport is something like running, you have to be a little forward and ask whether you can join someone or a group about to run. The people you can keep up with are your natural exercise partners.

If you're not a member of a club, finding an exercise partner is a little more difficult. Then you have to approach people with whom you work or your significant other. Most people are happy to walk with you, and some will run and bike with you. Cyclists seem to like group activity, and you can usually find a bike group to ride with. Check out listings at a local bike shop or the Sunday newspaper in the activities section.

Remember that just as you have or had many potential spouses out there for you, you have many potential exercise partners. If you do not find the right one on the first try, keep trying.

Use Your Foot Doctor

Your foot doctor is your first line of defense against lesions of the foot. He or she knows what the foot should look like and will notice problems very early when they're still reversible.

One of the most useful things the foot doctor can do is to cut your nails. It is too easy to accidentally cut your skin when you try to cut your own nails. If you have diabetes, the consequences can be serious.

Should you notice an abnormality, you must get to the foot doctor immediately. This is a situation where you are much better off erring on the side of too much rather than too little medical care. In my practice, I ask the patients about their feet at every visit and examine the feet of those who have been found to have neuropathy (see Chapter 5) in the past. If I discover a foot problem, the foot doctor sees it that day.

Doctors recently did the first hand transplantation, which seems to be going well, but as far as I know, there are no plans to do a foot transplantation. You better take good care of your feet because they have to last a lifetime. Your foot doctor can be your major ally in this endeavor.

Avoid Temptation

Ever since Adam and Eve, the problem of temptation has been on the front burner. I am not referring here to the temptation that they were involved in but, rather, the temptation to eat foods that will not further your major diabetic goal, which is to control your blood glucose. The opportunities for screwing up your diet are boundless. Just like your exercise partner, your "food partner" can make staying on your diet a lot easier for you.

First of all, he or she can prepare the right kinds of foods. To do this, your partner must know what to make and what to avoid (see Chapter 8). If you go to the dietitian, take your food preparer along. Numerous books of recipes and meals are written specifically for the person with diabetes. The first cookbook you should look at is *Diabetes Cookbook For Dummies* (published by Hungry Minds, Inc.), which I wrote with Fran Stach. That book would not have been written if it didn't offer a special feature — the recipes of some of the finest chefs in the United States and Canada. You can also go on the Internet to find some good choices; see Appendix C for a list of great Web sites to check out. You can even look inside this book (see Appendix A) for some great recipes.

Knowing how much food to make is just as important as what to make for your meals. Again, that information is available in books, especially those published by the American Diabetes Association.

I believe that the big problem in diabetes (as well as the nondiabetic obese population) is large portions of food. One of the simplest of diets is to eat the same foods but half as much. As I worked with the chefs in the various restaurants in this book, again and again they remarked to me that Americans eat much more food in a portion than Europeans. Americans have learned to avoid fat, but they eat too much carbohydrate. Your food preparer can make sure that the amount of food you eat is appropriate.

When it comes to eating out, your loved one can steer you to restaurants where you can choose foods that work for you. Once in the restaurant, he or she can point out the healthy choices. The best way to direct you is to set an example for you. Sticking to a diet is much easier if you see the same kinds of foods across the table.

If you're asked to dinner in someone's home, your loved one can help by telling your host and hostess in advance that you have diabetes and need to avoid eating certain foods. It is unwise, however, to turn your loved one into a nag. Don't ask that you be reminded each time you stray from your diet. That will lead to hostility.

Expand Your Education

The person who serves as your diabetes educator is the source of a huge amount of necessary and sometimes critical information. Every person with diabetes ought to go through a program of education once the initial shock of the diagnosis is past (see Chapter 1). You need to know a lot of information, and the diabetes educator is most highly qualified to teach it to you. Never hesitate to ask a question, no matter how basic you think it may be. You will be surprised by how many others want the same information. Things that seem obvious to the people who have followed those with diabetes for years are confusing to people who have just been given the diagnosis.

Of course, every caregiver should be a diabetes educator as well. Once you are past the formal diabetes education program, ask your physician, your dietitian, or any of the other people in your team (see Chapter 11) if you have questions or concerns.

Knowledge in diabetes is expanding so fast that great advances are arriving almost daily. Some of these advances may be just what you need for your diabetes. Keep aware of them by checking with your diabetes educators on a regular basis.

Enjoy Your Favorite Foods

Years ago when you got diabetes, it meant you had to make enormous changes in your diet. This was hard enough for people who ate the usual American diet, but much harder for people who came from another culture and had an entirely different diet. This has changed dramatically over the years. The new program is to take your usual diet and fit it into a diabetic eating plan. Unless your diet consists of many bottles of soda or beer each day, you should be able to find a diet plan for you that you find palatable.

The dietitian's job is to come up with a diabetic diet plan based upon **your** food choices, not those of the dietitian. If you have special dietary needs because of your culture, a dietitian must be able to accommodate those needs if they are reasonable.

Do not be satisfied with a printed sheet of paper with the heading "Diabetic Diet." The keyword in diabetic diets is individualization. It is not likely that you will stay on a diet that you do not enjoy.

Find Out about the Latest and Greatest

The specialist who knows the most about diabetes is the diabetologist, a physician with advanced training in diabetes care who maintains his or her edge by attending diabetes meetings regularly and keeping up with the literature by reading the most important clinical diabetes journals. In addition, in the modern world, an up-to-date specialist has to be aware of what is on the Internet and how to differentiate reality from hype. This person can be the source of information about the latest advances in diabetes and should be the person you go to when things are not going the way you want them to.

The pace of advances in diabetes is amazing. A general physician cannot keep up with them. A general physician has to worry about heart disease, lung disease, liver disease, and so on. The diabetes specialist concentrates on diabetes and that is to your benefit.

You have the right to insist on a visit to a diabetes specialist at least once a year just to check in and make sure that you are benefiting from the "latest and greatest." Be sure that you have your questions ready when you go. Write them down and check them off as you receive your answers.

Understand Your Medications

One of your most valuable and least utilized resources is your pharmacist. He or she is loaded with information about drug actions, interactions, side effects, proper dosage and administration, contraindications, and what to do in case of an overdosage. Every time you get a new medication, you can have your pharmacist run it against the medications you're already taking and see whether there might be any problems. Thanks to computers, this comparison should take only a few minutes. If you work with one drug store, you should be able to get a printout of your entire list of medications, which you can carry with you in case you ever need medical care.

Remember that the information in the computer tends to be all-inclusive. If a drug has ever had a side effect, no matter how rare, it will probably be in the computer. The drug manufacturer wants to be able to say that it warned you about every possibility. If a side effect or drug interaction is serious, you may want to discuss it with your physician before you start the new medication.

Your pharmacist also can tell you when a drug needs monitoring. For example, rosiglitazone requires liver function testing every two months for the first 12 months of use. If your doctor does not order the tests, the pharmacist will often remind you to remind the doctor.

Share This Book

If you really want your friends and loved ones to understand what you're going through, why not give them a copy of this book and ask them to read it? You can select the chapters that are most important to you. If they need to understand your diet, put a bookmark in Chapter 8. If they're unaware of the emotional adjustment you're going through, tell them to read Chapter 1. Your family and friends will probably be delighted to have a resource they can understand, and you can expect a lot more help from them.

When I began this book, I did so because I saw a need for information that could be understood by most people without the benefit of a medical school education. At the same time, I wanted you to have a little fun because "a spoonful of sugar helps the medicine go down." But I did not want to trivialize diabetes and hope I have not done so. If you believe I have succeeded in what I set out to do, share this book with others.

Part VI
Appendixes

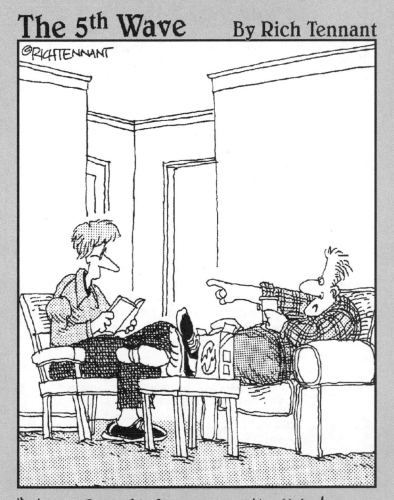

"C'mon, Darrel! Someone with diabetes shouldn't be lying around all day. Whereas someone with no life, like myself, has a very good reason."

In this part . . .

Appendix A is the *Diabetes For Dummies* Mini-Cookbook. Here, you find some of the most delicious and satisfying recipes that you can make. If you don't feel like making them, you find the name of the restaurant that has taken the time and effort to make sure that it offers excellent food for a person with diabetes. You can generally go to this restaurant and order that dish off the menu, knowing you will be on your diabetic diet.

Appendix B shows you how to use diabetic exchanges to figure out a proper diabetic diet. The appendix is based on the information presented in Chapter 8. You know what and how much food should be eaten to maintain normal weight and normal blood glucose levels, the key to prevention of complications.

Appendix C presents an introduction to the magnificent World Wide Web and the almost limitless resources to be found there about diabetes. You will be amazed at how much is given away for free on the Web. Some of it, however, is worth what you pay for it.

Appendix D is a glossary of terms you encounter as you read and hear about diabetes. You should be able to find any word that you do not understand in this glossary.

Appendix A

Mini-Cookbook

This appendix should make it clear to you that you can have great food from every ethnic corner of the world and still stay within the requirements of a diabetic diet. In a short appendix like this, I could not include every possible type of food, but tried to select the foods that most people enjoy either at home or in a restaurant. I chose the restaurants from among the best in the country, with an emphasis on San Francisco because that is where I reside and (happily) get to try them.

Sometimes it was necessary to alter a recipe slightly to keep it appropriate for a diabetic diet, but this was never done without the approval of the chef who created it. These chefs and these restaurants were a pleasure to work with and deserve great praise for their willingness to accommodate the needs of the diabetic patient.

Some recipes may take a little longer to prepare, but all are worth the time and the effort. In any case, you can go to the restaurant that provided the recipe, order that meal, and know that you are on your diabetic diet.

Keep in mind that all temperatures are in Fahrenheit.

Aqua

Situated in a grand post-1906 earthquake building on California Street, Aqua is located in the heart of San Francisco's bustling Financial District. At Aqua, owner Charles Condy and Executive Chef Michael Mina have joined forces to redefine dining and to pay elegant tribute to the flavors of the sea. The contemporary American design, combining a relaxed yet elegant ambiance, has set the stage for Chef Mina's imaginative menu.

Since becoming the Executive Chef of Aqua, Michael Mina's intensely flavorful and creative seafood cooking has earned him a reputation as one of the nation's most influential and respected chefs. Embracing a straightforward approach in coaxing lusty flavors and California's seasonal bounty, this young chef continues to capture hearts and palates of diners and critics. His culinary skills resulted in his designation as the James Beard Foundation's Rising Star Chef in 1997 and other prestigious awards have followed.

Aqua, 252 California Street, San Francisco, California. 415-956-9662.

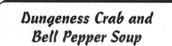

Dungeness Crab and Bell Pepper Soup

This soup is a wonderful start to any meal. Serve with some crusty French bread, so your friends can clean out their bowls.

Preparation time: *1 hour, 5 minutes*

Cooking time: *1½ hours*

Yield: *4 servings*

For Crab Stock

2 tablespoons olive oil

1 each whole dungeness crab, cut into 4 pieces

2 ounces brandy

2 tablespoons tomato paste

1 head garlic

2 quarts lobster stock (water may be used)

For Soup

3 red bell peppers

1½ red jalapeno with seeds

2 tablespoons olive oil

1 bay leaf

6 Roma tomatoes, split in half

1 large yellow onion, sliced in ½ to ¼ inch pieces

1 For crab stock: In a stockpot, heat oil until smoking. Add crab and cook 3 minutes until crab turns red in color. Add brandy and cook, stirring to dissolve any flavorful particles adhered to the bottom of the pot, until reduced by half, about 1 to 2 minutes. Add the garlic and tomato paste and cook, stirring, another 2 minutes. Add stock (or water) and bring to a boil. Reduce heat and simmer for 1 hour. Strain and reserve liquid.

2 *For soup:* Preheat oven to 300°. In a large bowl, toss soup ingredients together, evenly coating the vegetables with the olive oil. Spread out on sheet pan. Roast for 1 hour or until soft. Add pepper mixture to crab stock and simmer 30 minutes. Remove bay leaf. Puree in blender and strain. Add salt and pepper to taste.

Nutrient analysis per serving: *290 calories; 8 grams protein, 23 grams carbohydrate, 15 grams fat, 2 grams saturated fat, 50 milligrams cholesterol, 4 grams fiber, 935 milligrams sodium.*

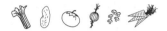

Warm Asparagus and Morel Salad

This dish is perfect as the first or second course to any meal. Try serving it after the Dungeness Crab and Bell Pepper Soup.

Preparation time: *1 hour*

Cooking time: *30 minutes*

Yield: *8 servings*

48 asparagus spears	*Salt and pepper to taste*
1 cup balsamic vinegar	*2 heads frisee*
8 ounces morel mushrooms	*1 to 2 tablespoons water*
1 tablespoon butter, plus 1 teaspoon to warm asparagus	*¼ cup olive oil*

1 Peel each piece of asparagus 2 inches from the top to the base (you won't need to do this if you're using young, thin asparagus). Cut each spear, leaving a 3- to 4-inch tip. Use remaining asparagus by slicing ¼-inch rounds Do not use woody part of asparagus. Keep tips and rounds separate.

2 Boil water, adding salt to taste. Add asparagus tips to boiling water. Once tender but still firm, about 2 minutes, place the asparagus in ice cold water to cool. Proceed by blanching asparagus rounds another 2 to 3 minutes. Use same process to cool. Set the cooling tips and rounds aside, keeping them separate.

(continued)

3 Over low heat, in a heavy-bottom saucepan, cook the vinegar for 20 to 30 minutes, never allowing it to reach a boil. Once the balsamic reaches a syrupy consistency, remove from heat. This process requires attention. It is quite easy to burn the balsamic.

4 Slice the morel mushrooms into ¼-inch rounds and place in warm water to remove excess dirt. Dry mushrooms to get rid of the moisture. In a medium sauté pan, heat the butter over medium heat. When bubbly, add the mushrooms. Cook, occasionally stirring gently, until soft, about 4 to 5 minutes. Season with salt and pepper to taste. Set aside.

5 Remove all outside leaves from the frisee, leaving only the inner white leaves. Separate the leaves from the stem, rinse under cold water, and spin or pat dry. Set aside.

6 To serve: Drizzle the balsamic glaze decoratively on each plate. In a medium sauté pan, warm the asparagus tips in the remaining butter mixed with 1 to 2 tablespoons water. Place the asparagus tips facing outward toward the rim of the plate. In the same sauté pan, heat the asparagus rounds with the morel slices. Then place the morels and asparagus rounds in a neat mound slightly overlapping the ends of the asparagus tips. In a medium bowl, mix the frisee with the olive oil. Finally, top the mushrooms and asparagus with the frisee.

Nutrient analysis per serving: 133 calories; 3 grams protein, 13 grams carbohydrate, 9 grams fat, 2 grams saturated fat, 4 milligrams cholesterol, 3 grams fiber, 37 milligrams sodium.

Grilled Swordfish with Worcestershire Vinaigrette and Roasted Vegetables

This dish is a delightful way to flavor both the fish and vegetables. It is a complete meal, but low enough in carbohydrate to include a couple of slices of French bread.

Preparation time: 40 minutes

Cooking time: 1 hour, 10 minutes

Yield: 8 servings

Vinaigrette

½ cup Worcestershire sauce

1 sprig rosemary, leaves only, chopped

⅛ cup chopped chives

1 clove garlic, minced

1 tablespoon balsamic vinegar

Juice of ¼ lemon

1 cup extra-virgin olive oil

Roasted Vegetables

8 new potatoes, cut in half

16 baby beets, well rinsed and ends trimmed

24 baby carrots, peeled

16 shiitake mushrooms, stems removed

16 shallots, unpeeled and cut in half

2 pounds red and yellow cherry tomatoes

3 tablespoons olive oil

8 swordfish, approximately 6 ounces each

Salt and pepper to taste

1 pound arugula

1 *For vinaigrette:* Mix all ingredients together. This vinaigrette should be made 24 hours in advance. The nutritional analysis reflects only 2 tablespoons.

2 *For roasted vegetables:* Heat oven to 375°. Place iron skillet in oven until hot. Keeping vegetables separate, in a large bowl, toss the potatoes, beets, carrots, mushrooms, shallots, tomatoes, 2 tablespoons olive oil, and salt and pepper, then transfer to hot skillet, and then roast until tender, about 45 minutes. You can do this ahead of time and then reheat the vegetables when you're ready to cook the fish.

3 *To serve:* Reheat the vegetables in the oven if done ahead of time. Preheat the grill. Season the swordfish on both sides and cook until medium rare, about 3 minutes per side.

4 In a large sauté pan, heat the remaining olive oil over high heat. Add the arugula and cook, tossing or gently mixing with kitchen tongs, just until the greens start to wilt, about 1 minute. Mix greens with the hot vegetables and place in the center of the plate, dividing vegetables evenly.

5 Place swordfish on top of vegetables. Drizzle 2 tablespoons vinaigrette over each portion.

Nutrient analysis per serving: *519 calories; 48 grams protein, 36 grams carbohydrate, 22 grams fat, 3 grams saturated fat, 126 milligrams cholesterol, 3 grams fiber, 544 milligrams sodium.*

Miso Marinated Seabass

This unique marinade adds a tremendous amount of flavor without the use of fat. You can add a tossed green salad with your favorite vinaigrette. This dish is also low in carbohydrate, so complete the meal with a cup of rice.

Preparation time: *45 minutes*

Cooking time: *5 minutes*

Yield: *8 servings*

(continued)

¼ pound brown sugar

¼ pound sugar

½ pound miso paste

¼ cup soy sauce

1 cup sake

1 cup rice wine vinegar

8 6-ounce portions Chilean sea bass

Vegetable oil

1 cup chicken consommé

1 cup snow peas

1 cup carrots, sliced thin and boiled in salted water 3 to 4 minutes

½ pound baby bok choy, boiled in salted water 1 to 2 minutes

5 each assorted radishes, thinly sliced

1 cup shiitake mushrooms, sliced

1 8-ounce package enoki mushrooms

1 *For marinade:* In a large bowl, mix together the sugars, miso paste, soy sauce, sake, and rice wine vinegar. Place the fish into the bowl, coat it with marinade, and cover the bowl. Refrigerate and marinate for 24 hours.

2 Preheat the broiler. Rub a shallow roasting pan (large enough to fit the fish in 1 layer) lightly with vegetable oil. Remove the sea bass fillets from the marinade, place them on the roasting pan, and place under the broiler. Cook until the fish begins to brown, about 2 to 3 minutes. Transfer the pan to the oven and cook through, about 5 minutes, depending on the thickness of the fillets.

3 Combine the consommé with snow peas, carrots, bok choy, radishes, and shiitake and enoki mushrooms in a medium sauté pan. Simmer, covered, until vegetables are warm. Season to taste. Place a pile of vegetables in the center of each large serving bowl, set a sea bass fillet on top, and spoon the consommé around.

Nutrient analysis per serving: 295 calories; 37 grams protein, 26 grams carbohydrate, 4 grams fat, .5 grams saturated fat, 82 milligrams cholesterol, 2 grams fiber, 1,295 milligrams sodium.

Marinated Grilled Duck Breast

Although duck is higher in fat than other types of poultry, it still can be served as a dish for special occasions. Round out this meal with a cup of wild rice and sautéed vegetables.

Preparation time: 30 minutes

Cooking time: 1 hour

Yield: 4 servings

1 cup balsamic vinegar

½ cup Worcestershire sauce

¼ cup honey

1 cup extra virgin olive oil

1 tablespoon chopped garlic

½ tablespoon lemon juice

½ bunch Italian parsley

½ bunch rosemary

½ bunch chives mushrooms

4 duck breasts

Salt and pepper to taste

1 *For marinade:* Place all ingredients, except for duck, in a large bowl and mix well. Score (make crisscross patterns with the tip of a sharp knife) skin side of the cleaned duck breast. Place the duck into the bowl, coat it with marinade, and cover the bowl. Refrigerate and marinate for 24 hours.

2 Preheat grill. Remove duck from marinade and pat dry with a clean towel. Season with salt and pepper. Grill for 10 minutes on skin side, turn, moving the breasts to cooler portions of the grill, and cook another 5 minutes, or until medium rare. To sear duck, place 2 nonstick skillets over medium-high heat. When hot, add the duck breasts, skin side down. Cook for 10 minutes. Reduce the heat, turn breasts over, and cook another 5 minutes or until medium rare. Slice just before serving.

Nutrient analysis per serving: 507 calories; 47 grams protein, 6 grams carbohydrate, 32 grams fat, 8 grams saturated fat, 177 milligrams cholesterol, 0 grams fiber, 300 milligrams sodium.

Border Grill

Situated in Santa Monica, California, the critically acclaimed Border Grill Restaurant features the bold foods of Mexico. The original restaurant has been joined by another Border Grill, this time in Las Vegas, and by Ciudad in downtown Los Angeles, which emphasize the cooking of Central and South America, Spain, and the Caribbean.

The restaurants are the inspiration of two women who are chefs, restauranteurs, cookbook authors, and television and radio personalities, Mary Sue Milliken and Susan Feniger. They are hosts of the Food Network's popular series, *Two Hot Tamales* and *Tamales World Tour.* They are natural teachers who share their passion for bold flavors and strong statements through many media. If you find, as I did, that their recipes make you hunger for more, look for their book *Mexican Cooking For Dummies* (IDG Books Worldwide, Inc.).

Border Grill, 1445 4th St., Santa Monica, California. 310-451-1655.

Cinnamon-Brandy Chicken

Looking for a different way of cooking chicken? Here is a wonderful recipe brimming with flavor and easy to prepare. Serve with the rice pilaf and roasted vegetable dishes, later in this section.

Preparation time: *30 minutes*

Cooking time: *40 minutes*

Yield: *6 servings*

½ cup brandy

1 tablespoon cinnamon

¼ cup honey

½ cup lemon juice

½ cup orange juice

4 garlic cloves, minced

1 teaspoon salt

½ teaspoon freshly ground black pepper

1 frying chicken, 2½ to 3 pounds, cut into pieces

2 tablespoons vegetable oil

1 In a medium bowl, mix the brandy, cinnamon, honey, lemon and orange juices, garlic, and salt and pepper. Add the seasoned chicken and toss to evenly coat. Cover and marinate in the refrigerator 8 hours or overnight.

2 Preheat oven to 350°. Remove the chicken, shaking off excess marinade. Pour the marinade into a small saucepan and bring to a boil. Boil until it begins to thicken and about 1 cup remains, 5 to 10 minutes.

3 Heat the oil in an ovenproof skillet over medium-high heat. Sear the chicken until golden on both sides. Pour the reduced marinade over the chicken and place in the oven. Bake about 20 minutes and serve.

Nutrient analysis per serving: *506 calories; 42 grams protein, 16 grams carbohydrate, 25 grams fat, 7 grams saturated fat, 134 milligrams cholesterol, 0 grams fiber, 502 milligrams sodium.*

Green Rice Pilaf

This dish can accompany the chicken in the preceding recipe, or it can be served with meat or fish.

Preparation time: *40 minutes*

Cooking time: *25 minutes*

Yield: *6 servings*

1½ tablespoons vegetable oil

1 small onion, finely diced

1 cup long-grain white rice

2 cups hot vegetable or chicken broth, preferably homemade

½ teaspoon salt

3 medium poblano chiles, roasted, peeled, seeded, and cut into strips

1 cup fresh or frozen peas

½ cup crumbled Mexican queso fresco or feta cheese

½ bunch Italian parsley leaves, finely chopped

½ bunch cilantro, finely chopped

1 Heat the oil in a heavy saucepan over medium heat. Add the rice and onion and cook, stirring frequently, about 7 minutes, until the onion is softened but not browned.

2 Add the hot broth, salt, and chiles and bring to a boil. Reduce to a simmer and cook, covered, about 10 minutes.

3 Add the peas and simmer 5 minutes longer. Remove from heat and let stand, covered, about 10 minutes.

4 Add the cheese, parsley, and cilantro, evenly mix, and fluff with a fork. Serve immediately.

Nutrient analysis per serving: *202 calories; 12 grams protein, 28 grams carbohydrate, 7 grams fat, 3 grams saturated fat, 1 milligram cholesterol, 2 grams fiber, 948 milligrams sodium.*

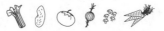

Red Roasted Root Vegetables

You can substitute any of your favorite root vegetables in this dish. It is a great side dish for chicken, fish, or meat.

Preparation time: *35 minutes*

Cooking time: *40 minutes*

Yield: *6 servings*

½ pound turnips, peeled and cut into 1-inch chunks

½ pound beets, peeled and cut into 1-inch chunks

½ pound carrots, peeled and cut into 1-inch chunks

½ pound butternut or other firm squash, peeled and cut into 1-inch chunks

1 onion, coarsely chopped

2 garlic cloves, minced

½ bunch fresh oregano leaves, coarsely chopped

⅓ cup olive oil

1 teaspoon salt

½ teaspoon freshly ground pepper

1 Preheat oven to 450°. In a large bowl, toss together all the ingredients until well mixed.

2 Arrange in a single layer in an enameled cast-iron casserole or baking dish. Cover and roast 30 to 40 minutes, stirring every 10 minutes. The vegetables are done when golden, lightly caramelized on the edges, and easily pierced with the tip of a knife.

Nutrient analysis per serving: *171 calories; 2 grams protein, 15 grams carbohydrate, 11 grams fat, 2 grams saturated fat, 0 milligrams cholesterol, 4 grams fiber, 432 milligrams sodium.*

Baked Apples

This dessert is a wonderful way to top off any meal. It is light, healthy, and low in calories.

Preparation time: *35 minutes*

Cooking time: *1 hour*

Yield: *6 servings*

1 cup plus 2 tablespoons apple juice

¼ cup raisins

¼ cup apple butter

¼ cup toasted chopped walnuts

2 tablespoons maple syrup

2 tablespoons brandy

6 medium apples, cored and the top third peeled

2 tablespoons unsalted butter

1 In a small saucepan, bring 2 tablespoons apple juice and the raisins to a simmer and remove from heat. Let sit for 10 minutes.

2 Preheat the oven to 350°. In a bowl, stir together the apple butter, walnuts, maple syrup, brandy, and raisins with their juice and mix well.

3 Stuff the apples with the raisin mixture. Place the apples in a small roasting pan and top each with a dab of butter. Pour the remaining cup of apple juice into the pan and bake 50 to 60 minutes, or until tender but not split or mushy.

Nutrient analysis per serving: 218 calories; 2 grams protein, 38 grams carbohydrate, 8 grams fat, 3 grams saturated fat, 11 milligrams cholesterol, 4 grams fiber, 2 milligrams sodium.

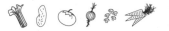

Baked Sea Bass

Here is a delightful way to season and bake fish. You can serve this with the rice pilaf and roasted vegetable dishes earlier in this section for a complete meal.

Preparation time: *45 minutes*

Cooking time: *15 minutes*

Yield: *6 servings*

6 4-ounce sea bass fillets

Salt and freshly ground pepper to taste

Salsa Verde

2 garlic cloves

2 jalepenos, stemmed, seeded, and chopped

½ bunch cilantro leaves, chopped

½ bunch Italian parsley leaves, chopped

6 green onions, white and light green only, trimmed and chopped

6 Tomatillos, husked, washed, and roasted

2 teaspoons dried oregano

⅓ cup clam juice or chicken broth

2 tablespoons fruity olive oil

1 teaspoon salt

Lemon wedges for serving

(continued)

1 Preheat the oven to 350°. Season the fish all over with salt and pepper and place in an oil-lined ovenproof baking dish.

2 To make salsa, combine all the ingredients in a blender or food processor and puree.

3 Pour the salsa over the fish in the pan and bake 8 to 12 minutes, until the thickest part of the fish is done. Serve with lemon wedges and salsa spooned on top.

Nutrient analysis per serving: 158 calories; 22 grams protein, 2 grams carbohydrate, 9 grams fat, 1 gram saturated fat, 8 milligrams cholesterol, .2 grams fiber, 499 milligrams sodium.

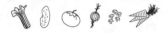

Charlie Trotter's

One of the most innovative restaurants in the country, Charlie Trotter's specializes in creative American cuisine with French and Asian overtones. It stresses the use of healthful, fresh foodstuffs. Naturally raised meats, game birds, organic fruits, and vegetables form the heart of Trotter's cooking.

Charlie Trotter's has won numerous awards and other recognition for the quality of its food, its décor, and its service. It received five stars from the *Mobil Travel Guide*, is listed in the very prestigious *Relais and Chateaux,* and was given the Grand Award by the *Wine Spectator* as The Best Restaurant in the World for Wine and Food (1998).

Owner and chef Charlie Trotter began to cook professionally in 1982. He trained in Europe and America with Norman Van Aken, Bradley Ogden, and Gordon Sinclair.

The recipes provided by Charlie Trotter tend to take a little more time to prepare than some of the other restaurants, but the results more than make up for the time spent. (If you like the recipes, you may want to check out Charlie Trotter's book, *Gourmet Cooking For Dummies,* Hungry Minds, Inc.)

Charlie Trotter's, 816 West Armitage, Chicago, Illinois. 773-248-6228.

Roasted Tomatoes Stuffed with Couscous, Chicken, Chanterelles, and Pinenuts

You can serve this dish as a main course for lunch or as a side dish for dinner. If you serve this as a main course for lunch, you can round out the meal with a couple of slices of French bread and a tossed salad with 1 tablespoon olive oil.

Preparation time: *1 hour, 15 minutes*

Cooking time: *15 minutes*

Yield: *4 servings*

8 small tomatoes

2 tablespoons basil oil

8 cloves garlic

8 thyme sprigs

8 bay leaves

8 large basil leaves

¼ cup, quartered chanterelle mushrooms

1 tablespoon olive oil

2 tablespoons sweet corn kernels

2 cups cooked couscous

2 tablespoons peeled, seeded, and diced tomatoes

2 tablespoons pinenuts

1 tablespoon peeled and finely diced cucumber

1 chicken breast, cooked and finely diced

2 teaspoons chopped chives

1 tablespoon chopped mixed herbs (tarragon, mint, basil)

Salt and pepper to taste

1 *For tomatoes:* Preheat oven to 250°. Cut a small *x* in the bottom of each tomato and drop into boiling water for 15 seconds. Remove the tomatoes from the water and peel off the skins. Cut a ¾-inch slice off the bottom of each tomato, reserving them for lids. Scoop out the seeds and center flesh. Rub the insides with 1 tablespoon basil oil and place a clove of garlic, a sprig of thyme, bay leaf, and basil leaf in each tomato. Place the tomatoes in a small baking pan or casserole, put the lids on, and roast for 10 to 12 minutes, or until the tomatoes just begin to soften. Remove and discard the garlic and herbs.

2 *For filling:* In a medium sauté pan, cook the mushrooms in a teaspoon of olive oil over medium heat for 3 minutes or until tender. Remove the mushrooms from the pan, add the corn kernels, and sauté for 2 minutes or until hot. Warm the couscous over a double broiler and stir in the mushrooms, tomatoes, pinenuts, cucumber, chicken, and corn until thoroughly incorporated. Stir in the remaining 2 teaspoons olive oil, chives, and herbs, and season to taste with salt and pepper.

3 Rub the outsides of the tomatoes with the remaining 1 tablespoon basil oil and return to the oven for 3 minutes. Place 2 tomatoes in the center of each plate. Spoon the filling loosely into each tomato, spooning the remaining filling around the base of the tomatoes.

Nutrient analysis per serving: *309 calories; 14 grams protein, 35 grams carbohydrate, 10 grams fat, 1 gram saturated fat, 18 milligrams cholesterol, 4 grams fiber, 504 milligrams sodium.*

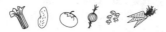

Scallops with Barley, Wild Mushroom Ragout, and Chicken Stock Reduction

This meal is low in carbohydrate, which allows you to have a couple of slices of bread or a serving of sherbet to round it out.

Preparation time: *1 hour*

Cooking time: *45 minutes*

Yield: *4 servings*

3 tablespoons chopped fennel	*6 tablespoons Madeira*
3 tablespoons canola oil	*Salt and pepper*
½ cup red wine	*1 teaspoon chopped parsley*
¼ cup peeled, seeded, and diced tomato	*1 teaspoon tarragon leaves*
3 cups chicken stock	*20 medium seas scallops*
1¼ pounds mixed wild mushrooms (shitake, cepe, portobello, and so on)	*2 cups cooked barley*

1 *For the reduction:* In a medium sauté pan, cook the fennel in 1 tablespoon canola oil for 5 minutes or until thoroughly softened. Add the red wine and stir continuously until the wine is reduced to a glaze. Add the tomato and chicken stock and cook over medium-low heat for 30 minutes or until reduced to 1 cup.

2 *For mushrooms:* Cut the mushrooms into large pieces (smaller ones can be used whole). In a medium nonstick sauté pan, heat 1 tablespoon canola oil over medium-low heat. Add the mushrooms and cook, tossing or stirring occasionally, for 10 minutes, or until mushrooms are tender and all the liquid is evaporated. Add the Madeira and cook until it is completely reduced. Season the mushrooms to taste with salt and pepper and add the parsley and tarragon. Set aside.

3 *For scallops:* Heat the remaining 1 tablespoon canola oil in a nonstick sauté pan over medium-high heat or until hot. Add the scallops and cook for 2 minutes, or until golden brown. Season the scallops with salt and pepper. Turn over the scallops and cook for 1 minute.

4 *To serve:* Place the cooked barley on each plate. Spoon some of the fennel sauce onto each plate, place a neat mound of mushrooms over the sauce, and surround with 5 scallops, leaning them against the mushrooms.

Nutrient analysis per serving: *398 calories; 27 grams protein, 36 grams carbohydrate, 20 grams fat, 5 grams saturated fat, 42 milligrams cholesterol, 2 grams fiber, 1,084 milligrams sodium.*

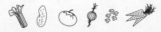

Peppered Tuna with Red Wine-Mushroom Broth, Brussel Sprouts, and Potato Gnocchi

This meal is low in total carbohydrate and total fat. You can complete the meal with a couple of slices of bread.

Preparation time: *1 hour, 30 minutes*

Cooking time: *2 hours*

Yield: *4 servings*

1½ pounds button mushrooms

3 cups water

1 small onion, peeled and chopped

1 stalk celery, chopped

6 cloves garlic, peeled and chopped

1½ tablespoons olive oil

1 small tomato, chopped

½ cup balsamic vinegar

1 bottle Cabernet Sauvignon or Zinfandel

2 tablespoons plus 1½ teaspoons butter

Salt and pepper to taste

1 egg yolk

2 medium potatoes, peeled, cooked, and diced

¾ to 1 cup flour

½ cup julienned leeks

20 Brussel sprouts

1 12-ounce tuna loin

2 teaspoons coarsely ground black pepper

1½ teaspoons canola oil

1 *For sauce:* Place the mushrooms and water in a saucepan and simmer for 25 minutes. Strain the liquid into a smaller saucepan, discarding the solids, and continue to simmer for 25 minutes or until reduced to about ¾ cup. In a medium nonstick sauté pan, cook the onion, celery, and garlic in ½ teaspoon olive oil over low-medium heat for 8 minutes, or until the onions are soft. Add the tomatoes and balsamic vinegar and reduce to a syrupy glaze. Add the wine and cook over low heat for 30 minutes. Strain through a fine-meshed sieve, discarding the solids and returning the sauce to the pan. Continue cooking at a low simmer for 30 to 40 minutes or until reduced to ½ cup. Combine the mushroom broth and reduced red wine in a small saucepan and bring to a boil. Remove from heat, whisk in 2 tablespoons butter, and season with salt and pepper. Set aside, keeping sauce warm.

2 *For gnocchi:* Work the egg yolk into the potatoes with a wooden spoon and knead in enough flour so that the dough is not sticky. Season with salt. Divide the dough into 4 portions. Roll each portion into a long cigar shape about ½ inch in diameter. Cut into ½-inch pieces and delicately pinch the pieces in the middle.

(continued)

3 *For leeks:* Place the leeks in a small colander or cooking basket and place them in boiling salted water for 5 minutes or until soft. Remove, drain, and season to taste with salt and pepper. Keep the water boiling for the Brussel sprouts.

4 *For Brussel sprouts:* Place a steaming basket or colander over the boiling water and steam the Brussel sprouts for 10 minutes, or until tender when the stem is pierced with a paring knife. Remove from pan and slice each one in half. Change the water, season with salt, and bring it to a boil to cook the gnocchi.

5 *For tuna:* Rub the tuna with the remaining 1 tablespoon olive oil and coat with ground peppercorns. Heat canola oil and remaining ½ teaspoon butter in a medium sauté pan over medium-high heat and sauté the tuna on all sides for 3 to 5 minutes total. The tuna should still be quite raw.

6 Drop the gnocchi into the gently boiling, salted water and cook for 3 to 4 minutes, or until they float at the surface. Using a skimmer, transfer them to a bowl and lightly drizzle with olive oil.

7 *To serve:* Cut the tuna in 16 even slices and arrange 4 slices in the center of each shallow bowl. Place a mound of the poached leeks in the center of the tuna. Spoon the sauce around the tuna and arrange gnocchi and Brussel sprouts around the bowl.

Nutrient analysis per serving: 427 calories; 28 grams protein, 45 grams carbohydrate, 14 grams fat, 7 grams saturated fat, 78 milligrams cholesterol, 6 grams fiber, 1572 milligrams sodium.

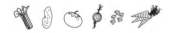

Steamed Whitefish with Haricotes Verts and Potato-Apple-Celery Puree

This dish allows for an extra serving of starch or fruit and 1 tablespoon fat. Why not share a dessert with your dinner companion?

Preparation time: 1 hour

Cooking time: 1 hour

Yield: 4 servings

1 cup chopped celery

2 cups chopped apples, preferably Granny Smith

1½ cups chopped potatoes, boiled

Salt and pepper to taste

2 cups celery juice

3 tablespoons plus 2 teaspoons butter

1½ cups haricots verts (French string beans)

6 tablespoons chopped fresh chives

2 tablespoons chopped fresh chervil

Canola oil

4 3-ounce pieces whitefish

1½ cups julienned Spanish onion

1 *For puree:* Place the celery and 1 cup apple in a medium saucepan, cover with water, and simmer over medium heat for 5 to 7 minutes, or until slightly soft. Drain and puree with the cooked potatoes, adding water as needed, until smooth. Place the puree in a nonstick pan and slowly dry over medium heat for 10 minutes, stirring continuously, until the puree has a thick consistency. Season to taste with salt and pepper. Set aside, covered, to maintain heat.

2 *For sauce:* Place the celery juice in a small saucepan with the remaining 1 cup apple and simmer over medium heat for 15 minutes. Strain through a fine-mesh sieve and season to taste with salt and pepper. Set aside.

3 *For onion:* In a small sauté pan, heat 2 teaspoons butter over medium-high heat for 12 minutes, tossing or stirring often, until golden brown. Set aside.

4 *For haricots verts:* Blanche the haricots verts in boiling salted water for 2 minutes, drain, and season to taste with salt and pepper.

5 *To finish the sauce:* Heat the sauce until simmering. Remove from heat and whisk in 3 tablespoons butter, 3 tablespoons chives, and 1½ tablespoons chervil until frothy. Keep warm.

6 *For fish:* Lightly brush the whitefish with canola oil. Season both sides with salt and pepper. Crust the top with the remaining 3 tablespoons chives and ½ tablespoon chervil. Place on a rack in a steamer and steam for 3 minutes, or until just cooked.

7 *To serve:* Spoon some of the puree in the center of each shallow bowl and top with a piece of steamed fish. Spoon the haricots verts and julienned onions around the fish and ladle the sauce around the bowl.

Nutrient analysis per serving: *350 calories; 22 grams protein, 44 grams carbohydrate, 11 grams fat, 6 grams saturated fat, 56 milligrams cholesterol, 5 grams fiber, 768 milligrams sodium.*

Sautéed Salmon with Caramelized Onion-Strewn Grits and Portobello Mushroom-Red Wine Sauce

This dish allows room for 2 additional servings of starches or fruits. You can top the meal off with a bowl of strawberries and an ounce of cream.

(continued)

Preparation time: 1 hour

Cooking time: 1 hour

Yield: 4 servings

½ chopped onion

⅓ cup chopped celery

⅓ cup chopped carrots

1½ tablespoons canola oil

⅓ cup chopped apple, preferably Granny Smith

⅓ cup peeled and chopped orange

2 cups Burgundy wine

1 cup Port

2 roasted portobello mushrooms

2½ tablespoons butter

Salt and pepper to taste

1 red onion, julienned

2 tablespoons chopped chives

1 tablespoon lemon juice

2 cups cooked white grits

4 4-ounce pieces salmon, skin on

Freshly ground black pepper

1 *For sauce:* In a medium nonstick pan, cook the onions, celery, and carrots in ½ tablespoon canola oil over high heat for 10 minutes, or until golden brown and caramelized. Add the apple, orange, Burgundy, and Port and simmer over medium heat for 30 minutes. Strain through a fine-meshed sieve and return to the saucepan. Simmer for 15 minutes, or until reduced to about ½ cup. Coarsely chop 1 portobello mushroom, place in the blender with the reduced red wine, and puree for 2 minutes, or until smooth. Place the mushroom puree in a small saucepan and warm over medium heat. Remove from heat and whisk in 2 tablespoons butter and season to taste with salt and pepper. Set aside and keep warm.

2 *For grits:* Cook the red onion in a hot sauce pan with the remaining ½ tablespoon butter for 5 to 8 minutes, or until golden brown and caramelized. Fold the onion, chives, and lemon juice into the cooked grits and season to taste with salt and pepper.

3 *For salmon:* Season the salmon with salt and pepper and score the skin side with a sharp knife or razor blade. Place skin side down in a hot sauté pan with the remaining 1 tablespoon canola oil and cook for 2 to 3 minutes on each side, or until golden brown and cooked medium.

4 *To serve:* Thinly slice the remaining portobello mushroom. Place a mound of grits in the center of each plate and top with some of the sliced portobello. Place a piece of the salmon on the mushrooms and spoon the sauce around the plate. Top with freshly ground black pepper.

Nutrient analysis per serving: 376 calories; 20 grams protein, 29 grams carbohydrate, 16 grams fat, 6 grams saturated fat, 64 milligrams cholesterol, 2 grams fiber, 1,157 milligrams sodium.

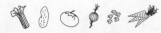

Fringale

Fringale has been called the perfect French bistro. The owners, Gerald Hirigoyen and J.B. Lorda, consider it a California/Basque bistro. By whatever designation, the food is straightforward and flavorful, and the social atmosphere is full of character and energy. The high quality of the food is in contrast to the moderate prices of everything on the menu. Much of the menu can be enjoyed not only for taste but also for the healthful qualities of the food.

Partner Gerald Hirigoyen is also the chef. He trained in the Basque region of France and in Paris with some of the great names in French cuisine. He came to San Francisco in 1980 and ran the kitchens of several fine restaurants, but in 1991, he decided to go out on his own and start this restaurant. He has received numerous awards and much recognition for the quality of his food. *Food and Wine* called him one of 1994's "Best New Chefs in America."

Fringale Restaurant, 570 Fourth Street, San Francisco, CA. 415-543-0573.

Onion Pie with Roquefort and Walnuts

This dish is a feast for the eyes as well as the tongue. Serve as a main course for lunch. A fresh fruit salad and French roll are perfect complements to this meal.

Preparation time: *1 hour*

Cooking time: *15 minutes*

Yield: *8 servings*

2 tablespoons olive oil

2 white onions, very thinly sliced

¼ cup water

3 ounces Roquefort cheese, crumbled into small pieces

Salt and freshly ground pepper to taste

½ cup walnuts, coarsely chopped

1 tablespoon Melted butter

2 puff pastry sheets (11 x 15-inch sheets), fresh or thawed frozen

1 egg, lightly beaten

8 slices of prosciutto (about .5 ounce each)

Mixed greens to garnish

1 Place a baking sheet with sides in a freezer.

(continued)

2 In a sauté pan over medium-high heat, warm the olive oil. Add the onions and sauté until golden brown (about 10 minutes). Add the water and continue to sauté until all the moisture evaporates, about 5 minutes longer. Reduce heat to medium-low. Add the Roquefort cheese and continue cooking, stirring occasionally, until melted, about 5 more minutes. Season only lightly with salt, if needed, and add pepper to taste. Stir in the walnuts and then spread the mixture out onto the chilled sheet pan. Place in the freezer until the onions cool down completely (about 10 minutes).

3 Preheat oven to 450° and evenly brush a sheet pan with melted butter.

4 Place the puff pastry on a cutting board. Using the rim of a small plate about 5 inches in diameter as a guide, cut the pastry into 8 rounds. Discard scraps.

5 Place the rounds onto the prepared baking sheet. Brush the outer rims and tops with the beaten egg. Evenly distribute the cooled onion mixture in the middle of each of the 8 rounds, leaving 1 inch uncovered all around the edges. Place 1 prosciutto slice on top of each mound of the onion mixture. Fold over the pastry round to create a half-moon shape. Pinch down firmly around the edges to seal in the filling. Brush the top of each pie with more of the beaten egg. Using a sharp knife, pierce the top of each pie with a small slit.

6 Bake until the pastry is pale golden and fully puffed, about 20 to 25 minutes.

Nutrient analysis per serving: *454 calories; 13 grams protein, 26 grams carbohydrate, 34 grams fat, 7 grams saturated fat, 47 milligrams cholesterol, 1 gram fiber, 562 milligrams sodium.*

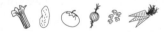

Lemon and Pastis Grilled Prawns with Couscous Salad

This meal is perfect for lunch or for dinner on warm summer evenings. Round out the meal with a fresh roll, a chilled vegetable dish, and fresh fruit dessert.

Preparation time: *1 hour, 15 minutes*

Cooking time: *15 minutes*

Yield: *6 servings*

Prawns

3 tablespoons Ricard or Pernod (the pastis)

3 tablespoons freshly squeezed lemon juice

4 garlic cloves, finely sliced

6 sprigs of fresh thyme

½ teaspoon sea salt

¼ teaspoon freshly ground pepeper

¼ teaspoon mild cayenne powder

5 tablespoons extra-virgin olive oil

6-inch bamboo skewers

1 pound fresh gulf prawns (23 to 25 prawns), peeled, and remove the vein in the back of each prawn

Couscous Salad

1 cup water

1 cup couscous

1 cup cucumber, peeled and finely diced

1 cup finely diced pineapple

1 large shallot, minced

4 tablespoons freshly chopped parsley

3 tablespoons fresh chopped mint

3 tablespoons fresh lemon juice

3 tablespoons extra-virgin olive oil

Salt and pepper to taste

Pinch of mild cayenne

1 *Marinade for prawns:* Combine pastis, lemon juice, garlic, thyme, salt, pepper, cayenne, and olive oil in a mixing bowl; set aside. Insert 1 skewer, lengthwise, though the body of each prawn, starting with the tail end first, and working the skewer up though the head. In a shallow glass casserole, lay all the skewered prawns in a single layer. Pour the marinade over the prawns; making sure that they're thoroughly coated. Cover with plastic wrap and set aside in a refrigerator for 2 to 3 hours, turning them over after 1 to 1½ hours.

2 *For the couscous:* Bring 1 cup water to a rolling boil. Add the couscous, stir, cover, and remove from heat. Allow to sit for 5 to 6 minutes and then fluff with a fork. Spread the couscous on a tray and place in a refrigerator to cool. In a large mixing bowl, combine the cucumber, pineapple, and shallots. Add the cooled couscous, parsley, mint, lemon juice, and olive oil and mix together until well combined. Season with salt and pepper to taste.

3 Preheat an indoor or outdoor grill (to a hot temperature, but not smoking). Place a small bed of couscous on the center of each plate to be served. Grill the prawns for 1 to 2 minutes on each side, depending on the size of the prawn. Remove from grill and place on top of the couscous salad. Sprinkle with a pinch of cayenne and serve immediately.

Nutrient analysis per serving: *303 calories; 17 grams protein, 14 grams carbohydrate, 20 grams fat, 3 grams saturated fat, 115 milligrams cholesterol, 1 gram fiber, 311 milligrams sodium.*

Lemon Braised Sea Bass with Star Anise and Baby Spinach

This meal is low in total carbohydrate and total fat, so you can complete the meal with a couple of servings of carbohydrate (such as a serving of French bread and rice) and a tossed green salad with vinaigrette dressing.

(continued)

Preparation time: 30 minutes

Cooking time: 15 minutes

Yield: 4 servings

4 sea bass fillets (about 4 ounces each)

Salt and freshly ground pepper to taste

1 teaspoon olive oil

¼ cup finely diced celery root

⅓ cup finely diced fennel

¼ cup finely diced carrot

3 garlic cloves, peeled and chopped

4 star anise

¼ cup freshly squeezed lemon juice

1½ cups water

⅓ cup finely diced cucumber

⅓ cup finely diced tomato

⅛ cup finely diced apple

4 cups baby spinach leaves

2 teaspoons extra-virgin olive oil

Pinch mild cayenne powder

2 tablespoons fresh chopped chives

2 tablespoons fresh chopped parsley

1 Preheat oven to 475°. Rub both sides of the sea bass fillets with salt and pepper and set aside.

2 Heat 1 teaspoon olive oil in a large sauté pan (preferably nonstick) over high heat. Add the celery root, fennel, carrot, garlic, and star anise and sauté until slightly caramelized, 4 to 5 minutes. Soften the caramel with the lemon juice and cook for 1 minute.

3 Lay the sea bass fillets on top of the vegetables, add the water, and cover the pan. Place the pan into the preheated oven just until the fish is cooked though (5 to 6 minutes). Remove the pan from oven and remove the fillets of fish and set them aside, covered to keep warm.

4 Add the cucumber, tomato, and apple to the sauté pan and place over high heat. Bring to a boil and cook for 1 to 2 minutes. Add the spinach, extra-virgin olive oil, mild cayenne, and salt and pepper to taste. Cook just until the spinach wilts (30 seconds to 1 minute).

5 *To serve:* In 4 shallow soup bowls, spread an even amount of the vegetables and juice from the pan. Lay a fillet on top of the vegetables in each bowl and place a star anise on top to garnish. Sprinkle the chives and parsley over the top of each dish and serve immediately.

Nutrient analysis per serving: 236 calories; 31 grams protein, 17 grams carbohydrate, 6 grams fat, 1 gram saturated fat, 77 milligrams cholesterol, 3 grams fiber, 240 milligrams sodium.

Drunken Pork Shoulder with Cabbage and Pears

This dish is a complete meal within itself. Luckily, it's low in carbohydrate, which leaves room for a couple of slices of French bread to dunk in this delicious sauce.

Preparation time: *3 hours*

Cooking time: *1 hour*

Yield: *6 servings*

Bouquet garni (a seasoning)

2 white onions, diced

2 carrots, peeled and diced

2 celery stalks, diced

3 garlic cloves

30 whole black peppercorns

5 cups dry red wine, such as Cabernet or Merlot

Salt to taste

2 pounds boneless pork shoulder, cut into 1-inch cubes

2 tablespoons olive oil

4 cups veal stock or chicken stock

1 head green cabbage, thinly sliced

1 tablespoon unsalted butter

¼ vanilla bean, split in half lengthwise

3 ripe but firm pears, such as Comice, cored, peeled, and cut into ¾-inch cubes

3 tablespoons chopped fresh parsley

1 In a large nonaluminum (nonreactive) dish, combine the bouquet garni, onions, carrots, celery, garlic, peppercorns, 4½ cups red wine, and salt to taste. Stir to mix. Add pork and turn to coat evenly. Cover with plastic wrap and marinate for at least 5 hours or as long as overnight.

2 Drain the meat and vegetables in a sieve, capturing the marinade into a small saucepan. Bring the marinade to a boil, remove from heat, and set aside. Separate the meat from the vegetables and set both aside.

3 In a sauté pan over high heat, warm 2 tablespoons olive oil. Pat the meat dry with paper towels. Working in small batches, add the meat to the pan and brown on all sides, about 2 minutes. Transfer the meat to a large saucepan.

4 To the same sauté pan used for browning meat, add the reserved vegetables and sauté over medium-high heat until they begin to brown, about 5 minutes.

5 Transfer the vegetables to the saucepan holding the meat. Add the reserved red wine marinade. Bring to a boil over high heat and boil until reduced by half, about 10 minutes. Add the veal stock and return to a boil. Reduce the heat to medium and simmer, uncovered, until the pork is tender, 50 to 60 minutes.

(continued)

6 Meanwhile, fill another large saucepan two-thirds full with water, add a pinch of salt, and bring to a boil. Add the cabbage, return to a boil, and cook until wilted, about 2 minutes. Drain the cabbage, rinse with cold water, and drain again. In a frying pan over medium heat, melt the butter. Add the cabbage and sauté for 2 minutes. Remove from heat and set aside.

7 In another small saucepan, combine the remaining ½ cup red wine, the vanilla bean, and pears and bring to a boil. Reduce the heat to medium and simmer, turning the fruit every few minutes, until tender, 5 to 10 minutes.

8 Drain the meat and vegetables in a sieve, capturing the juices in a bowl. Cover the juices to keep them warm. Separate the pork from the vegetables; discard the vegetables.

9 *To serve:* Arrange a bed of the cabbage on a warmed platter. Place the pork on top of the cabbage and pour the juices over the top. Scatter the poached pear cubes around the meat. Garnish with the parsley and serve at once.

Nutrient analysis per serving: 610 calories; 32 grams protein, 25 grams carbohydrate, 30 grams fat, 10 grams saturated fat, 156 milligrams cholesterol, 5 grams fiber, 718 milligrams sodium.

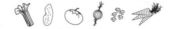

Marinated Chicken in Red Wine with Braising Greens, Parsnips, and Cippolini Onions

This dish allows room for 2 additional servings of starches. You may want to include a couple of servings of bread to soak up this wonderful sauce!

Preparation time: 30 minutes

Cooking time: 1 hour, 20 minutes

Yield: 4 servings

4 chicken thighs, without skin

4 chicken breasts, split, without skin

2 cups red wine

1 small onion, chopped

2 garlic cloves, chopped

6 sprigs thyme

1 tablespoon whole black peppercorns

Kosher salt and freshly ground black pepper to taste

2 tablespoons olive oil

1 cup veal stock

8 cippolini onions, peeled

8 baby carrots, peeled

2 medium parsnips, peeled and cut into large matchsticks

3 tablespoons unsalted butter

2 pounds braising greens, such as green chard, with stems removed and leaves torn into large pieces

2 tablespoons finely chopped parsley

1 In a large bowl, combine the chicken thighs, breasts, red wine, onion, garlic, thyme, black peppercorns, and salt and pepper to season. Cover with plastic wrap and refrigerate for at least 6 hours, preferably overnight.

2 Preheat oven to 450°. Separate the chicken from the marinade and set both aside.

3 Warm 1 tablespoon olive oil in a large casserole. Add the 4 chicken thighs and sauté until browned, about 5 minutes. Pour the marinade into the casserole with the thighs, add the veal stock, and bring to a boil. Once it boils, reduce heat and let the ingredients simmer for 25 to 30 minutes.

4 Warm 1 tablespoon olive oil in a large sauté pan over high heat. Add breasts and sauté until browned, about 3 to 4 minutes. Season with salt and pepper to taste and place in the oven until cooked, about 10 minutes.

5 Place the cippolini onions in a small pan with enough water to cover, bring to a boil, and cook until soft and tender, about 20 minutes. Strain and set aside. Fill a saucepan two-thirds full of water, bring to a boil, add baby carrots, and cook until tender, about 6 to 8 minutes. Strain and set aside. Place parsnips in a saucepan with enough water to cover, bring to a boil, and cook until tender, about 10 to 12 minutes. Strain and set aside.

6 When the chicken thighs are done, separate them from the marinade and set aside. Using a fine meshed sieve, strain the marinade into a small saucepan and discard the vegetables.

7 Bring the marinade to a boil and reduce by half. Turn off the heat, swirl in 1 tablespoon butter in a steady motion until completely incorporated, and season with salt and pepper to taste.

8 To prepare braising greens, combine ⅓ cup water, 1 tablespoon butter, the braising greens, and salt and pepper to taste in a large saucepan. Cover and cook over high heat just until wilted, about 5 minutes.

9 In a separate sauté pan, warm 1 tablespoon butter and then add the onion mixture and salt and pepper to taste and sauté until nicely caramelized, about 6 minutes. Add the parsley and set aside.

10 To assemble the dish, using a slotted spoon, place a small bed of the braising greens in the center of each plate. Lay one chicken thigh and one breast on top of the greens. Evenly scatter the cippolini onions, carrots, and parsnips on top of the chicken and spoon the sauce on top of and around the edges of the dish.

(continued)

Nutrient analysis per serving: 596 calories; 49 grams protein, 30 grams carbohydrate, 25 grams fat, 9 grams saturated fat, 195 milligrams cholesterol, 5 grams fiber, 936 milligrams sodium.

Gaylord India Restaurant

A bit of India in San Francisco — Gaylord is synonymous with delicious and authentic Indian food, served with true Indian hospitality. Located atop world famous Ghirardelli Square in San Francisco, the setting is one of relaxed elegance, with magnificent views of San Francisco Bay and the Marin County Headlands. At Gaylord, master chefs specialize in North Indian cuisine including centuries-old techniques of tandoori cooking.

Head chef Santok Kaler has been at Gaylord for 14 years. He was trained in the Punjab in India, the home of North Indian cooking.

Gaylord India Restaurant, Ghirardelli Square, 900 North Point, San Francisco, California. 415-771-8822.

Seekh Kabab (Barbecued Lamb on Skewer)

Spices are a wonderful way of adding full flavor to a dish without using extra fats. This dish can be served as an entrée or as an appetizer. Combine this recipe with 1 cup rice to provide the necessary carbohydrate. Two servings of vegetables, one of which could be the Saag, the last recipe in this section, round out the meal.

Preparation time: *30 minutes*

Cooking time: *10 minutes*

Yield: *6 servings*

1 medium onion

1-inch fresh ginger

2 garlic cloves

2 teaspoons water

1 teaspoon salt

¼ teaspoon cayenne pepper

½ teaspoon coriander powder

½ teaspoon cumin powder

¾ teaspoon garam masala (available in Indian food stores)

1 pound lean ground lamb

1 In a blender or mini-food processor, grind onion, ginger, and garlic with 2 teaspoons water. Transfer to a medium bowl and mix in salt, cayenne pepper, coriander powder, cumin powder, and garam masala.

2 Add the ground lamb and mix until thoroughly combined. Let stand for 20 to 30 minutes in the refrigerator.

3 Preheat oven to 375°. Divide the mixture into 6 equal portions. Lightly oil the skewers. Shape the lamb mixture into sausage shapes on the skewers, about 1 inch thick. Place skewers on a rack over a pan and bake for 15 to 20 minutes or until done. To broil, place skewers 3 to 4 inches from heat and cook approximately 7 minutes per side. Serve hot with lemon garnish.

Tip: *If using wood or bamboo skewers, soak them overnight in water and oil them lightly. This step prevents burning the skewers while cooking.*

Nutrient analysis per serving: *144 calories; 12.6 grams protein, 2 grams carbohydrate, 9 grams fat, 42 milligrams cholesterol, 0.2 grams fiber, 419 milligrams sodium.*

Chicken Tikka Kabab (Barbecued Chicken Kebab)

Marinades can add great flavor to a meal without extra fat and/or sodium. Make this dish early in the day and grill right before serving. Combine this recipe with 1 cup rice to provide the necessary carbohydrate. Two servings of vegetables, one of which could be the Saag, the last recipe in this section, round out the meal.

Preparation time: *30 minutes*

Cooking time: *10 minutes*

Yield: *6 servings*

2 tablespoons chopped ginger	*½ teaspoon red pepper*
2 tablespoons chopped garlic	*½ teaspoon ground turmeric*
¼ cup nonfat yogurt	*¼ cup lemon juice*
½ teaspoon ground white pepper	*2 teaspoons vegetable oil*
½ teaspoon ground cumin	*Salt to taste*
¼ teaspoon ground nutmeg	*3 whole chicken breasts, boned, skinned, and cut into 18 pieces*
¼ teaspoon cardamom	

(continued)

1 Combine the ginger, garlic, white pepper, yogurt, cumin, nutmeg, cardamom, red pepper, turmeric, and lemon juice in a blender or food processor. With the motor running, drizzle in the oil.

2 Add the chicken pieces to the marinade. Mix thoroughly to coat. Cover and let marinade for 3 to 4 hours in the refrigerator.

3 Preheat oven to 375°. Place chicken breasts on a skewer about 1 inch apart. Place skewers on a rack over a pan and bake for about 10 to 12 minutes or until cooked. To broil, place skewers 3 to 4 inches from the heat and broil approximately 5 minutes per side. Serve hot with lemon garnish.

Nutrient analysis per serving: *197 calories; 31.6 grams protein, 2.2 grams carbohydrate, 6 grams fat, 1.52 grams saturated fat, 14 milligrams cholesterol, .1 gram fiber, 8 milligrams sodium.*

Tandoori Fish Tikka (Barbecued Fish Kebabs with Black Pepper)

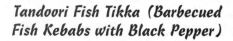

This dish works well with fresh salmon, swordfish, or sea bass. Combine this recipe with 1 cup rice to provide the necessary carbohydrate. Two servings of vegetables, one of which could be the Saag, the last recipe in this section, round out the meal.

Preparation time: *15 minutes*

Cooking time: *10 minutes*

Yield: *8 servings*

2 pounds firm flesh fish (fillet and cut into 1½-inch cubes), such as swordfish, tuna, or halibut

2 teaspoons vegetable oil

1 teaspoon salt

1 teaspoon ground black pepper

1 teaspoon ground cumin pepper seed

¼ teaspoon turmeric

2 garlic cloves, chopped

1 teaspoon fresh lemon juice

1 In a medium bowl, combine the fish with the vegetable oil, salt, pepper, cumin, turmeric, and garlic. Mix to evenly coat fish with marinade, cover, and refrigerate for 3 to 4 hours.

2 Preheat oven to 400°. Pierce the fish with skewers. Place on a rack over a pan. Bake for 8 to 10 minutes or until done. Fish should be firm to the touch. It is done when it easily flakes with a fork. To grill or broil, set skewers 3 inches from the heat, turning once during cooking, until cooked through, about 6 minutes per side.

3 Sprinkle with lemon juice. Serve hot.

Nutrient analysis per serving (recipe with salmon): 182 calories; 21.1 grams protein, 0 grams carbohydrate, 10.3 grams fat, 2.0 grams saturated fat, 20 milligrams cholesterol, 0 grams fiber, 341.5 milligrams sodium.

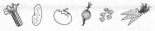

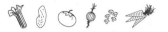
Toor Dal (Pigeon Peas)

This dish is very similar to split pea soup only with a beautiful golden color. Take 2 or 3 servings of Toor Dal to replace the rice in the previous dishes.

Preparation time: 15 minutes

Cooking time: 45 minutes

Yield: 8 servings

1 cup toor dal (a type of pea)	*1 teaspoon coriander powder*
4 cups water	*¼ teaspoon cumin powder*
1 teaspoon salt	*¼ teaspoon cumin seeds*
¼ teaspoon turmeric	*1 tablespoon fresh cilantro*
1 teaspoon vegetable oil	
Pinch of asafetida (found in Indian food stores)	

1 Clean the dal by washing it in water. Remove and discard water. Repeat process until dal is thoroughly cleaned.

2 In a heavy skillet, add the dal, 4 cups water, salt, and turmeric. Bring to boil over medium-high heat. Reduce heat, cover with lid, and simmer for 30 minutes, skimming off foam as it rises to the top and stirring occasionally. The dal should be tender and soupy.

3 In a small fry pan, heat the vegetable oil to a near smoking point. Add the asafedita, coriander, and cumin seeds. Cook for a few seconds, until seeds are golden brown. Remove from heat and add the cumin powder. Add to dal and stir. Garnish with chopped cilantro. Serve hot.

Nutrient analysis per serving: 90 calories; 5 grams protein, 15 grams carbohydrate, 63 gram fat, 1 gram saturated fat, 0 milligrams cholesterol, 3 grams fiber, 287 milligrams sodium.

Saag (Spinach)

Here's a sure way of jazzing up a bland vegetable. This can provide one of the servings of vegetables in the previous lamb, chicken, and fish dishes.

Preparation time: *15 minutes*

Cooking time: *15 minutes*

Yield: *6 servings*

2 10-ounce bags of fresh spinach, trimmed and washed

2 teaspoons vegetable oil

½ teaspoon cumin seeds

10 garlic cloves sliced into ¼-inch slices

2 dried red chiles

Salt to taste

1 In a large saucepan of boiling salted water, blanch the spinach in batches for 30 seconds or until wilted. Drain and refresh in cold water. Squeeze the moisture from leaves and chop finely.

2 Heat the vegetable oil over medium heat in a nonstick pan. Add the cumin seeds and stir for 5 seconds. Add garlic and fry until soft, 2 to 3 minutes. Add the chiles and cook another minute. Add the spinach, toss well, and sauté until heated thoroughly and liquid in the pan has evaporated (approximately 2 to 3 minutes). Season with salt. Serve hot.

Nutrient analysis per serving: *34.2 calories; 2.7 grams protein, 3.4 grams carbohydrate, 1.5 grams fat, 0.2 gram saturated fat, 0 milligrams cholesterol, 2 grams fiber, 63 milligrams sodium.*

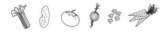

Greens

When residents of the San Francisco Bay area think of great vegetarian food, Greens is the first name that comes to mind. Greens uses the freshest ingredients, many of which come from the Zen Center's Green Gulch Farm, across the Golden Gate Bridge in Marin County. This brief trip results in no loss of freshness for the fine seasonal organic produce.

Chef Annie Somerville came to Greens in 1981 and became Executive Chef in 1985. In her 18th year of cooking at Greens, she continues to create outstanding dishes with a balance of colors, flavors, and contrast of textures. In addition to the Green Gulch and Start Route Farms in Marin County, she uses artisan cheeses from West Marin and Sonoma Counties. She has authored the award-winning book *Field of Greens: New Vegetarian Recipes from the Celebrated Greens Restaurant.*

Greens, Fort Mason, San Francisco, California. 415-771-6222.

Romaine Hearts with Sourdough Croutons and Parmesan Cheese

This is a wonderful dish to begin any meal. Combine it with the next recipe for Summer Minestrone and a bowl of fresh fruit, and you will be in vegetarian heaven.

Preparation time: *10 minutes*

Cooking time: *10 minutes*

Yield: *4 servings*

4 small heads of Romaine lettuce	*¼ teaspoon salt*
2 garlic cloves, finely chopped	*1½ tablespoons vinegar or lemon juice*
6 tablespoons extra-virgin olive oil, divided	*8 Geata or Nicoise olives, pitted and coarsely chopped*
4 thick slices of sourdough bread, cut into ½-inch cubes, about 1½ cups	*1 ounce Parmesan cheese, grated, about ⅓ cup*
1¼ teaspoon minced lemon zest	*Freshly ground pepper to taste*

1 Discard the outer leaves of the Romaine and use the whole leaves and the hearts, which should be pale green or yellow and firm. Wash the leaves, dry them in a spinner, and wrap loosely in a damp towel and refrigerate.

2 Preheat the oven to 375°. Add 1 garlic clove to 1 tablespoon olive oil and toss with the cubed bread. Spread the cubes on a baking sheet and bake for 7 to 8 minutes, until golden brown. Set aside to cool.

3 Make the vinaigrette. Combine the lemon zest, salt, garlic, and vinegar. Then whisk in 5 tablespoons olive oil.

4 When you're ready to serve the salad, place the lettuce in a large bowl. Add the olives and toss with the vinaigrette, coating all the leaves. Add the croutons and Parmesan; toss again. Sprinkle with freshly ground pepper and serve.

Nutrient analysis per serving: *355 calories; 9 grams protein, 31 grams carbohydrate, 23 grams fat, 4 grams saturated fat, 6 milligrams cholesterol, 3 grams fiber, 696 milligrams sodium.*

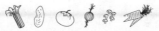

Summer Minestrone

This soup can be a complete meal. Serve with some crusty, fresh French bread, the salad in the preceding recipe, and a bowl of strawberries and an ounce of cream.

Preparation time: *30 minutes*

Cooking time: *1 hour*

Yield: *6 servings*

½ cup dried red beans, about 3 ounces, sorted and soaked overnight

6 cups cold water

2 bay leaves

2 fresh sage leaves

1 fresh oregano sprig

1 tablespoon extra-virgin olive oil

1 medium red onion, diced, about 2 cups

½ teaspoon salt

¼ teaspoon dried basil

Pepper to taste

6 garlic cloves, finely chopped

1 small carrot, diced, about ¼ cup

1 small red bell pepper, diced, about ¾ cup

1 small zucchini, diced, about ¾ cup

¼ cup red wine

2 pounds fresh tomatoes, peeled, seeded, and coarsely chopped, about 3 cups, or one 28-ounce can tomatoes with juice, coarsely chopped

¼ cup small pasta, cooked al dente, drained, and rinsed

½ bunch of fresh spinach or chard, cut into thin ribbons and washed, about 2 cups packed

2 tablespoons chopped fresh basil

Grated Parmesan cheese

1 Drain and rinse beans. Place in a 2-quart saucepan with the water, 1 bay leaf, sage leaves, and oregano. Bring to a boil; reduce heat and simmer, uncovered, until the beans are tender, about 30 minutes. Remove the herbs.

2 While the beans are cooking, heat the oil in a soup pot. Add the onion, ½ teapoon salt, dried herbs, and a few pinches of pepper. Sauté the onion over medium heat until soft, 5 to 7 minutes. Add the garlic, carrots, peppers, and zucchini and sauté for 7 to 8 minutes, stirring often. Add the wine and cook for 1 to 2 minutes, until the pan is almost dry. Add the tomatoes and then add the pasta, spinach or chard, and beans with their broth. Season with salt and pepper to taste. Add the basil just before serving. Garnish each serving with a generous tablespoon of Parmesan cheese.

Nutrient analysis per serving: *98 calories; 4 grams protein, 17 grams carbohydrate, 2 grams fat, 0 grams saturated fat, 1 milligram cholesterol, 2 grams fiber, 652 milligrams sodium.*

Sweet Pepper and Basil Frittata

You can serve this dish right out of the oven as a main course or let it cool and serve as a light lunch. You can also refrigerate the dish and cut it into small squares to serve as an hors d'oeuvre. You can serve it with the Almond-Currant Couscous, the next recipe in this group, and a tossed salad as a complete meal.

Preparation time: *30 minutes*

Cooking time: *25 minutes*

Yield: *10 servings*

2 tablespoons light olive oil	*6 eggs*
1 medium yellow onion, thinly sliced, about 2 cups	*3 ounces Fontina cheese, grated, about 1½ cups*
¾ teaspoon salt and pepper	*2 ounces Parmesan cheese, grated, about ¾ cup*
4 medium sweet peppers, preferably a combination of red and yellow, thinly sliced, about 4 cups	*¼ cup fresh basil leaves, bundled and thinly sliced*
4 garlic cloves, finely chopped	*3 tablespoons balsamic vinegar*
1 bay leaf	

1 Preheat oven to 475°. Heat 1 tablespoon olive oil in a large skillet; add the onion, ½ teaspoon salt, and a few pinches of pepper. Sauté the onion over medium heat until it begins to soften, about 4 to 5 minutes. Add the sweet peppers, garlic, and bay leaf; stew the onion and peppers together for about 15 minutes, until the peppers are tender. Set the vegetables aside to cool. Remove the bay leaf.

2 Beat the eggs in a bowl and add the onion-pepper mixture, cheeses, and basil. Season with ¼ teaspoon salt and ⅛ teaspoon pepper.

3 In a 9-inch nonstick sauté pan with an ovenproof handle, heat the remaining tablespoon of olive oil until almost smoking. Swirl the oil around the side of the pan to coat. Turn the heat down to low and then immediately pour the frittata mixture into the pan. The pan should be hot enough so that the eggs sizzle when they touch the oil. Cook the frittata over low heat for 2 to 3 minutes, until the sides begin to set; transfer to the oven and bake, uncovered, for 6 to 8 minutes, until firm and the eggs are completely cooked.

(continued)

4 Loosen the fritatta gently with a rubber spatula; the bottom will tend to stick to the pan. Place a plate over the pan, flip it over, and put it on a plate. Brush the bottom and sides with the vinegar and cut into wedges. Serve warm or at room temperature.

Nutrient analysis per serving: 149 calories; 9.6 grams protein, 45 grams carbohydrate, 10 grams fat, 4 grams saturated fat, 159 milligrams cholesterol, 1 gram fiber, 349 milligrams sodium.

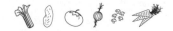

Almond-Currant Couscous

Here is a side dish that almost tastes like dessert, an excellent source of delicious carbohydrate.

Preparation time: 10 minutes

Cooking time: 20 minutes

Yield: 4 to 6 servings

¼ cup whole almonds, unskinned, toasted	¼ teaspoon salt
2 tablespoons unsalted butter	½ teaspoon cinnamon, preferably freshly ground
1½ cups instant couscous	
1½ cups water	¼ cup dried currants

1 Chop the toasted almonds when they have cooled.

2 In a medium skillet with a tight-fitting lid, melt the butter. Add the couscous grains and almonds and stir over medium heat for 4 to 5 minutes, until the grains are fragrant and heated through. Turn off the heat.

3 While toasting the couscous, bring the water to a boil in a small saucepan. Add the salt, cinnamon, and currants; give a quick stir and pour over the couscous. Cover the skillet and let sit for 5 minutes (or follow the package directions). Fluff the couscous with a fork and season with salt if needed. Serve immediately or hold in a warm oven until you're ready to serve it.

Nutrient analysis per serving: 262 calories; 7 grams protein, 39 grams carbohydrate, 8 grams fat, 3 grams saturated fat, 10 milligrams cholesterol, 3 grams fiber, 300 milligrams sodium.

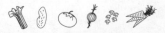

Rhubarb-Strawberry Cobbler

This wonderful dessert is a snap to make. You can make it with less sugar (⅓ cup) if you use strawberries alone. You need 3 baskets of berries, about 5 cups washed, hulled, and cut into halves or left whole if small. You can serve it warm topped with a touch of whipped cream.

Preparation time: *40 minutes*

Cooking time: *40 minutes*

Yield: *6 servings*

Cobbler filling

1¼ pounds rhubarb

1 pint basket of strawberries, about 1½ cups

¼ cup sugar

2½ tablespoons unbleached white flour

Zest of 1 small orange

Cobbler topping

1½ cups unbleached white flour

¼ teaspoon salt

1 tablespoon baking powder

2 tablespoons sugar

4 tablespoons unsalted butter

1 cup heavy cream

1 Preheat oven to 375°. Wash the rhubarb well, cutting off any brown spots or leaves still on the stalks. If the stalks are especially thick, cut them in half lengthwise before slicing ½ inch thick so that all the pieces are approximately the same size.

2 Wash the strawberries, pat dry, and hull them. Cut them into halves or leave whole if small.

3 Toss the fruit with the sugar, flour, and zest; place in an 8-inch square baking dish, a 9-inch round cake pan, or 6 to 8 individual ovenproof dishes.

4 Make the cobbler topping by combining the dry ingredients. Cut in the butter with a food processor, electric mixer, a pastry blender, or 2 knives until it resembles coarse meal. Add the cream and mix lightly, just until the dry ingredients are moistened.

5 Cover the fruit with tablespoon-size dollops of cobbler topping, using all the topping. Bake for 25 to 30 minutes, until the topping is browned and cooked through and the fruit is bubbling. Individual cobblers take about 20 minutes.

Nutrient analysis per serving: *328 calories; 5 grams protein, 60 grams carbohydrate, 8 grams fat, 5 grams saturated fat, 21 milligrams cholesterol, 2 grams fiber, 425 milligrams sodium.*

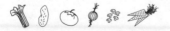

Harbor Village

Acclaimed by *Gourmet Magazine* as a "gold cup restaurant commanding the respect of Chinese gastronomics," Harbor Village was serving award-winning food in Hong Kong for many years before coming to San Francisco and later Los Angeles. In an environment that reminds you of the fine restaurants of Hong Kong, the Chinese chefs prepare dim sum that has been called the finest in the United States. The seafood is prepared fresh from their fish tanks. Dishes are made up of fresh local ingredients, yet the result is exotic delicacies such as abalone, shark's fin, and bird's nest soup. The service is just as good as the food.

Executive chef Andy Wai runs a kitchen staff of 40 in San Francisco. He learned his craft in the finest Hong Kong restaurants, finally cooking at Harbor Village's parent restaurant in Hong Kong, Tsui Hang Village. From there, he came to San Francisco in 1989 where he has been the recipient of numerous awards for his creativity.

Harbor Village, Four Embarcadero Center, Lobby Level, San Francisco, California. 415-781-8833.

Chicken Soup with Watercress and Tofu

You can serve this dish as the first course to any meal. Try serving it with any of the recipes later in this section.

Preparation time: *20 minutes*

Cooking time: *45 minutes*

Yield: *8 servings*

1 teaspoon vegetable oil

Chicken bones of 1 chicken, cut into quarters

Chicken pieces of 1 chicken, finely chopped

1 ounce fresh ginger

4 ounces pork, boneless shoulder, cut in strips

8 red dates, quartered

8 pieces shiitake mushrooms

1 small carrot, diced

½ teaspoon chicken powder, or ½ bouillon cube

2½ quarts water

1 bunch watercress, cleaned and trimmed of stems

1 container tofu, drained and cut into ½-inch cubes

½ teaspoon salt

Pinch white pepper

1 Heat the oil in a wok over high heat. Add the chicken bones and ginger. Stir-fry for about 2 minutes.

2 In a large pot, add the chicken, pork, red dates, shitake mushrooms, carrots, chicken powder or bouillon, and water.

3 Bring soup to boil, reduce heat, and simmer for 30 minutes, skimming any foam from the top. Using a skimmer, carefully remove the chicken bones. Then add the watercress and tofu and simmer for 10 more minutes. Season with salt and pepper.

Nutrient analysis per serving: *103 calories; 8.4 grams protein, 6.6 grams carbohydrate, 5 grams fat, .7 gram saturated fat, 9 milligrams cholesterol, 1.4 grams fiber, 176 milligrams sodium.*

Shiitake Mushrooms with Baby Bok Choy

This recipe makes a great vegetable side dish for any of the entrees in this section.

Preparation time: *30 minutes*

Cooking time: *15 minutes*

Yield: *4 servings*

½ piece of ginger root, peeled and smashed

Pinch of sugar

Pinch of salt

1 tablespoon plus 1 teaspoon vegetable oil

4 cups water

2 bunches baby bok choy

1 teaspoon minced ginger

Salt to season

1 cup chicken stock

1 tablespoon oyster sauce

1 tablespoon dark mushroom soy sauce

1 tablespoon sherry

1 teaspoon sugar

½ pound shitake mushrooms, cleaned, stemmed, and poached until tender

1 tablespoon cornstarch mixed with ½ cup cold water

1 Place the smashed ginger root, a pinch of sugar and salt, 1 teaspoon vegetable oil, and water in a large pot and bring to a boil. After 1 minute, using a skimmer, remove the ginger. Set aside to cool slightly and then mince.

2 Add the baby bok choy to the simmering water and cook for 1 minute. Drain. Set aside.

(continued)

3 Heat the remaining vegetable oil in a wok and add the baby bok choy and minced ginger. Season with salt and stir-fry for 1 minute. Arrange the baby bok choy on a platter.

4 Pour the chicken stock, oyster sauce, soy sauce, sherry, and 1 teaspoon sugar into a hot wok and bring to a boil. Add the shitake and cook until they are heated through. Stir the corn starch-water mixture into the mushrooms in the wok, simmering 2 to 3 minutes, until thickened.

5 Pour the sauce over the baby bok choy on the platter and serve immediately.

Nutrient analysis per serving: 98 calories; 7.3 grams protein, 22 grams carbohydrate, 4.7 grams fat, 2.5 grams saturated fat, 0 milligrams cholesterol, 4 grams fiber, 1,294 milligrams sodium.

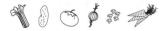

Minced Chicken in Lettuce Cup

This entrée is the perfect complement to the watercress and tofu soup recipe earlier in this section. Just add a bowl of rice, and you have a complete meal.

Preparation time: 20 minutes

Cooking time: 15 minutes

Yield: 4 servings

2 chicken breasts, skinned, boned, and finely chopped	*½ small fresh chili pepper, seeded and minced*
1 egg yolk	*1 teaspoon soy sauce*
2 teaspoons water	*2 tablespoons cooking sherry*
1 teaspoon cornstarch	*1 teaspoon oyster sauce*
Pinch of salt	*¼ teaspoon powdered chicken bouillon*
½ head Romaine or iceberg lettuce	*¼ teaspoon sugar*
1 tablespoon cooking oil	*¼ cup golden chives, chopped*
3 tablespoons Chinese sausage or ground pork Italian sausage	*3 tablespoons pinenuts*
2 cloves garlic, minced	*Hoisin sauce*
	Pickled ginger, finely minced

1 Place the chopped chicken breasts into a bowl. Add the egg yolk, water, cornstarch, and a pinch of salt. Marinate for 15 minutes.

2 Separate the lettuce leaves, keeping them whole, wash, pat dry, and set aside.

3 Heat a wok over high heat. When very hot, add the cooking oil. When the oil is wavy, add the minced chicken; stir fry, separating the pieces with a spatula, until chicken is cooked, 1 to 2 minutes.

4 Add the Chinese sausage, garlic, and chili pepper and stir-fry for 2 minutes. Then stir in the soy sauce, sherry, oyster sauce, powdered chicken bouillon, and sugar. Add the golden chives and pinenuts and stir-fry for about 2 to 3 minutes. Present on a platter with the lettuce leaves and sauces on the side.

5 To serve, spread a little hoisin sauce and ginger on a lettuce leaf. Top with 1 to 2 spoonfuls of the chicken mixture (depending on the size of the leaf), wrapping the lettuce leaf around the stuffing.

Nutrient analysis per serving: *276 calories; 17 grams protein, 11 grams carbohydrate, 19 grams fat, 1.5 grams saturated fat, 9 milligrams cholesterol, 1 gram fiber, 720 milligrams sodium.*

Steamed Rock Cod

This dish is also a perfect complement to the soup and vegetable dish recipes, earlier in this section. Round the meal out with either a bowl of rice or noodles.

Preparation time: *15 minutes*

Cooking time: *15 minutes*

Yield: *6 servings*

½ cup water	*Pinch white peper*
2 tablespoons light soy sauce	*3½ pounds fresh whole rock cod*
4 teaspoons vegetable oil	*1 quart water (for steaming)*
1 teaspoon oyster sauce	*1 slice fresh ginger*
½ teaspoon sugar	*Salt and pepper to taste*
½ teaspoon chicken powder	*2 ounces scallions, finely chopped*
Sesame oil to taste	*¼ cup chopped fresh cilantro*

(continued)

1 Mix ½ cup water, the soy sauce, 2 teaspoons vegetable oil, oyster sauce, sugar, chicken powder, sesame oil, and white pepper in a medium saucepan. Heat the sauce, but do not boil. Keep warm over low heat.

2 In a Chinese steamer or a large pot fitted with a colander and a tight-fitting lid, bring 1 quart water to a boil. Lightly brush the cod with the remaining vegetable oil and season with salt and pepper. Place the fish into the steamer or colander and place a slice of ginger over top. Steam for 12 to 15 minutes, until firm and opaque in the center.

3 Using a large spatula, carefully remove the fish from steamer; sprinkle with chopped scallions and cilantro; pour the warm sauce over the fish and serve immediately.

Nutrient analysis per serving: 340 calories; 55 grams protein, 2 grams carbohydrate, 11 grams fat, 2 grams saturated fat, 154 milligrams cholesterol, .5 gram fiber, 285 milligrams sodium.

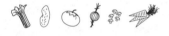

Stir-Fried Clams in Black Bean Sauce

You can serve this dish along with the soup and bok choy recipe, earlier in this chapter. This dish is so low in fat that even if served along with soup and bok choy, you still have some room for additional fat.

Preparation time: 15 minutes

Cooking time: 15 minutes

Yield: 10 servings

½ cup fresh black beans

3 cloves garlic

2 cloves shallots

1 chili pepper

4 pounds fresh Manila clams, scrubbed

1 teaspoon sesame oil

Pinch red pepper

1 teaspoon cooking sherry

2 teaspoons cornstarch with ½ cup chicken stock

½ teaspoon oyster sauce

1 teaspoon MSG (optional)

1 teaspoon sugar

Pinch white pepper

2 tablespoons light soy sauce

1 Mince black beans, garlic, shallots, and chili pepper. Set aside.

2 Bring 1 cup water to a boil in a 6-quart pot with a tight-fitting lid. Add the clams, cover, and simmer for 10 to 15 minutes, until all the clams have opened. Scoop the clams into a bowl and cover to keep warm.

3 Heat a wok over high heat. Add the sesame oil, black beans, and red pepper and cook, stirring, for 1 minute. Add the sherry, stock, oyster sauce, MSG, sugar, white pepper, soy sauce, and clams. Cook until sauce thickens, about 2 minutes.

Nutrient analysis per serving: 224 calories; 25 grams protein, 12 grams carbohydrate, 8 grams fat, 1 gram saturated fat, 62 milligrams cholesterol, 1 gram fiber, 355 milligrams sodium.

Il Fornaio

Il Fornaio *(eel for-NIGH-oh)* means "the baker" in Italian. The company began as a baking school outside Milan, Italy, in 1972, created in response to the disappearing art of centuries-old Italian baking. In 1981, Il Fornaio came to the United States and has since grown to include some of the most successful restaurants and bakeries in America. Today, you can enjoy Il Fornaio's authentic Italian food and baked goods at any of 21 locations in California, Portland, Seattle, Las Vegas, Denver, and Atlanta. For more information, you can visit www.ilfornaio.com on the Web.

Head chef Edmondo Sarti comes from the Emilia-Romagna section of Italy, which includes the great cuisine of Bologna. He learned to cook at his Uncle Salvatore's knee, going on to culinary school in Cervia, Italy. He apprenticed in the finest Italian restaurants and was offered a position at Valentino Restaurant in Los Angeles where he met his wife. Italy's loss became San Francisco's gain when he took a position as head chef at Il Fornaio.

Il Fornaio, 1265 Battery Street, San Francisco, California. 415-986-0100.

Scallopine Al Funghi (Veal with Mushrooms)

This recipe makes delicious use of veal, but you can substitute chicken breasts for the veal. Just marinate the chicken with chopped sage and rosemary. Try using different types of mushrooms, which gives the recipe a different taste: bottom mushrooms, shitake, chanterelle, or porcini. A half cup of any pasta (or, if you prefer, a slice of bread and a quarter cup of pasta) provides the necessary carbohydrate.

(continued)

Preparation time: 25 minutes

Cooking time: 15 minutes

Yield: 4 servings

8 2- to 3-ounce veal scallops

Salt and pepper to taste

1 tablespoon flour

2 tablespoons butter

2 tablespoons olive oil

1 chopped garlic clove

1 cup sliced mixed mushrooms

½ cup white wine

10 leaves Italian parsley

¼ cup vegetable stock

1 Place the veal scallops two at a time between sheets of plastic wrap and pound them with a meat mallet until ¼ inch thick. Season them with salt and pepper. Cover the veal scallops with flour, shaking off excess. Heat the butter in a sauté pan. Add the veal and cook for 2 minutes on each side. Transfer veal to a plate.

2 In the same pan add the oil, garlic, mushrooms, white wine, and parsley. Cook for a few minutes and add the veal and stock. Simmer for about 5 minutes.

3 Set veal on a plate and top with the mushroom sauce.

Nutrient analysis per serving: 442 calories; 49 grams protein, 2 grams carbohydrate, 22 grams fat, 7 grams saturated fat, 179 milligrams cholesterol, .5 gram fiber, 175 milligrams sodium.

Maniche Al Pollo (Elbow Pasta with Chicken)

This recipe is fairly concentrated in calories but is a delicious way to give chicken an Italian flavor. It's a complete meal as written, but you can eat less pasta and replace it with a piece of bread if you prefer.

Preparation time: 10 minutes

Cooking time: 20 minutes

Yield: 4 servings

2 tablespoons olive oil

12 ounces skinless chicken breasts, diced

Salt and pepper to taste

4 garlic cloves, sliced

½ cup white wine

10 ounces elbow pasta

4 sundried tomatoes

4 cups fresh broccoli florets

4 tablespoons Parmesan cheese

1 Heat the oil in large sauté pan over high heat. Add the diced chicken and salt and pepper. Sauté 2 to 3 minutes, or until cooked through. Add the garlic and lightly brown. Add the wine and cook until sauce is reduced to 1 to 2 tablespoons.

2 Boil the pasta according to directions. Three minutes before the pasta is ready, add the sundried tomatoes and broccoli. Drain and toss with the chicken, sauce, and Parmesan cheese.

Nutrient analysis per serving: *561 calories; 41 grams protein, 66 grams carbohydrate, 24 grams fat, 3 grams saturated fat, 70 milligrams cholesterol, 2.5 grams fiber, 283 milligrams sodium.*

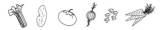

Spaghetti Gamberi E Zucchine (Spaghetti with Prawns and Zucchini)

The delicious taste of prawns is combined with a favorite Italian vegetable. This recipe is a complete meal. If you prefer to have a slice of bread, reduce the amount of pasta in the dish.

Preparation time: *20 minutes*

Cooking time: *20 minutes*

Yield: *4 servings*

4 tablespoons extra-virgin olive oil

16 ounces clean prawns or shrimp

Salt and pepper to taste

4 cloves garlic, sliced

4 small Italian zucchini, diced

4 ripened Roma tomatoes, peeled and diced

20 leaves Italian parsley

1 pinch chili flakes

4 tablespoons brandy

½ cup white wine

12 ounces spaghetti or other pasta

1 In a large sauté pan, heat the oil over high heat. Add the prawns and season with salt and pepper to taste. Sauté about 1 minute per side and then add the garlic and zucchini. Cook, tossing or gently stirring, for another minute. Add the tomatoes, parsley, chili flakes, brandy, and wine. Simmer 4 to 5 minutes, until the sauce thickens and the zucchini is tender.

(continued)

2 Boil the spaghetti in salted water. Drain and toss with shrimp sauce.

Nutrient analysis per serving: 562 calories; 31 grams protein, 60 grams carbohydrate, 15 grams fat, 2 grams saturated fat, 229 milligrams cholesterol, 3 grams fiber, 297 milligrams sodium.

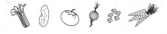

Branzino Al Fornaio (Sea Bass in the Il Fornaio Manner)

You can have a piece of bread with this recipe to get a complete meal. You can replace the sea bass with halibut, stripped bass, or red snapper for a change in taste. You can also add a serving of another vegetable.

Preparation time: 20 minutes

Cooking time: 20 minutes

Yield: 4 servings

1½ pounds sea bass fillet	*2 Roma tomatoes, diced*
Salt and pepper to taste	*¼ cup black olives, pitted*
2 tablespoons olive oil	*¼ cup white wine*
2 tablespoons butter	*2 cups steamed spinach*
¼ of an onion, diced	*¾ cup water*
2 cups potatoes, peeled and sliced	

1 Preheat oven to 375°. Season sea bass fillet with salt and pepper. Heat the oil and butter over high heat in a large sauté pan with a tight-fitting lid. Add the sea bass, cook for 2 minutes per side, and then add the onions, potatoes, tomatoes, and olives. Season with salt and pepper. Pour in the white wine and cook until almost completely reduced. Add the water, cover, and place in the oven for 15 to 20 minutes.

2 Check at 10 minutes and add a little more water if necessary. When done, serve over steamed spinach.

Nutrient analysis per serving: 316 calories; 25.5 grams protein, 18.4 grams carbohydrate, 16.2 grams fat, 5.4 grams saturated fat, 63 milligrams cholesterol, 4 grams fiber, 241 milligrams sodium.

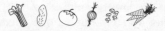

Risotto Ai Vegetali (Italian Rice with Vegetables)

A serving of this recipe provides all the carbohydrates for a full meal. It contains the vegetables you need as well. It lacks protein, which you can make up with a few ounces of chicken or fish. Use whatever vegetable is in season, including zucchini, artichokes, asparagus, or mushrooms. Be aware of the number of servings you have when you make this dish. Overeating is easy if you're not careful!

Preparation time: *10 minutes*

Cooking time: *1 hour*

Yield: *10 servings*

3 tablespoons butter

1 large shallot, diced

3 cups seasonal vegetables, diced

2 cups Italian Arborio rice

½ cup white wine

8 cups vegetable stock

½ tablespoon grated Parmesan cheese

Salt and pepper to taste

1 In a 4- to 6-quart heavy-bottom saucepan, heat 1 tablespoon butter over low-medium heat. Stir in the shallots and cook slowly for 4 minutes or until onions are soft and clear, but not brown. Increase the heat to medium, add all the vegetables, and cook, stirring, for 1 to 2 minutes. Stir in the rice and cook, gently stirring, for 1 to 2 minutes. Pour in the white wine and cook until it is almost completely reduced. Add the stock, 1 cup at a time, and cook at a low boil, stirring often, until absorbed. Each cup must be absorbed before the next is added. After 15 minutes, taste a grain of rice — it should have a slight resistance to the bite. If it seems too hard, add a little bit more stock and continue cooking for a couple more minutes.

2 When rice is ready, remove from heat. Add remaining butter and Parmesan cheese. Add salt and pepper to taste and mix with a wooden spoon until creamy in texture.

Nutrient analysis per serving: *204 calories; 4.6 grams protein, 34 grams carbohydrate, 5 grams fat, 2.3 grams saturated fat, 9 milligrams cholesterol, 1.6 grams fiber, 625 milligrams sodium.*

Bavarese Bianca Con Frutta (White Gelatin with Fruit)

This recipe is a dessert treat that should not be eaten too often, but it shows you that you can enjoy such treats in moderation and still follow your diabetic diet. Because the recipe is mostly carbohydrate and fat, it replaces those energy sources in your meal. The meal itself should be a few ounces of meat, fish, or poultry with a couple of servings of vegetables.

Preparation time: *20 minutes*

Cooking time: *None*

Yield: *4 servings*

1 envelope plain gelatin	¼ cup sugar
1½ cups 1 percent milk	1 cup mixed berries
½ cup cream	4 mint leaves

1 In a small bowl, mix together the gelatin and milk; let sit 5 minutes, until gelatin is dissolved. In a double boiler, bring the milk, cream, and sugar to a boil, stirring continuously to dissolve sugar. Remove from heat and allow to cool slightly.

2 Line four 3-ounce espresso cups with clear plastic wrap. Pour mixture into cups and refrigerate overnight or at least 6 hours.

3 Turn over the cups onto a plate. Remove plastic wrap and garnish with berries and mint leaves.

Nutrient analysis per 2 tablespoons: *259 calories; 6 grams protein, 28 grams carbohydrate, 13 grams fat, 9 grams saturated fat, 56 milligrams cholesterol, 1.3 grams fiber, 64 milligrams sodium.*

Windows on the World

Before its destruction on September 11, 2001, Windows on the World featured some of the most spectacular views in New York City from its location on the 106th and 107th floors of the World Trade Center. It was a dramatic, unrivaled setting for dinner, entertainment, and private occasions. The interior décor rivaled the views in its glamour and elegance. The American food served did justice to the unique setting. The freshest ingredients, contributed by area farmers and growers, were combined to produce distinctive dishes.

Chef/Director Michael Lomonaco led this and several previous kitchens to the top level of culinary accomplishment. He received numerous awards for creative cooking, including being proclaimed one of New York's Great Chefs by the James Beard Foundation. In Lomonaco's philosophy, great cooking is the ability to prepare foods creatively yet with simplicity, allowing the natural essence of the ingredients to shine through.

Manhattan Clam Chowder

This soup is a wonderful start to any meal. Make sure that you have some crusty French bread on the table, so you and your friends can clean out the soup bowl.

Preparation time: *45 minutes*

Cooking time: *1 hour, 30 minutes*

Yield: *6 servings*

1 tablespoon olive oil	*2 tablespoons chopped garlic*
2 tablespoons fresh slab bacon or fat back, diced	*¼ teaspoon cayenne powder*
4 carrots, peeled and diced, about 2 cups	*1 cup plum tomatoes, drained and crushed*
1 large onion, peeled and diced, about 1 cup	*2 quarts water*
4 celery stalks, diced, about 1 cup	*2 russet potatoes (about ¾ pound), cleaned, peeled, and diced*
3 tablespoons fresh oregano	*2 dozen chowder clams steamed open, chopped, cleaned, and juices reserved*
3 tablespoons fresh thyme leaves	*Salt and freshly ground black pepper to taste*
2 bay leaves	

1 In a heavy-bottomed soup pot, heat the olive oil, add the bacon or fat back, and cook until its fat begins to render, about 5 minutes.

2 Add the carrots, onions, and celery to the pot and cook, stirring often, over low heat until tender, about 15 minutes.

3 Add the oregano, thyme, bay leaves, garlic, and cayenne and stir to combine.

(continued)

4 Add the crushed tomatoes and water and bring to a boil. Reduce the heat and simmer for 1 hour.

5 Add the potatoes and continue to simmer for another half hour. Stir in the chopped clams with their juice and continue to cook for 2 minutes.

6 Season with salt and freshly ground pepper. Serve hot, with chowder crackers and freshly grated horseradish as a garnish.

Nutrient analysis per serving: 77 calories; 4 grams protein, 10 grams carbohydrate, 3 grams fat, .7 gram saturated fat, 92 milligrams cholesterol, 2 grams fiber, 604 milligrams sodium.

Chicken Thighs Braised in Apple Cider

This meal is low in carbohydrate as well as calories. You can even enjoy a couple of servings of starch. Why not serve with the potato gnocchi (recipe follows) and a fresh dinner roll? Top off the meal with a serving of strawberries and dollop of cream.

Preparation time: 30 minutes

Cooking time: 1 hour

Yield: 6 servings

6 chicken dark meat leg-thigh sections, skin and excess fat removed

Salt and pepper to taste

2 tablespoons olive oil

1 large onion, diced, about 1 cup

3 carrots, diced

2 Granny Smith apples, peeled, cored and cut into eighths

1 tablespoon curry powder

1 tablespoon flour

¼ cup applejack brandy or extract

½ cup apple cider

½ cup hot chicken stock

1 Preheat oven to 350°. Season chicken thighs with salt and pepper. Heat a large skillet or casserole over medium heat with the olive oil. Add the chicken thighs and cook 4 to 5 minutes, until well browned. Then turn and brown on the other side. When chicken is browned, remove and set aside.

2 Add the onion to the skillet and cook over medium heat to a golden brown before adding the carrot. Cook the carrot for 2 to 3 minutes, add the apple slices, and begin to caramelize.

3 Sprinkle the curry powder over the vegetables and apple and then sprinkle on the flour in the same way. Stir to combine well and begin to toast the curry-flour combination for 1 minute.

4 Add the chicken back to the pan and carefully pour in the applejack by removing the pan from the heat for a moment. Let the brandy bubble and begin to evaporate in the hot casserole before returning it to the heat.

5 Add the apple cider and chicken stock, bring quickly to a boil, reduce the heat to a slow simmer, cover the pan with a tight-fitting lid, and place in the oven for 35 minutes. When chicken is fully cooked, remove from oven, carefully ladle off any grease, and serve.

Nutrient analysis per serving: *236 calories; 14 grams protein, 16 grams carbohydrate, 10 grams fat, 2 grams saturated fat, 48 milligrams cholesterol, 3 grams fiber, 618 milligrams sodium.*

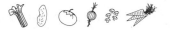

Potato Gnocchi with Spring Peas and Proscuitto

This recipe makes a wonderful side dish, or you can serve it as a main course. If you choose to serve the gnocchi as an entrée, serve it with a tossed green salad, a fresh dinner roll, and fresh fruit for dessert.

Preparation time: *1 hour, 30 minutes*

Cooking time: *15 minutes*

Yield: *6 servings*

1 pound Yukon gold potatoes, unpeeled

2 quarts water

1 egg

2 egg whites

1 cup flour

1 teaspoon salt

1 teaspoon ground black pepper

½ cup chicken broth, lowfat, low salt

¼ cup heavy cream

½ pound fresh peas, shelled and blanched in boiling water 2 minutes

1 tablespoon butter

¼ pound proscuitto, julienne

1 Put the potatoes in a pot with water. Bring the water to a boil and cook the potatoes at a strong simmer for 20 minutes or until tender. Drain the water from the pot and let the potatoes cool for only a few minutes before you begin to pull the skins from the potatoes. Discard the potato skins and, while still hot, pass the potatoes through a ricer into a bowl.

(continued)

2 *For gnocchi:* To the diced potatoes, add the whole egg and egg whites, season with salt and pepper, and using a rubber spatula or wooden spoon, mix until just combined. Add the flour in 2 stages so that only the amount that is necessary will be used to bind the potato. Add the second half of the flour (and some additional flour available if necessary) and mix well to form dough. Divide the dough in half and, on a floured work surface, roll the first half of dough into a log 1 inch thick. Cut the log into ½-inch thick round pieces. Lay the pieces out and, with your thumb, make an indentation on one side. Set aside and refrigerate until needed.

3 *For sauce:* Heat the chicken broth and cream together in a saucepan, add the peas, and allow to simmer several minutes. Remove from heat and add the butter to the cream, whisking to incorporate well. Stir in the proscuitto. Set aside, keeping sauce warm.

4 *For gnocchi:* Cook the gnocchi as you would pasta in several quarts of boiling, salted water. They cook very quickly and are cooked when they float to the surface, about 2 to 3 minutes.

5 *To serve:* Pour the sauce over the drained gnocchi, stir gently in a large serving bowl and serve immediately.

Nutrient analysis per serving: *241 calories; 10 grams protein, 32 grams carbohydrate, 8 grams fat, 4 grams saturated fat, 64 milligrams cholesterol, 2 grams fiber, 614 milligrams sodium.*

Asparagus and Wild Leek Tart with Goat Cheese and Red Pepper Vinaigrette

This finished dish resembles a piece of art and tastes even better than it looks. Complete the meal with a tossed salad and dish of fresh fruit.

Preparation time: *1 hour, 30 minutes*

Cooking time: *25 minutes*

Yield: *6 servings*

½ pound wild leeks (ramps) or scallions

3 tablespoons unsalted butter

Salt and pepper to taste

½ cup chicken broth

1 pound pencil asparagus

½ package phyllo dough

⅓ cup extra-virgin olive oil

6 ounces goat cheese

½ small red pepper, ribs and seeds removed

1 teaspoon mustard

¼ cup white wine vinegar

2 tablespoons walnut oil

1 Trim the root ends and tops of the leeks, leaving 3 inches of green. Rinse thoroughly under cold running water. Heat the butter in a medium sauté pan over medium heat. When the butter begins to foam, add the leeks, season with salt and pepper, and cook gently for 3 to 4 minutes. Add the broth to the wild leeks and simmer until all the broth has evaporated, but be careful not to burn the leeks. Remove from the sauté pan and allow to cool.

2 Wash the asparagus and cut off the bottom of the stems that are greenish-white and tough. Bring a pot of water to boil, add 1 tablespoon salt, submerge the asparagus for 30 seconds to blanch. Remove the asparagus from the pot and quickly submerge in iced water to shock. Set the asparagus aside.

3 Preheat oven to 375°. Prepare a space to work with the phyllo dough: Wrap the dough and cover with a cloth; have a brush, the olive oil, and a cookie sheet ready. Begin by lightly brushing the center of the cookie sheet with a film of olive oil. Next, lay the first sheet of dough on the cookie pan, brush the dough lightly with oil, overlap widthwise the next sheet over the half of the first so that now the 2 sheets make a pastry sheet 50 percent wider (not longer) than the original dimension of the pastry. Don't be concerned if the lengthwise ends of the dough are overflowing from the edges of the pan: All the edges of the dough will be rolled up to form the edges of the tart. Brush the second sheet of dough with oil and lay another sheet squarely over the first so that, in alternating this pattern, you build your pastry base. Continue to alternate the dough sheets, brushing each layer with oil, until you have used half of the package of dough. Gather the edges of the phyllo dough between the tips of your fingers and begin to roll them toward the center to form the sides of the tart. Roll uniformly inward until the rolled edge is even all around and the round tart resembles a pizza. Leave a pastry base of 10 to 12 inches into which the vegetables and cheese will go after the tart shell is partially baked. Place the empty tart into the oven and bake for 6 minutes. Remove the pastry from the oven and allow to cool for 10 minutes. You can do this pastry preparation over the course of several hours or even a day or two ahead if the partial cooking is reserved until the last moment and the pastry is covered with plastic wrap and refrigerated.

4 To fill the tart, crumble the goat cheese and spread it evenly over the base of the tart. Next add an even layer of wild leeks, followed by the asparagus, which should be fanned, tips out, from the center of the tart. Season the tart lightly with salt and pepper, place into the 375° oven, and bake for 15 minutes or until the cheese has softened and the crust becomes a rich golden brown.

5 While the tart is baking (or ahead of time if possible), prepare the vinaigrette. Place the red pepper, mustard, vinegar, ¼ teaspoon salt, and black pepper in a food processor. Pulse to chop the red pepper to a fine dice. When the pepper has been pulsed enough, begin to drizzle in the walnut oil to create an emulsified dressing. Serve the tart with drizzle of red pepper vinaigrette.

Nutrient analysis per serving: *514 calories; 11 grams protein, 44 grams carbohydrate, 28 grams fat, 9 grams saturated fat, 31 milligrams cholesterol, 3 grams fiber, 668 milligrams sodium.*

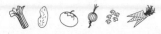

Buckwheat Groats and Mushroom Griddle Cakes

This recipe is a refreshing change from the standard, starch-based side dishes, such as rice, potatoes, or pasta. You can also serve it as a main dish along with a green salad, roll, and bowl of raspberries.

Preparation time: *30 minutes*

Cooking time: *1 hour*

Yield: *6 servings*

1 tablespoon olive oil

1 small onion, about ½ cup

1 cup kasha or buckwheat groats

1 whole egg

2 cups hot chicken stock

1 teaspoon salt

2 tablespoons butter

3 tablespoons flour

¼ cup milk

½ cup sautéed mushrooms, roughly chopped

½ teaspoon cayenne pepper

Vegetable oil

1 Heat the olive oil in a large skillet over medium heat. Add the onion and cook until translucent.

2 In a bowl, combine the buckwheat groats and egg and stir to thoroughly coat the groats. Pour the groats into the hot pan with the onion and stir rapidly to toast the grains and keep them separate.

3 Add the chicken stock and salt and bring to a boil. Reduce heat, cover, and simmer for 30 minutes.

4 When the kasha has cooked, add the butter and stir until the butter has been absorbed. Stir in the flour, milk, mushrooms, and cayenne. Heat a griddle pan with a thin coating of vegetable oil and, using a ladle, begin to make small griddlecakes. Cook until the bottoms of the griddlecakes brown lightly before turning to brown the second side.

Nutrient analysis per serving: *224 calories; 9 grams protein, 27 grams carbohydrate, 10 grams fat, 4 grams saturated fat, 49 milligrams cholesterol, 1 gram fiber, 930 milligrams sodium.*

Appendix B

Exchange Lists

● ●

In This Appendix

▶ Listing the foods

▶ Using exchanges to create your diet

● ●

*I*n this appendix, you discover the method that dieticians have been using for many years to help their clients eat the right number of calories from the correct energy sources while permitting them to vary their foods.

Listing the Foods

Thousands of different foods are available, but each one can be broken down on the basis of the energy source (carbohydrate, protein, or fat) that is most prevalent in the food. Fortunately, the food content of one type of fish — salmon, for example — is just about the same as another type of fish, like halibut. Therefore, a diet that calls for one fish exchange can use any one of a number of choices or exchanges. You can exchange one for the other, so your diet is never boring.

Listing all food sources in this space isn't possible. But for a list of just about all foods you might eat, purchase "The Official Pocket Guide to Diabetic Exchanges" from the American Diabetes Association at 800-232-6733 or through the ADA Web site in Appendix C.

The starches list

The starch exchanges are listed in Tables B-1 and B-2. Each exchange contains 15 grams of carbohydrate plus 3 grams of protein and 0 to 1 grams of fat, which amounts to 80 kcalories per exchange. If the produce contains whole grains, it has about 2 grams of fiber.

Table B-1	Starch Exchanges	
Cereals, Grains, Pasta	*Bread*	*Dried Beans, Peas, Lentils (Higher in Fiber)*
Bran cereals, ½ cup	Bagel, ½	Beans and peas, ⅓ cup (cooked)
Cooked cereals, ½ cup (cooked)	Breadsticks, 2	Lentils, ⅓ cup (⅔ ounce total)
Grape Nuts, 3 tablespoons	English muffin, ½	Baked beans, ¼ cup
Grits (cooked), ½ cup	Frankfurter, ½ bun	
Pasta (cooked), ½ cup	Hamburger roll, ½	Lima beans, ½ cup
Puffed cereal, 1½ cups	Pita, 6 inches across, ½	Peas, green, ½ cup
Rice (cooked), ⅓ cup	Raisin bread, 1 slice	
Shredded wheat, ½ cup	Tortilla, 6 inches, 1 slice	
	White bread, 1 slice	
	Whole wheat bread, 1 slice	

Table B-2	More Starch Exchanges	
Crackers/Snacks	*Starchy Vegetables*	*Starchy Foods with Fats*
Animal crackers, 8	Corn, ½ cup	Chow mein noodles, ½ cup
Graham crackers, 3	Corn on the cob, 1	Cornbread, 2 ounces
Matzoh, ¾ ounce	Potato, baked, 1	French fries, 10 (3 ounces)
Melba toast, 5 slices	Potato, mashed, ½ cup (add a fat exchange)	Muffin, 1
Popcorn (no fat), 3 cups	Squash, winter, ¾ cup	Pancake, 4 inches, 2
Pretzels, ¾ ounce	Yam, sweet potato, ⅓ cup	Waffle, 4½ inches, 1
Whole wheat cracker, 4		
Saltine-type cracker, 6		

Meat and meat substitutes list

One exchange contains no carbohydrate, 7 grams of protein, and 1 to 8 grams of fat. Thus the kcalories vary from 35 to 100 per exchange.

Lean meat and substitutes:

- Beef: Lean, such as round, sirloin, and flank steak, tenderloin, 1 ounce
- Pork: Lean, such as fresh, canned, cured, or boiled ham, 1 ounce
- Veal: All cuts but veal cutlets, 1 ounce
- Poultry: Chicken, turkey, and Cornish hen (no skin), 1 ounce

Fish:

- All fresh and frozen fish, 1 ounce
- Crab, lobster, scallops, shrimp, and clams, 2 ounces
- Oysters, 6 medium
- Tuna (canned in water), 1 cup
- Sardines (canned), 2 medium

Wild game:

- Venison, rabbit, and squirrel, 1 ounce
- Pheasant, duck, and goose, 1 ounce

Cheese:

- Any cottage cheese, ¼ cup
- Grated Parmesan, 2 tablespoons
- Diet cheeses, 1 ounce

Other:

- Egg whites, 3 whites
- Egg substitutes, ¼ cup

Medium-fat meat and substitutes:

- Beef: Ground, roast, steak, and meat loaf, 1 ounce
- Pork: Chops, loin, and cutlets, 1 ounce
- Lamb: Chops, leg, and roast, 1 ounce

✔ Veal: Cutlet, 1 ounce

✔ Poultry: Chicken with skin, ground turkey, 1 ounce

✔ Fish: Tuna in oil, salmon (canned), ¼ cup

✔ Cheese: Skim or part-skim milk cheese like ricotta (¼ cup) and mozzarella and diet cheeses (1 ounce)

High-fat meat and substitutes:

✔ Beef: Prime cuts like ribs and corn beef, 1 ounce

✔ Pork: Spareribs, ground pork, and pork sausage, 1 ounce

✔ Lamb: Ground, 1 ounce

✔ Fish: Any fried fish, 1 ounce

✔ Cheese: All regular like Swiss, American, Cheddar, and Monterey, 1 ounce

✔ Other: Luncheon meat like bologna and salami, 1 ounce; sausage, knockwurst, and bratwurst, 1 ounce; frankfurter, 1 frank; and peanut butter, 1 tablespoon

Fruit list

Each exchange in Table B-3 contains carbohydrate (60 kcalories) but no protein or fat. The list includes fresh, frozen, canned, and dried fruit and juice.

Table B-3	Fruit Exchanges	
Fruit	*Dried Fruit*	*Fruit Juice*
Apple, 4 oz	Apple, 4 rings	Apple, ½ cup
Applesauce, ½ cup	Apricots, 7 halves	Cranberry, ⅓ cup
Apricots, 4	Dates, 2½	Grapefruit, ½ cup
Apricots (canned) ½ cup	Figs, 1½	Grape, ⅓ cup
Banana (9 inches), ½	Prunes, 3	Orange, ½ cup
Blackberries, ¾ cup	Raisins, 2 tablespoons	Pineapple, ½ cup
Blueberries, ¾ cup		Prune, ⅓ cup
Cantaloupe, ⅓ melon (5-inch diameter)		

Fruit	Dried Fruit	Fruit Juice
Cherries, 12		
Cherries (canned), ½ cup		
Figs, 2		
Fruit cocktail, ½ cup		
Grapefruit, ½		
Grapes, 15		
Honeydew, ⅛ melon		
Kiwi, 1		
Mango, ½		
Nectarine, 1		
Orange, 1		
Papaya, 1 cup		
Peach, 1		
Peaches (canned), ½ cup		
Pear, 1 small		
Pears (canned), ½ cup		
Persimmon, 2		
Pineapple, ½ cup		
Pineapple (canned), ⅓ cup		
Plum, 2		
Raspberries, 1 cup		
Strawberries, 1¼ cups		
Tangerine, 2		
Watermelon, 1¼ cups		

Milk list

Each exchange has 12 grams of carbohydrate and 8 grams of protein. Each exchange may have 0 to 8 grams of fat, so the kcalorie count is 90 to 150.

Skim and very lowfat milk list: Add 0 kcal for fat content

- Skim milk, 1 cup
- ½ percent milk, 1 cup
- 1 percent milk, 1 cup
- Nonfat or lowfat buttermilk, 1 cup
- Evaporated skim milk, ½ cup
- Dry nonfat milk, ⅓ cup dry
- Plain nonfat yogurt, ¾ cup
- Nonfat or lowfat fruit-flavored yogurt sweetened with aspartame

Reduced fat milk list: Add 45 kcalories for fat content

- 2 percent milk, 1 cup
- Plain lowfat yogurt, ¾ cup
- Sweet acidophilus milk, 1 cup

Whole milk list: Add 72 kcalories for fat content

- Whole milk, 1 cup
- Evaporated whole milk, ½ cup
- Goat's milk, 1 cup
- Kefir

Vegetable list

Each exchange has 5 grams of carbohydrate and 2 grams of protein, which equals 25 kcalories. Vegetables have 2 to 3 grams of fiber. Remember that the starchy vegetables like lentils, corn, and potatoes are on the starches list, earlier in this chapter. The serving size for all is ½ cup of cooked vegetables and 1 cup of raw vegetables.

- Artichoke (½ medium)
- Asparagus
- Beans (green, wax, Italian)
- Bean sprouts
- Cabbage
- Carrots

- Cauliflower
- Eggplant
- Greens (collard, mustard)
- Kohlrabi
- Okra
- Onions
- Pea pods
- Peppers (green)
- Rutabaga
- Sauerkraut
- Summer squash
- Turnips
- Water chestnuts
- Zucchini

Fats list

These foods have 5 grams of fat and little or no protein or carbohydrate per portion. The calorie count is, therefore, 45 kcalories. The important thing in this category is to notice the foods that are high in cholesterol and saturated fats and avoid them. See Table B-4.

Table B-4	Fat Exchanges
Unsaturated Fats	*Saturated Fats*
Avocado, ⅛ medium	Butter, 1 teaspoon
Salad dressing, 1 tablespoon	Bacon, 1 slice
Margarine, 1 teaspoon	Coconut, 2 tablespoons
Salad dressing, lowfat, 2 tablespoons	Cream, 2 tablespoons
Margarine, diet, 1 tablespoon	Cream, sour, 2 tablespoons
Mayonnaise, 1 teaspoon	Cream, heavy, 1 tablespoon
Almonds, 6	Cream cheese, 1 tablespoon
Cashews, 1 tablespoon	Salt pork, ¼ ounce

(continued)

Table B-4 *(continued)*

Unsaturated Fats	Saturated Fats
Pecans, 2 whole	
Peanuts, 10 large	
Walnuts, 2 whole	
Seeds (pine nuts, sunflower) 1 tablespoon	
Seeds (pumpkin) 2 teaspoons	
Oil (corn, olive, soybean, sunflower, peanut), 1 teaspoon	
Olives, 10 small	

Other carbohydrates

This new list (as of 1997) contains cakes, pies, puddings, and other foods with lots of carbohydrate (and often fat). They're considered to have 15 grams of carbohydrate and a variable amount of fat and given the kcalorie value of 60 per exchange. Examples are too numerous to list but include, for example:

- Ice cream, ½ cup
- Brownies, 2-inch square

Free foods

These foods contain less than 20 calories per serving, so you can eat as much of them as you want without worrying about overeating and without worrying about serving size.

- **Drinks:** Bouillon, sugar-free drinks, club soda, coffee, and tea
- **Salad greens:** Endive, any type of lettuce, Romaine, and spinach
- **Nonstick pan spray**
- **Sweet substitutes:** Sugar-free candy, sugar-free gum, sugar-free jam or jelly, and sugar substitutes such as saccharin and aspartame
- **Fruit:** Cranberries, unsweetened, and rhubarb
- **Vegetables:** Cabbage, celery, cucumber, green onion, hot peppers, mushroom, and radish

✓ **Condiments:** Catsup (1 tablespoon), horseradish, mustard, pickles (unsweetened), low-calorie salad dressing, taco sauce, and vinegar

✓ **Seasonings:** Basil, lemon juice, celery seeds, lime, cinnamon, mint, chili powder, onion powder, chives, oregano, curry, paprika, dill, pepper, flavoring extracts (vanilla, for example), pimiento, garlic, spices, garlic powder, soy sauce, herbs, wine (used in cooking), lemon, and Worcestershire sauce

Using Exchanges to Create a Diet

Having all foods in exchange lists makes it easy to create a diet with great variation. You can find typical diets in the ADA booklet, but remember that they generally permit more carbohydrate than I do. The following menus have been adjusted to reflect the lower carbohydrate and higher protein that I recommend. Here are the amounts for diets of 1,500 and 1,800 kcalories. See Table B-5.

Table B-5	1,500 kcalories
Breakfast	*Lunch*
1 fruit exchange	3 lean meat exchanges
1 starch exchange	1 vegetable exchange
1 medium fat meat exchange	2 fat exchanges
1 fat exchange	1 starch exchange
1 lowfat milk exchange	2 fruit exchanges
Dinner	*Snack*
4 lean meat exchanges	1 bread exchange
2 starch exchanges	½ lowfat milk exchange
2 vegetable exchanges	1 lean meat exchange
1 fruit exchange	
2 fat exchanges	
½ lowfat milk exchange	

This diet provides 150 grams of carbohydrate, 125 grams of protein and 45 grams of fat, keeping it in line with the 40 percent carbohydrate, 30 percent protein, and 30 percent fat program.

Translating this into food, you can have the menu in Table B-6 on one day:

Table B-6	A Sample Menu
Breakfast	*Lunch*
½ cup apple juice	3 ounces skinless chicken
1 piece of toast	½ cup cooked green beans
1 teaspoon margarine	4 walnuts
1 egg	1 slice bread
1 cup skim milk	1 cup applesauce
Dinner	*Snack*
4 ounces lean beef	¼ cup cottage cheese
1 piece bread	½ English muffin
½ cup peas	½ cup skim milk
1 cup broccoli	
⅓ cantaloupe	
2 tablespoons salad dressing	
salad of free foods	
4 ounces lowfat yogurt	

For an 1,800 kcalorie diet, you would have the menu in Table B-7:

Table B-7	1,800 kcalories
Breakfast	*Lunch*
1 fruit exchange	3 lean meat exchanges
1 starch exchange	1 vegetable exchange
1 medium fat meat exchange	2 fat exchanges
2 fat exchanges	2 starch exchanges
1 lowfat milk exchange	2 fruit exchanges
	½ lowfat milk exchange

Dinner	Snack
4 lean meat exchanges	2 bread exchanges
2 starch exchanges	2 lean meat exchanges
2 vegetable exchanges	½ lowfat milk exchange
1 fruit exchange	
3 fat exchanges	

This diet provides 180 grams of carbohydrate, 135 grams of protein, and 60 grams of fat, again maintaining the 40:30:30 division of calories.

Using the example of the 1,500 kcalorie diet, you should be able to make up an 1,800 kcalorie diet at this point.

Appendix C
Dr. W. W. Web

• •

In This Appendix

▶ Starting at my Web site

▶ Checking the general sites about diabetes

▶ Looking at companies that make diabetes products

▶ Combining athletics and diabetes

▶ Browsing government diabetes sites

▶ Using nongovernmental sites that help to search government sites

▶ Searching Web pages in other languages besides English

▶ Viewing sites for the visually impaired

▶ Finding out about diabetic dogs and cats

▶ Reading books and Web sites on diabetic eating

• •

*I*n just a few years, the World Wide Web has gone from little or no information to more than anyone can digest. This appendix presents the best places for you to check. You should be able to get answers to just about any questions that you have, but you must be cautious about the source of the advice. Do not make any major changes in your diabetes care without checking with your physician. In Chapter 19, you find advice about how to differentiate between useful and useless information on the Web. Any Web site I discuss in this section can be relied upon, but sometimes free advice is worth no more than you pay for it. Remember that the Web is constantly changing and growing, so these addresses are valid at least on the day I list them.

My Web Site

You can start your search at my Web page:

```
www.drrubin.com
```

You can find general information and advice about diabetes, daily tips, new developments, and answers to questions. You also find all of the sites listed in this appendix so that you need only click on them to see them for yourself.

General Sites

These sites tell you about diabetes from A to Z. They run the gamut from well-known organizations to individual doctors who specialize in diabetes. Sometimes the sites get a little technical. That is when you need to return to this book for clarification.

The American Diabetes Association

This huge site has just about everything you need to know about diabetes and then some. It may be a little technical in places, but that's probably because you got into the professional section by mistake. You can order all its publications from here.

```
www.diabetes.org
```

Online Diabetes Resources by Rick Mendosa

Rick Mendosa, who has diabetes himself, has cataloged just about everything there is on the Web concerning diabetes. It's a huge undertaking, and he manages to bring it off beautifully. He also has some excellent articles that he has written on various topics in diabetes.

```
www.mendosa.com/diabetes.htm
```

National Diabetes Education Program

The federal government is sponsoring the National Diabetes Education Program to improve treatments and outcomes for people with diabetes, to promote early diagnosis, and to prevent the onset of diabetes. It is a vast undertaking.

```
137.187.36.5/health/diabetes/ndep/ndep.htm
```

National Diabetes Education Initiative

The federal government is determined to teach physicians about the importance of meeting the standards of diabetes care and how to go about doing this. You can learn a lot by looking at its programs.

```
www.ndei.org
```

Medscape Diabetes and Endocrinology Home Page

You can find numerous articles about diabetes from the medical literature as well as free access to the files of the National Library of Medicine.

```
endocrine.medscape.com/Home/Topics/endocrinology/
           endocrinology.html
```

The Diabetes Monitor

The Diabetes Monitor is the creation of diabetes specialist Dr. William Quick. He discusses every aspect of diabetes, including the latest discoveries.

```
www.diabetesmonitor.com
```

Juvenile Diabetes Foundation

The JDF prides itself on its contribution to research in diabetes, and this site reflects that. You can find what you want to know about the latest government programs that emphasize finding a cure for diabetes.

```
www.jdfcure.org
```

Children with Diabetes

This site is the creation of a father of a diabetic child and has an enormous database of information for the parents of children with diabetes.

```
www.childrenwithdiabetes.com
```

Diabetes Information at Mediconsult.com

If you're looking for information about proper use of drugs, this site is the place to go. In addition, you can find answers to all your diabetes questions.

```
www.mediconsult.com/mc/mcsite.nsf/conditionnav/
```

```
diabetes~sectionintroduction
```

Joslin Diabetes Center

The Joslin Diabetes Center has been one of the world's leading pioneers in diabetes care and the information to be found reflects this. It also tells you how you can join Joslin, do research, or go to diabetes camp.

```
www.joslin.org
```

Canadian Diabetes Association

If you're a Canadian, you will want to visit this site because a lot of its information, obviously, pertains to the special needs of the Canadian with diabetes. However, the information is general. A major benefit is that the information is in French as well as English.

```
www.diabetes.ca
```

The International Diabetes Federation

This organization of over 100 countries meets every three years and can be a source for knowledgeable diabetes experts around the world.

```
www.idf.org
```

Ask NOAH about Diabetes

This site provides a large amount of information in both English and Spanish. It comes from the New York Online Access to Health, a partnership of New York institutions.

```
www.noah-health.org/
```

Sites of Companies That Make Diabetes Products

This section helps you find the companies that are making the products that you need to control your diabetes. If you have questions about the proper use of a drug or a device, you can usually find it here. But keep in mind that the companies are very limited (by the FDA) with respect to the uses of their products. Often doctors are using drugs in ways that have been proven to be successful but have not yet received FDA approval.

Glucose meters

These companies are making the meters that are used by the largest number of people with diabetes. You can expect that they will be around when you start having problems after a year or two of use.

- **Abbott Laboratories:** www.abbott.com
- **Bayer:** www.bayerdiag.com
- **Home Diagnostics Inc.:** www.homediagnosticsinc.com
- **LifeScan:** www.lifescan.com
- **Roche:** www.roche.com

Lancing devices

A company that has a very large share of the market for lancing devices is **Owen Mumford,** which you can find at www.owenmumford.com.

Insulin pumps

Three companies dominate the market for insulin pump devices. They are

- **Animas:** www.animascorp.com
- **Disetronic Holding AG:** www.disetronic.com
- **MiniMed Technologies:** minimed.com

Insulin

Three companies also dominate the insulin market in the United States.

- **Aventis:** www.aventis.com/main/
- **Eli Lilly and Company:** www.lilly.com/diabetes
- **Novo Nordisk:** www.novo-nordisk.com

Insulin syringes

If you want to find the major company for syringes, go to **Becton Dickinson and Company** at www.bd.com/diabetes.

Insulin jet injection devices

Jet injection devices provide "painless" insulin injection. A number of companies are trying to monopolize this market, including:

- **Activa Brand Products:** www.advantajet.com
- **Bioject, Inc:** www.bioject.com
- **Antares Pharma (formerly Medi-Ject Corporation):** www.mediject.com
- **Vitajet Corp:** www.vitajet.com

Companies and their oral medications

This list contains only six companies at present, but the market for oral medications is heating up and there will be several more in the not-too-distant future.

- **Bristol-Myers Squibb-Glucophage, Glucovance, Glucophage XR:** www.bms.com
- **Aventis-Amaryl:** www2.aventis.com/homepage/homepage.htm
- **Eli Lilly-Taked-Actos:** www.lilly.com/diabetes/
- **Pfizer Inc.-Glucotrol:** www.pfizer.com
- **Pharmacia & Upjohn Inc.-Micronase and Glynase and Glyset:** www.pnu.com
- **Glaxo SmithKline-Avandia:** www.gsk.com

Diabetic Exercise and Sports Association

The Diabetes Exercise and Sports Association is a place where you can find out about many different kinds of exercise, how much you can and should do, and whether there are any limitations because of the diabetes. You will find others who share your interests. You can find this group at

www.diabetes-exercise.org

Government Web Sites

These sites provide lots of authoritative information in their many online publications about diabetes while telling you all about the latest government programs to eradicate the disease.

National Institute of Diabetes and Digestive and Kidney Disease

This site is loaded with great publications about diabetes. Find it at

```
www.niddk.nih.gov/health/diabetes/diabetes.htm
```

Centers for Disease Control

If you want to know all the latest statistics about every aspect of diabetes, go to this site at

```
www.cdc.gov/nccdphp/ddt/ddthome.htm
```

Healthfinder Web Site

Healthfinder is a service of the U.S. Department of Health and Human Services. It has information about many important diseases and has a large section about diabetes at

```
www.healthfinder.gov
```

PubMed Search Service of the National Library of Medicine

This is where you go to use the National Library of Medicine. It's easy to use and gives you (for free) a large number of the latest scientific papers on any medical topic of interest. Find it at

```
www.ncbi.nlm.nih.gov/PubMed
```

Nongovernment Web Site for Searching the National Library

MedFetch is an excellent site for creating repeated searches on a topic like diabetes over time. The information arrives by e-mail.

```
www.medfetch.com
```

Diabetes Information in Other Languages

Not everyone speaks and reads English. Here, you find diabetes educational sites in many languages. The following ones account for only the most common languages, but you can find many others.

- **French:** `www.sante-ujf-grenoble.fr/SANTE/alfediam/mellitis.html`
- **German:** `www.uni-leipzig.de/~diabetes`
- **Italian:** `www.publinet.it/diabete`
- **Korean:** `www.diabetes.or.kr`
- **Russian:** `www.diabet.ru`
- **Spanish:** `www.saludlatina.com/diabetes`

Sites for the Visually Impaired

Because diabetes has such a major impact on vision, when the disease is not controlled, you can find huge quantities of information on every issue relating to visual impairment at these sites.

American Foundation for the Blind

The American Foundation for the Blind has resources, information, reports, talking books, and limitless other facts and wisdom about dealing with visual impairment at

```
www.afb.org
```

Blindness Resource Center

This site points you in the right direction for information on every aspect of blindness. It is a guide to other sites about visual impairment.

```
www.nyise.org/text/blindness.htm
```

Diabetes Division of the National Federation of the Blind

This national organization is another major source of information about every aspect of blindness at

```
www.nfb.org/diabetes.htm
```

Diabetic Retinopathy Foundation

The Diabetic Retinopathy Foundation is a not-for-profit organization whose mission is to support research and public awareness, which leads to the prevention of one of the world's major causes of blindness — diabetic retinopathy. Find it at

```
www.retinopathy.org/
```

Animals with Diabetes

Yes, your dog and cat and many other animals can get diabetes. Here are sites for those two animals.

Dogs

This site tells you everything you need to know to manage your canine with diabetes.

```
www.petdiabetes.org/
```

Cats

This site is packed with helpful information for the cat owner who has a diabetic cat.

`pricemd.com/felinediabetes.com`

Recipe Web Sites for People with Diabetes

You can find a number of excellent recipes on World Wide Web sites. You can generally count on the recipes in books to contain the nutrients they list, but on the Web, you need to evaluate the site before accepting the recipes. You can trust the sites that I list here. These are the best of the currently available Web sites that provide recipes appropriate for a person with diabetes. Things change so frequently on the Web that it's difficult to keep up to date, so check back often.

- ✔ The nutrition section of the American Diabetes Association Web site begins at `www.diabetes.org/nutrition`. Here you find discussions of nutrition as well as lots of recipes.

- ✔ Children with Diabetes includes a large amount of information on meal planning, sugar substitutes, and the food guide pyramid, as well as many recipes at `www.childrenwithdiabetes.com/d_08_000.htm`.

- ✔ The Joslin Diabetes Center points out that "There is no such thing as a diabetic diet" among many other topics on nutrition at `www.joslin.org/education/library/index.html`.

- ✔ Ask NOAH About Diabetes supplies links to many important articles about diabetic nutrition as well as diabetic recipes at `www.noah-health.org/`.

- ✔ Olen Publishing has a Food Finder site that lists the nutritional values for the food in about 20 major fast food restaurants at `www.olen.com/food`.

- ✔ The Vegetarian Resource Group maintains a large site filled with information for vegetarians who have developed diabetes at `www.vrg.org/journal/diabetes.htm`.

- ✔ The Food and Drug Administration provides a long article about diabetic nutrition at `vm.cfsan.fda.gov/~lrd/cons1194.txt`.

- ✔ *Diabetic Gourmet Magazine* offers a valuable site that contains information about diagnosis and treatment as well as numerous recipes that you can use at `diabeticgourmet.com`.

Appendix D

Glossary

Acarbose: An oral agent that lowers blood glucose by blocking breakdown of carbohydrates in the intestine.

ACE inhibitor: A drug that lowers blood pressure but is especially useful when diabetes affects the kidneys.

Acetone: A breakdown product of fat formed when fat rather than glucose is being used for energy.

Advanced glycosylation end products (AGEs): Combination of glucose and other substances in the body. Too much may damage various organs.

Alpha cells: Cells in the Islets of Langerhans within the pancreas that make glucagon, which raises blood glucose.

Algorithm: In diabetes care, a step-by-step plan for determining how much insulin to use for the blood level of glucose and the intake of carbohydrates.

Amaryl: An oral agent that lowers glucose by raising insulin levels.

Amino acids: Compounds that link together to form proteins.

Amyotrophy: A form of diabetic neuropathy causing muscle wasting and weakness.

Angiography: Using a dye to take pictures of blood vessels to detect disease. In diabetes, angiography is often used in the eyes.

Antibodies: Substances formed when the body detects something foreign such as bacteria.

Antigens: Substances against which the antibody forms.

Artificial pancreas: A large machine that can measure blood glucose and release appropriate insulin.

Atherosclerosis: Narrowing of arteries due to deposits of cholesterol and other factors.

Autoimmune disorder: Disease in which the body mistakenly attacks its own tissues.

Autonomic neuropathy: Diseases of nerves that affect organs not under conscious control, such as the heart, lungs, and intestine.

Avandia: One of a new class of oral antidiabetic agents that lowers glucose by reducing insulin resistance.

Background retinopathy: An early stage of diabetic eye involvement that does not reduce vision.

Beta cell: A cell in the Islets of Langerhans in the pancreas, which makes the key hormone, insulin.

Blood urea nitrogen (BUN): A substance in blood that reflects kidney function.

Body mass index: A number derived by dividing the weight in kilograms by the height times the height in meters giving a result that reflects both factors.

Borderline diabetes: Formerly used to mean mild or early diabetes but no longer used.

Carbohydrate: One of the three major energy sources, the one usually found in grain, fruits, and vegetables and the one most responsible for raising the blood glucose.

Carbohydrate counting: Estimating the amount of carbohydrate in food in order to determine insulin needs.

Cataract: A clouding of the lens of the eye often found earlier and more commonly in people with diabetes.

Charcot's foot: Destruction of joints and soft tissue in the foot leading to an unusable foot as a result of diabetic neuropathy.

Cholesterol: A form of fat that is needed in the body for production of certain hormones. Can lead to atherosclerosis if present in excessive levels. Butter and egg yolks are high in cholesterol.

Conventional diabetes treatment: Usually referring to treatment in type 1 diabetes where only one or two shots of insulin are given daily.

Continuous subcutaneous insulin infusion (CSII): Continuous delivery of insulin under the skin, usually by an insulin pump, to mimic the way the body provides insulin.

Creatinine: A substance in blood that is measured to reflect the level of kidney function.

Dawn phenomenon: The tendency for blood glucose to rise early in the morning due to secretion of hormones that counteract insulin.

Diabetes Control and Complications Trial (DCCT): The decisive study of type 1 diabetes that showed that intensive control of blood glucose would prevent or delay complications of diabetes.

Diabetic ketoacidosis: An acute loss of control of diabetes with high blood glucose levels and breakdown of fat leading to acidification of the blood with nausea, vomiting, and dehydration, which can lead to coma and death.

Diabetologist: A physician who specializes in diabetes treatment.

Dialysis: Artificial cleaning of the blood when the kidneys are not working.

Endocrinologist: A physician who specializes in diseases of the glands, including the adrenal glands, the thyroid, the pituitary, the parathyroid glands, the ovaries, testicles, and pancreas.

Euglycemia: A state in which the blood glucose remains in the normal range.

Exchange plan: A dietary plan where foods that are similar in type are grouped together so that a diet can substitute any one for any other within that group. The seven groups are starches and breads, meats and meat substitutes, fruits, milks, vegetables, fats, and other carbohydrates.

Fiber: A substance in plants that can't be digested, so it provides no energy but can lower fat and blood glucose if it dissolves in water and is absorbed or can help prevent constipation if it does not dissolve in water and remains in the intestine.

Fructose: The sugar found in fruits, vegetables, and honey. It has calories but is more slowly absorbed than glucose.

Gastroparesis: A form of autonomic neuropathy involving nerves to the stomach so that food is held in the stomach.

Gestational diabetes mellitus: Diabetes that occurs during a pregnancy, usually ending at delivery.

Glimeperide: *See Amaryl.*

Glucagon: A hormone made in the alpha cell of the pancreas that raises glucose and can be injected in severe hypoglycemia.

Glucose: The body's main source of energy in the blood and cells.

Glucophage: An oral agent for diabetes that lowers glucose by blocking release from the liver.

Glycemic index: The extent to which a given food raises blood glucose usually compared to white bread. Low glycemic index foods are preferred in diabetes.

Glycogen: The storage form of glucose in the liver and muscles.

Glycosuria: Glucose in the urine.

Glycosylated hemoglobin: *See Hemoglobin A1c.*

Glyset: An oral hypoglycemic drug that lowers blood glucose by blocking breakdown of complex sugars and starches.

Hemoglobin A1c: A measurement of blood glucose control reflecting the average blood glucose for the last 60 to 90 days.

High density lipoprotein (HDL): A particle in blood that carries cholesterol and helps reduce arteriosclerosis.

Honeymoon phase: A period of variable duration, usually less than a year, after a diagnosis of type 1 diabetes when the need for injections of insulin is reduced or eliminated.

Humalog insulin: *See Lispro insulin.*

Hyperglycemia: Levels of blood glucose greater than 110 mg/dl fasting or 140 mg/dl in the fed state.

Hyperinsulinemia: More insulin than normal in the blood often found early in type 2 diabetes.

Hyperlipidemia: Elevated levels of fat in the blood.

Hyperosmolar syndrome: Very high glucose in type 2 diabetes associated with severe dehydration but not excessive fat breakdown and acidosis. It can lead to coma and death.

Hypoglycemia: Levels of blood glucose lower than normal, usually less than 60 mg/dl.

Impaired glucose tolerance (IGT): Levels of glucose between 140 and 200 mg/dl after eating, not normal but not quite high enough for a diagnosis of diabetes.

Impotence: Loss of the ability to have or sustain an erection of the penis.

Insulin: The key hormone that permits glucose to enter cells.

Insulin dependent diabetes: Former name for type 1 diabetes.

Insulin glargine: *See Lantus.*

Insulin pump: Device that slowly pushes insulin through a catheter under the skin but can also be used to give a large dose before meals.

Insulin reaction: Hypoglycemia as a consequence of too much injected insulin for the amount of food or exercise.

Insulin resistance: Decreased response to insulin found early in type 2 diabetes.

Insulin resistance syndrome: A combination of hypertension, increased visceral fat, high triglycerides, low HDL cholesterol, often obesity, and high uric acid associated with increased heart attacks.

Intensive diabetes treatment: Using three or four insulin injections based upon measurement of blood glucose along with very careful diet and exercise to approximate the normal range of glucose.

Islet cells: The cells in the pancreas that make insulin, glucagon, and other hormones.

Juvenile diabetes mellitus: Previous term for type 1 diabetes.

Ketones or ketone bodies: The breakdown products of fat metabolism.

Ketonuria: Finding ketones in the urine with a test strip.

Lancet: A sharp needle to prick the skin for a blood glucose test.

Lantus: A new insulin that provides a constant basal level 24 hours a day.

Laser treatment: Using a device that burns the back of the eye to prevent worsening of retinopathy.

Lente insulin: An intermediate-acting insulin that works in 4 to 6 hours and is gone by 12 hours.

Lipoatrophy: Indented areas where insulin is constantly injected.

Lipohypertrophy: Nodular swelling of the skin where insulin is constantly injected.

Lispro insulin: A very rapid-acting form of insulin, active within 15 minutes of injection.

Low density lipoprotein (LDL): A particle in the blood containing cholesterol and thought to be responsible for atherosclerosis.

Macrosomia: The condition of a large baby born when the mother's diabetes is not controlled.

Macrovascular complications: Heart attack, stroke, or diminished blood flow to the legs in diabetes.

Metformin: *See Glucophage.*

Microalbuminuria: Loss of small but abnormal amounts of protein in the urine.

Microvascular complications: Eye disease, nerve disease, or kidney disease in diabetes.

Miglitol: *See Glyset.*

Monounsaturated fat: One form of fat from vegetable sources like olives and nuts that does not raise cholesterol.

Morbidity rate: The rate at which sickness occurs compared with those who remain well.

Mortality rate: The rate at which death occurs compared with the total population.

Neovascularization: Formation of new vessels, especially from the retina of the eye.

Nephropathy: Damage to the kidneys.

Neuropathic ulcer: An infected area usually on the leg or foot resulting from damage that was not felt.

Neuropathy: Damage to parts of the nervous system.

Noninsulin dependent diabetes: Earlier name for type 2 diabetes.

NPH insulin: An intermediate-acting insulin, which starts to work in 4 to 6 hours and ends by 12 hours.

Ophthalmologist: A doctor who specializes in diseases of the eyes.

Oral hypoglycemic agent: A glucose-lowering drug taken by mouth.

Pancreas: The organ behind the stomach that contains the Islets of Langerhans.

Periodontal disease: Gum damage, which is more common in uncontrolled diabetes.

Peripheral neuropathy: Pain, numbness, and tingling, usually in the legs and feet.

Podiatrist: A person who specializes in treating the feet.

Polydipsia: Excessive intake of water.

Polyunsaturated fat: A form of fat from vegetables that may not raise cholesterol but lowers HDL.

Polyuria: Excessive urination.

Postprandial: After eating.

Prandin: An oral drug that lowers glucose by causing insulin secretion.

Precose: *See Acarbose.*

Proliferative retinopathy: Undesirable production of blood vessels in front of the retina.

Protein: A source of energy for the body made up of amino acids and found in meat, fish, poultry, and beans.

Proteinuria: Abnormal loss of protein from the body into the urine.

Receptor: Places on cells that bind to substances like insulin to permit the substance to do its job.

Regular insulin: A fast-acting form of insulin, active in one to two hours and gone by four to six hours.

Repaglinide: *See Prandin.*

Retina: The part of the eye that senses light.

Retinopathy: Disease of the retina.

Rezulin: The first of the class of glucose-lowering agents that reverses insulin resistance. Liver problems have caused its removal from the drug market.

Rosiglitazone: *See Avandia.*

Saturated fat: A form of fat from animals that raises cholesterol.

Secondary diabetes: Diabetes caused by some other disease, which raises glucose or blocks insulin.

Somogyi effect: A rapid increase in blood glucose in response to hypoglycemia.

Sulfonylureas: The earliest class of glucose-lowering agents, which works by stimulating insulin secretion.

Synthetic: Produced by artificial means.

Triglycerides: The main form of fat in animals.

Troglitazone: *See Rezulin.*

Ultralente insulin: A long-acting insulin that lasts for 24 to 36 hours.

Visceral fat: The fat accumulation that results in increased waist measurement.

Vitrectomy: Removal of the gel in the center of the eyeball because there has been leakage of blood and formation of scar tissue.

VLDL: The main particle in the blood that carries triglyceride.

Index

high blood pressure *(continued)*
  and kidney disease, 61, 62
  low-salt diet for, 64
  medications for, 64, 65, 183, 184, 341
  medications for, causing diabetes, 42
  medications for, causing erectile
    dysfunction, 85
  and peripheral vascular disease
    (PVD), 80
  weight loss improving, 128
high density lipoprotein (HDL). *see* HDL
Hispanic Americans. *see* Mexican
    Americans
history
  of diabetes treatments, 20–21, 225
  of the term diabetes mellitus, 17
HMO (Health Maintenance
    Organization), 220–221
Home Diagnostics Inc., meters produced
    by, 335
HONcode principles, 236
honeymoon phase, 29, 202, 203, 344
hormones
  alcohol's effect on, 49
  builder, 19
  causing diabetes, 41, 42
  causing insulin resistance, 232
  definition of, 19
  growth, 42
  thyroid, 42, 138, 183
Humalog insulin, 172
hunger
  as symptom of hypoglycemia, 47
  as symptom of type 1 diabetes, 28
hydrochlorothiazide, 42, 65
hydrocortisone, 42
hydroDiuril, 183
hyperbilirubinemia, 99
hypercholesterolemia, 80
hyperglycemia
  caused by underdosing insulin before
    exercise, 153
  definition of, 344
  fasting, 165

hyperinsulinemia, 344
hyperlipidemia, 344
hyperosmolar syndrome
  causes of, 55
  definition of, 54, 344
  symptoms of, 54–55
  treatment of, 56
hypertension. *see* high blood pressure
hyperthyroidism, 42
hypnosis, 241
hypoglycemia
  in babies after diabetic pregnancy, 98
  caused by alcohol, 49, 139
  caused by exercise, 49, 153, 159
  caused by injected insulin (insulin
    reaction), 48, 153, 172, 176, 177, 345
  caused by repaglinide, 169
  caused by sulfonylureas, 48, 49,
    162–164
  causes of, 48–50
  in children, 202, 204–205
  definition of, 27, 46, 345
  in elderly people, 214, 215
  family and friends helping with, 50,
    257–258
  myths about effects of, 254
  patient stories about, 48
  somogyi effect in response to, 348
  symptoms of, 47–48
  treatment of, 50, 344

• *I* •

ibuprofen, 74
icons used in this book, 4
IGT (impaired glucose tolerance), 19, 36,
    128, 345. *see also* glucose intolerance
Il Fornaio restaurant, 307–312
imipramine, 74
impaired fasting glucose, 18
impaired glucose tolerance (IGT), 19, 36,
    128, 345. *see also* glucose intolerance
implanted insulin pump, 230

PubMed Search Service of the National
Library of Medicine Web site, 337
pupil, abnormalities in, 76. *see also* eyes
PVD (peripheral vascular disease),
79–80
pyridoxine, 137

• *Q* •

quality of life, 14–16, 253
Quick, Dr. William, Web site by, 333

• *R* •

radiculopathy-nerve root
involvement, 74
rapid breathing, 51
rapid heartbeat
as symptom of hyperosmolar
syndrome, 55
as symptom of hypoglycemia, 47
receptor, 348
recipes. *see also* diet; food
desserts. *see* dessert recipes
meat. *see* meat recipes
poultry. *see* poultry recipes
rice and grain dishes. *see* rice and grain
recipes
salad. *see* salad recipes
seafood. *see* seafood recipes
soup. *see* soup recipes
vegetable dishes. *see* vegetable recipes
Web site resources for, 340
Regranex Gel, 82
regular insulin, 348
repaglinide, 169, 170
resistin, 232
resources. *see* publications; Web site
resources
respiratory distress syndrome, 99
responsibilities of managing
treatment, 186

restaurants
Aqua, in San Francisco, 268–273
Border Grill, in Santa Monica, 273–278
Charlie Trotters, in Chicago, 278–284
following diabetic diet in, 196, 246, 249,
260
Fringale, in San Francisco, 285–292
Gaylord India Restaurant, 292–296
Greens, in San Francisco, 296–301
Harbor Village, in San Francisco,
302–307
Il Fornaio, in San Francisco, 307–312
Windows on the World, in New York,
312–318
retina, 66, 348
retinal aneurysms, 67
retinal detachment, 68, 69
retinal hemorrhages, 67
retinopathy
background retinopathy, 67–68, 342
causing blindness, 66, 67, 68
definition of, 348
examinations for, 67
exercise and, 152, 159
incidence of, 68
laser surgery for treatment of,
68–69, 346
other complications associated with, 68
during pregnancy, 91
proliferative retinopathy, 68, 347
risk factors for, 68
vitrectomy for treatment of, 69
Web site resources for, 339
Rezulin, 167, 348
riboflavin, 137
rice and grain recipes
Almond-Currant Couscous, 300
Buckwheat Groats and Mushroom
Griddle Cakes, 318
Green Rice Pilaf, 275
Risotto Ai Vegetali (Italian Rice with
Vegetables), 311

Notes

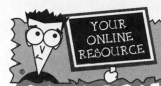
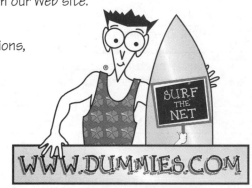
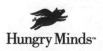

FOR DUMMIES
BOOK REGISTRATION

Register This Book and Win!

We want to hear from you!

Visit **dummies.com** to register this book and tell us how you liked it!

- Get entered in our monthly prize giveaway.

- Give us feedback about this book — tell us what you like best, what you like least, or maybe what you'd like to ask the author and us to change!

- Let us know any other *For Dummies* topics that interest you.

Your feedback helps us determine what books to publish, tells us what coverage to add as we revise our books, and lets us know whether we're meeting your needs as a *For Dummies* reader. You're our most valuable resource, and what you have to say is important to us!

Not on the Web yet? It's easy to get started with *Dummies 101: The Internet For Windows 98* or *The Internet For Dummies* at local retailers everywhere.

Or let us know what you think by sending us a letter at the following address:

For Dummies Book Registration
Dummies Press
10475 Crosspoint Blvd.
Indianapolis, IN 46256

™

..FOR
DUMMIES

**BESTSELLING
BOOK SERIES**